The Evidence for Orthopaedic Surgery

Edited by

David Limb & Stuart M Hay

Publisher

tfm Publishing Limited
Castle Hill Barns
Harley
Shrewsbury
SY5 6LX
UK

Tel: +44 (0)1952 510061
Fax: +44 (0)1952 510192
E-mail: nikki@tfmpublishing.com
Web site: www.tfmpublishing.com

Design and layout: Nikki Bramhill
Cartoon on front cover: Barry Foley

First Edition   © 2007

ISBN 1 903378 36 2

Printed by Gutenberg Press Ltd., Gudja Road, Tarxien, PLA 19, Malta.

Tel: +356 21897037; Fax: +356 21800069.

Contents

Contributors

Rami J Abboud BEng MSc PhD MIEEE ILTM Deputy Head of Division and Director of IMAR, Institute of Motion Analysis & Research (IMAR), Division of Surgery & Oncology, Tayside Orthopaedic & Rehabilitation Technology (TORT) Centre, Ninewells Hospital & Medical School, Dundee, Scotland

Robin Allum FRCS Consultant, Orthopaedic Surgery, Wexham Park Hospital, Slough, UK

Andrew Amis PhD DSc Professor, Department of Mechanical Engineering, Imperial College London, UK and Department of Orthopaedic Surgery, Imperial College London, UK

Robert Bethune MRCS Research Fellow, St. Mary's Hospital, London, UK

Jan Borremans Neurosurgeon (GMC) Specialist Registrar in Spinal Injuries, National Spinal Injuries Centre, Stoke Mandeville Hospital, Aylesbury, UK

Simon Carter FRCS Consultant Orthopaedic Oncologist, Royal Orthopaedic Hospital, Birmingham, UK

Graham Cheung MRCS Specialist Registrar, Orthopaedic Surgery, Robert Jones and Agnes Hunt Orthopaedic Hospital, Oswestry, UK and The Royal Shrewsbury Hospital, Shrewsbury, UK

James Davenport MRCS (Eng) Clinical Research Fellow, University Hospital, Queen's Medical Centre, Nottingham, UK

W. Dilworth Cannon MD Professor of Clinical Orthopaedics, University of California, San Francisco Department of Orthopaedic Surgery, San Francisco, USA

Roger Emery MS FRCS Reader, Orthopaedic Surgery, Department of Orthopaedic Surgery, Imperial College London, UK

Mark S Falworth FRCS (Tr & Orth) Specialist Registrar, Orthopaedic Surgery, Wexham Park Hospital, Slough, UK

David Ford FRCS (Orth) Consultant Orthopaedic Surgeon and Specialist in Hand Surgery, Robert Jones and Agnes Hunt Orthopaedic Hospital, Oswestry, UK and The Royal Shrewsbury Hospital, Shrewsbury, UK

Brian Freeman DM FRCS (Tr & Orth) Consultant Spinal Surgeon, University Hospital, Queen's Medical Centre, Nottingham, UK

Brian Gardner BM BCH MA (Oxon) FRCS FRCP (Lond & Edin) Consultant Surgeon in Spinal Injuries, National Spinal Injuries Centre, Stoke Mandeville Hospital, Aylesbury, UK

Peter V Giannoudis MD EEC (Orth) Professor, Trauma & Orthopaedics, Academic Department of Trauma & Orthopaedics, School of Medicine, St. James's University Hospital, Leeds, UK

Sheila Gibbs SRP MSc MRCSHC Senior Clinical Gait Analyst, Institute of Motion Analysis & Research (IMAR), Division of Surgery & Oncology, Tayside Orthopaedic & Rehabilitation Technology (TORT) Centre, Ninewells Hospital & Medical School, Dundee, Scotland

Joanna C Gibson MCSP Clinical Specialist Physiotherapist, Liverpool Upper Limb Unit, Royal Liverpool University Hospital, Liverpool, UK

Jonathan J Gregory BSc MB ChB MRCS Specialist Registrar, Orthopaedic Surgery, Robert Jones and Agnes Hunt Orthopaedic Hospital, Oswestry, UK and The Royal Shrewsbury Hospital, Shrewsbury, UK

Ulrich Hansen PhD Lecturer, Department of Mechanical Engineering, Imperial College London, UK

Paul J Harwood MRCS Specialist Registrar, Orthopaedic Surgery, The General Infirmary at Leeds, Leeds, UK

Stuart M Hay MB ChB FRCS FRCS (Orth) Consultant Orthopaedic Surgeon and Specialist in Shoulder and Elbow Surgery, Robert Jones and Agnes Hunt Orthopaedic Hospital, Oswestry, UK and The Royal Shrewsbury Hospital, Shrewsbury, UK

Andreas Hinsche FRCSEd (Tr & Orth) Consultant Orthopaedic Surgeon, Queen Elizabeth Hospital, Gateshead, UK

James S Huntley MA (Hons) DPhil MB BChir MRCS Lecturer and Honorary Specialist Registrar, Royal Hospital for Sick Children, Edinburgh, Scotland

Patrick Kluger Surgeon for Trauma and Orthopaedics (GMC) Consultant in Spinal Injuries, National Spinal Injuries Centre, Stoke Mandeville Hospital, Aylesbury, UK

Simon M Lambert BSc FRCS FRCSEd (Orth) Consultant Orthopaedic Surgeon, Royal National Orthopaedic Hospital Trust and Honorary Senior Lecturer, Institute of Musculoskeletal Science, University College, London, UK

David Limb BSc FRCSEd (Orth) Senior Lecturer, Trauma and Orthopaedic Surgery, University of Leeds and Honorary Consultant, Leeds Teaching Hospitals Trust, Leeds, UK

Nick London MA MD FRCS (Tr & Orth) Consultant Trauma & Orthopaedic Surgeon, Harrogate District Hospital, Harrogate, UK

Jesus Lozano BS Medical Student, University of California, San Francisco School of Medicine, San Francisco, USA

C. Benjamin Ma MD Assistant Professor in Residence, University of California, San Francisco Department of Orthopaedic Surgery, San Francisco, USA

Malcolm F Macnicol MB ChB BSc (Hons) FRCS MCh FRCSEd (Orth) Consultant Orthopaedic Surgeon, Royal Hospital for Sick Children, Edinburgh, Scotland

Ajay Malviya MS (Orth/Traum) MRCS Specialist Registrar, Orthopaedic Surgery, The Freeman Hospital, Newcastle upon Tyne, UK

Andrew McCaskie MD FRCS FRCS (Orth) Professor of Trauma and Orthopaedic Surgery, The Freeman Hospital, Newcastle upon Tyne, UK

David JJ Miller MB ChB MRCS Specialist Registrar, Robert Jones and Agnes Hunt Orthopaedic Hospital, Oswestry, UK and The Royal Shrewsbury Hospital, Shrewsbury, UK

Vasilios Moutzouros MD Chief Resident, Orthopaedic Surgery, New England Baptist Hospital, Boston, USA

Nagarajan Muthukumar D Orth FRCS (Tr & Orth) Consultant Trauma & Orthopaedic Surgeon, Hull & East Yorkshire NHS Trust, Hull, UK

Paul Norman MA MSc MB FRCPath Consultant Microbiologist, Department of Microbiology, The Northern General Hospital, Sheffield, UK

Martyn J Parker MD FRCS (Ed) Orthopaedic Research Fellow, Peterborough and Stamford Hospital NHS Foundation Trust, Peterborough District Hospital, Peterborough, UK

Simon Pickard FRCS (Orth) Consultant Orthopaedic Surgeon and Specialist in Hand Surgery, Robert Jones and Agnes Hunt Orthopaedic Hospital, Oswestry, UK and The Royal Shrewsbury Hospital, Shrewsbury, UK

Martyn Porter FRCS (Tr & Orth) Consultant Orthopaedic Surgeon, Centre for Hip Surgery, Wrightington Hospital, Lancashire, UK

Matthew Revell BSc MB BS FRCS (Tr & Orth) 5th Cavendish Hip Fellow, Lower Limb Arthroplasty Unit, Department of Orthopaedics, The Northern General Hospital, Sheffield, UK

John C Richmond MD Chairman, Department of Orthopaedic Surgery, New England Baptist Hospital, Boston, USA

David I Rowley B Med Biol MD FRCS Professor of Orthopaedics, Institute of Motion Analysis & Research (IMAR), Division of Surgery & Oncology, Tayside Orthopaedic & Rehabilitation Technology (TORT) Centre, Ninewells Hospital & Medical School, Dundee, Scotland

Lech Rymaszewski FRCS (Ed) FRCS (Eng) MSc Consultant Orthopaedic Surgeon, Glasgow Royal Infirmary, Glasgow, UK

Kalpesh Shah MS Orthopaedics MRCS Specialist Registrar, Trauma & Orthopaedics, Glasgow Royal Infirmary, Glasgow, UK

Nikhil Shah FRCS (Tr & Orth) Consultant Orthopaedic Surgeon, North Manchester General Hospital, Manchester, UK

David Stanley MB BS BSc (Hons) FRCS Consultant Upper Limb Surgeon, The Elbow and Shoulder Unit, The Northern General Hospital, Sheffield, UK

Ian Stockley MD FRCS Consultant Orthopaedic Surgeon, Lower Limb Arthroplasty Unit, Department of Orthopaedics, The Northern General Hospital, Sheffield, UK

Peter A Templeton FRCS (Orth) Consultant in Orthopaedic Surgery, The General Infirmary at Leeds, Leeds, UK

Alan J Thurston ED MSc (Oxon) FRACS FNZOA Associate Professor of Orthopaedic and Hand Surgery, Wellington School of Medicine & Health Sciences, Wellington, New Zealand and Consultant Hand Surgeon, Wellington Hospital, Wellington, New Zealand

Christopher Tzioupis MD Trauma Fellow, Trauma & Orthopaedics, Academic Department of Trauma & Orthopaedics, School of Medicine, St. James's University Hospital, Leeds, UK

The Editors

David Limb BSc FRCSEd (Orth)

David Limb is a Senior Lecturer in Trauma and Orthopaedic Surgery at the University of Leeds and Honorary Consultant to the Leeds Teaching Hospitals Trust, with a special clinical interest in shoulder surgery. He has editorial board positions with the *Journal of Bone and Joint Surgery* and *Current Orthopaedics*. He is Chairman of the CPD Committee of the British Orthopaedic Association, an examiner for the Intercollegiate Board in Trauma and Orthopaedic Surgery and a member of the Specialist Advisory Committee in Trauma and Orthopaedic Surgery.

Stuart M Hay MB ChB FRCS FRCS (Orth)

Stuart Hay is a Consultant Orthopaedic Surgeon working at the Robert Jones and Agnes Hunt Orthopaedic Hospital in Oswestry and the Royal Shrewsbury Hospital. His area of specialist interest is surgery of the shoulder and the elbow, particularly arthroscopic surgery. He qualified from Edinburgh University, then spent orthopaedic training in Leicester, Sheffield as a Registrar and University Lecturer, then as a Fellow at the Melbourne Shoulder and Elbow Clinic. He is a member of the court of examiners for the Intercollegiate Faculty of Sport and Exercise Medicine. In his spare time he sleeps.

Dedications

David's dedication:
To Cath and the boys

Stuart's dedication:
To Fiona, Bruce, Emily and Angus, who inspire me

Introduction

Using evidence-based medicine in orthopaedic surgery

David Limb BSc FRCSEd (Orth), Senior Lecturer
Trauma and Orthopaedic Surgery [1] and Honorary Consultant [2]
Stuart M Hay MB ChB FRCS FRCS (Orth), Consultant Orthopaedic
Surgeon and Specialist in Shoulder and Elbow Surgery [3]

1 UNIVERSITY OF LEEDS AND 2 LEEDS TEACHING HOSPITALS TRUST, LEEDS, UK
3 ROBERT JONES AND AGNES HUNT ORTHOPAEDIC HOSPITAL, OSWESTRY, UK
AND THE ROYAL SHREWSBURY HOSPITAL, SHREWSBURY, UK

The concept of evidence-based medicine has particular relevance in orthopaedics. We are far removed from the sort of pharmaceutical study in medicine that facilitates randomised controlled trials, which prove whether or not a new treatment is better than the one it replaces. That is not to say that randomised controlled trials have no place in our craft specialty; they do, and they remain the gold standard. There are difficulties in constructing randomised controlled trials for surgical procedures. Differences between the technical abilities of surgical teams, the facilities and equipment available and even the specifics of supply and manufacture can make a significant difference in one unit meaningless in another. Most of the major advances in orthopaedic surgery, including the development of successful joint replacement surgery and the skeletal stabilisation of trauma victims, occurred before the concept of evidence-based medicine was born. This does not mean that evidence-based practice has no place; quite the opposite. In the absence of a plethora of randomised trials, distillation of the literature becomes critical in assessing how to manage change.

What is evidence-based medicine?

Evidence-based medicine demands that the care of individual patients is based on the best evidence currently available, taking into account the expertise of the clinician and the preferences of the patient. It is therefore a collaborative venture and not something that is dictated by the contents of the medical press. However, the best evidence is provided by well conducted research that is relevant to the clinical context.

Why use evidence-based medicine?

A consideration of what is meant by evidence-based medicine soon answers this question. However, the pace of scientific research in many areas is fast, and it is not uncommon for it to be proceeding on more than one front. At best the efforts of any individual to keep pace with the literature lead to selective reading. To keep abreast of it all would consume more time than is found in the working week, or indeed in the entire week. Does this therefore make the practice of evidence-based medicine an untenable ideal?

Introduction

Fortunately, there are other factors that make it easier for us to practice evidence-based medicine.

The reasons include:

- the development of electronic databases such as Medline, EMBASE and CINAHL, which make the comprehensive search through millions of articles possible (Table 1);
- electronic libraries and access to these through educational institutions, enabling access to articles without the need to locate a paper copy;
- free web access to back catalogues of major journals (e.g. the *Journal of Bone and Joint Surgery*, British Volume);
- the development of reference management software that can import reference lists from the above databases;
- the development of rigorous methods of systematic review and meta-analysis, developed by the Cochrane Collaboration, the Oxford Centre for Evidence-based Medicine and, in the orthopaedic field, McMaster University in Canada;
- the emergence of publications and journals dedicated to the dissemination of evidence-based reviews. The reader will not have to look far to find one example!

How do you practice evidence-based medicine?

The process starts with the patient and the question that has presented itself during the consultation. Usually this is a clinical problem and this has to be translated into an answerable question. It is often helpful to think about the patient group of interest (e.g. in patients under 50), the intervention to be considered (... is surface replacement of the hip ...), the alternative for comparison (... better than total

Table 1. Sources of EBM information.

Electronic databases:

Cochrane Central Register of Controlled Trials (CENTRAL)	http://www.cochrane.org
MEDLINE - (USA) 3900 journals	http://www.ncbi.nlm.nih.gov
EMBASE - (Europe) 4000 journals	http://www.embase.com
CINAHL - nursing and allied health literature	http://www.cinahl.com
SIGLE - grey literature: research reports, thesis, conference	http://internet.unib.ktu.lt/physics/sources/Reports.htm
proceedings, technical reports	http://www.stn-international.de/

General sources:

Centre for evidence-based medicine	http://www.cebm.net/index.asp
EBM on-line (subscription service)	http://ebm.bmjjournals.com
Centre for evidence-based medicine	http://www.cebm.utoronto.ca
Bandolier	http://www.jr2.ox.ac.uk/bandolier
EBM Toolkit	http://www.med.ualberta.ca/ebm/ebmintro.htm
Evidence-based medicine (University of Massachusetts)	http://library.umassmed.edu/EBM
Healthweb	http://healthweb.org/browse.cfm?subjectid=39
Netting the evidence	http://www.shef.ac.uk/scharr/ir/netting
LHS Peoria, Illinois	http://www.uic.edu/depts/lib/lhsp/resources/ebm.shtml
Centre for Health Evidence	http://www.cche.net/usersguides/main.asp

Table 2. Levels of evidence.

Level	Type of evidence
Ia	Evidence obtained from systematic review or meta-analysis of randomised controlled trials
Ib	Evidence obtained from at least one randomised controlled trial
IIa	Evidence obtained from at least one well-designed controlled study without randomisation
IIb	Evidence obtained from at least one other type of well-designed quasi-experimental study
III	Evidence obtained from well-designed non-experimental descriptive studies, such as comparative studies, correlation studies and case studies
IV	Evidence obtained from expert committee reports or opinions and/or clinical experience of respected authorities

Table 3. Grades of evidence.

Grade of evidence	Evidence
A	At least one randomised controlled trial as part of a body of literature of overall good quality and consistency addressing the specific recommendation (evidence levels Ia and Ib)
B	Well-conducted clinical studies but no randomised clinical trials on the topic of recommendation (evidence levels IIa, IIb, III)
C	Expert committee reports or opinions and/or clinical experience of respected authorities. This grading indicates that directly applicable clinical studies of good quality are absent (evidence level IV)

hip replacement …), and the outcome with which to judge the intervention (… in terms of five-year survivorship?).

The question then forms the basis for electronic searching and the starting point for most medical searches is Medline. It is valuable to search both Medline and Embase, however, as Medline contains primarily North American journals, whilst Embase includes more European titles. The number of abstracts returned by the search depends on the quality of the question asked, and sifting through the results can be a time-consuming process if the search terms have been left too broad.

Papers identified in the search should be assessed for quality. The validity of the study group, sample size and applicability of the results are all considered. The perceived strength of study designs has been used to construct a hierarchy of evidence - various versions of this concept are in use, most grading randomised controlled trials, or meta-analyses including randomised trials, as the highest level of evidence and an isolated case report as the lowest. Our contributors have used the hierarchy illustrated in Tables 2 and 3, which is widely used in evidence-based medicine.

It has been a formidable challenge, therefore, for our contributors to wade through the sea of evidence and pick out significant advances that represent a true step forward in our knowledge. In some cases the function has been to point out that the evidence underpinning a current trend is in fact very weak, and the reader may chose to avoid being swept along by the tide of enthusiasm. Where a statement or recommendation is made in the text, the level of supporting evidence is indicated. Please interpret these sensibly - not all aspects of surgical practice can be assessed in a randomised, controlled fashion and we still have no evidence from randomised trials that parachutes reduce the death rate in people who jump out of aeroplanes!

Chapter 1

Sources of infection in the operating theatre

Alan J Thurston ED MSc (Oxon) FRACS FNZOA

Associate Professor of Orthopaedic and Hand Surgery [1]

Consultant Hand Surgeon [2]

1 WELLINGTON SCHOOL OF MEDICINE & HEALTH SCIENCES, WELLINGTON, NEW ZEALAND
2 WELLINGTON HOSPITAL, WELLINGTON, NEW ZEALAND

Introduction

Surgical wound infections account for 20% [1,2] to 38% [3] of all nosocomial infections, which mostly occur because of contamination of the wound during surgery. The cost of an infection to the patient may range from a few extra days absence from work, to considerable pain and immobility. The cost to the hospital may also be considerable [4,5]. Surgical site infections result in delayed wound healing, increased hospital stays, unnecessary pain and in extreme cases the death of the patient [6,7]. The stay in hospital increases by an average of between four and ten days and prevents the admission of other patients for care and treatment [8]. The resources required to treat an infected total joint replacement (TJR) are four times greater than for the primary procedure [9]. In 1964, Sir John Charnley reported deep infection rates in TJR of 9.5% [10].

Improvements in theatre techniques, antibiotics, theatre clothing and ventilation have reduced this rate to as low as 0.3% [11]. However, it is still the contamination of the environment in the operating theatre (OT) by personnel and patients that continues to contribute to postoperative infections. Wound contamination occurs firstly, by direct fallout from the environment and secondly, by contaminated equipment and gloved hands that, initially, were contaminated by the environment [12]. The contamination of surgical instruments exposed to the air in an OT can be 1.18 times higher than that of instruments covered with a sterile guard. The exposure time has a positive correlation with bacterial contamination rate [13]. Whyte et al have estimated that a reduction in the airborne bacteria in the OT of about 13-fold would reduce the wound contamination by about 50% [14]. From a study by Duhaime et al it was concluded that bacteria most often associated with shunt infections are airborne in the OT, rather than originating from the patient's skin [15]. A number of studies exemplify the need to reduce the bacterial counts in the air in OTs to a minimum.

Lidwell et al have shown that there is a good correlation between the air contamination and prosthetic joint sepsis rate. From their data they concluded that the largest proportion of bacteria found in the wound after the prosthesis had been inserted reached it by the airborne route [16]. In another study by the same group, in those patients that developed deep sepsis, the strains of *Staphylococcus aureus* isolated from the infected joints were traced to carriers among the OT staff for seven out of the 14 infections and as a possible source for another five. They stressed that very small numbers of *S. aureus* were needed to initiate an infection [17].

As Charnley and the MRC trial confirmed, clinical infection rates correlate directly with bacterial air counts [18]. This has also been stated by Ritter in a review of bacterial contamination in the OT [12]. Wound contamination can be reduced by a number of practices including:

- limiting the number of personnel in the OT;
- disrupting the flow of bacteria to the wound;
- filtering bacteria from the theatre air;
- disinfecting the air and the wound;
- use of systemic antibiotics;
- removing bacteria by physical methods such as disinfection and surgical technique [18].

Methodology

A comprehensive search of the current literature from 1966 to 2005 was carried out electronically using Medline and Pubmed. Relevant papers were identified and analysed. A search of the Cochrane database of systematic reviews produced papers on surgical masks, the wearing of jewellery and surgical glove perforations. A review of the American Association of Operating Room Nurses (AAORN) Recommended Practices Committee's recommendations was used to identify current recommendations for safe practice in the OT. The published versions of these recommendations do not provide the evidence on which the recommendations are based.

Theatre staff

Sources of contamination

In the OT most infections are a result of bacteria carried by theatre staff [18-20]. Experimental data have shown that live micro-organisms are shed from hair, exposed skin and mucous membranes of the OT staff [21-27], but few controlled trials have

evaluated the relationship of these sources with the risk of surgical wound infection. Coagulase-positive staphylococcus is carried in the nasal passages in 40% of theatre staff and in the perineum of 12% [18]. Sneezing disperses approximately 390,000 bacteria, coughing 710 and speaking 100 words in a minute 36 organisms [28]. Sheretz *et al* have shown that few *S. aureus* are dispersed from the upper respiratory tract (URT) in the absence of a URT infection. After experimental induction of a rhinovirus URT infection, the dispersal of *S. aureus* without a surgical mask increased 40-fold; dispersal was significantly reduced when a surgical mask was worn (p< or = 0.015) [29].

Numbers of staff

Several reports of increased airborne contamination in the OT with increased numbers of staff have been published [12, 30-33]. The level of microbial contamination in the OT is directly proportional to the number of personnel present [34-36] and to their movement [37]. In a well-designed scientific study Fitzgerald and Washington measured the contamination of the air in the OTs at the Mayo Clinic. They concluded that, apart from other findings, the contamination can be reduced by limiting the movements in and out of the OT during a surgical procedure and limiting the total number of people in the OT to ten [35] **(IIb/B)**. Duvlis and Drescher also found that the concentration of airborne bacteria depended primarily on the number of persons present in the OT, the air exchange rate per hour and the room volume. Persons in sterile dress were found to have much less influence than did persons in unsterile dress [31] **(III/B)**.

Clothing

Cotton has a pore size of 80μm and does not prevent the escape of squames [38]. Woven synthetic fibres such as polyester are almost 1000 times better at filtering squames [39]. Compared with conventional surgical clothing, polypropylene coveralls reduce the bacterial contamination of the air of a conventionally ventilated OT by 62% [40-43] **(Ib/A)** and disposable OT gowns are superior to cotton and can reduce infection rates by more than 60% [26]. From a prospective, intervention study, Andersen and Solheim reported a 50% reduction in the bacterial contamination of the air in the OT when occlusive clothing was worn [44] **(IIb/B)**. A similar finding was reported from another prospective intervention study by Tammelin *et al* when they found that special scrub suits made of tightly woven material significantly reduced total counts of bacteria in the air compared to conventional scrub suits (p=0.002) [45] **(IIb/B)**. This was corroborated by the study reported by Friberg *et al* in which they found that the mean surface counts were 20-70cfu/m^2/h and the air counts 1-2cfu/m^3 in disposable clothing experiments, whilst the use of cotton clothing resulted in higher counts of 100-200cfu/m^2/h (wound p>0.05, patient p>0.05, instruments p<0.01) and 4cfu/m^3 (p<0.02-0.001) [46] **(IIb/B)**. Mitchell *et al* found that the lowest levels of microbial contamination of the air in the OT occurred when both the unscrubbed and scrubbed theatre staff wore clothes of non-woven fabric [47] **(IIb/B)**. Ayliffe has stated (based on the work of Whyte *et al* [48]) that bacterium-impervious clothing that fits tightly at the neck, ankles and wrists considerably reduces bacterial dispersion [34] **(IV/C)**. This precludes the wearing of a boiler suit or cover-all over street clothing in the OT.

Ritter has gone further and has recommended that, during joint replacement surgery, all OT personnel including anaesthetic staff, circulating nurses, visitors, and the OT team must wear inclusive (*sic*) gowns [12] **(IV/C)**. The American Association of Operating Room Nurses (AAORN) recommends that "All persons who enter the restricted or semi restricted areas of the surgical suite should wear ... approved, clean and freshly laundered attire made of multi use fabric or limited-use non-woven fabric ... that should be laundered in an approved and monitored laundry". It has been reported that bacterial colony counts are higher when clothing is stored and then reused after lunch [49] **(IV/C)**. Home laundering is precluded as an acceptable method of cleaning surgical attire [50] **(IV/C)**. Whereas the Association of periOperative Registered Nurses (AORN) opposes the practice, the American Centers for Disease Control and Prevention (ACDC) describes it as an unresolved issue [51].

In a prospective, randomised trial Brown *et al* found that bacterial air counts were 4.4 times higher during preparation and draping for hip or knee arthroplasty using an unscrubbed and ungowned person holding the leg than during the operation itself. With the leg holder scrubbed and gowned during preparation and draping, the air counts were reduced but were still 2.4-fold greater than intra-operatively. They recommend that the leg should be held by a scrubbed and gowned member of the team. More importantly, they considered that instrument packs should be opened only after skin preparation and draping have been completed [52] **(Ib/A)**.

The use of cover gowns outside the OT suite was investigated by Mailhot *et al* in a prospective, randomised trial. Bacterial colony counts on scrub suits were higher after lunch when scrub suits were worn without cover gowns outside the OT during lunch, and when they were removed before lunch, stored in a locker, and put on again after lunch. From this study, they concluded that wearing cover gowns outside the OT exerts a protective effect against bacterial contamination. This protective effect was comparable to that seen when subjects changed into fresh scrub suits after lunch [49, 53] **(Ib/A)**.

Footwear

Up to 15% of the air contamination in an OT comes from the floors [54], so it is incumbent on theatre staff to maintain strict cleanliness of the floors. Theatre overshoes do not reduce OT floors' bacterial counts [55] **(IIb/B)**. In a study carried out by Hambraeus and Malmborg, they found that the contamination of a floor due to walking was about 16 times higher than contamination of the floor due to sedimentation only. They recommended that a footwear regimen is vital in areas where floors are cleaned frequently during the day as in OTs [56] **(IIb/B)**.

Bacterial contamination of the floor of a corridor leading into an OT suite from the changing room was studied by Nagai *et al*. The recovery of bacteria showed a peak at the changing room and decreased with increasing distance from the site. When the site of exchange of shoes was moved further away from the clean area, the peak of contamination moved to the new site and bacterial contamination decreased in the clean area. They concluded that exchange of footwear should occur as far from the OT as possible [57] **(IIb/B)**. The corollary from this study is that footwear that has been used out of the OT suite should not be worn in the OT.

Agarwal *et al* examined OT boots for the presence of blood by visual inspection, then the presence or absence of blood was confirmed by a specific biochemical test. They reported that 44% of all of the boots tested were contaminated with blood and that the majority was contaminated with bacteria. Sixty-three percent of surgeons had boots that were contaminated with blood and bacteria normally associated with skin or the environment. Comfort shoes with perforations on their upper surface and plastic boots commonly found in OTs were most heavily contaminated, whereas Wellington boots and clogs had less contamination [58] **(IIb/B)**.

Hats

Hair acts as a filter when uncovered and collects bacteria in proportion to its length, curliness and oiliness [59]. Shedding from hair has been shown to affect surgical infections and, therefore, complete hair cover is essential [59]. For many years the surgical team has worn hats to cover all hair. Recently, there has been some resistance from staff members other than the surgical team to keeping their hair completely covered. It is now common to see staff in the recovery unit, for instance, without their hair covered and staff in other areas with the theatre cap balanced alluringly on the back of the head and most of the hair uncovered.

The effect of different head coverings on airborne transmission of bacteria and particles in the surgical area was studied in a prospective intervention investigation by Friberg *et al,* comparing a squire-type disposable hood worn with a triple laminar face mask, a sterilised helmet aspirator system or no head cover at all. They reported that a proper head cover minimised the emission of apparently heavy particles and contained mainly streptococci, presumably of

respiratory tract origin. They concluded that, from a bacteriological point of view, disposable hoods of the squire type and face masks are equally as efficient as a helmet aspirator in containing the substantial emission of bacteria-carrying droplets from the respiratory tract occurring when head cover is omitted [60] **(IIb/B)**.

Schonholtz has stated that "Surgical attire for all personnel must provide for complete coverage of hair and arms" [30]. The AAORN Recommended Practices Committee has stated "Personnel should cover head and facial hair, including sideburns and necklines, when in the semi restricted and restricted areas of the surgical suite." This includes a low-lint surgical hat that confines all hair. Skullcaps that fail to cover the side hair above the ears and at the nape of the neck should not be worn [50] **(IV/C)**.

Masks

Surgical facemasks were originally developed in 1897 to contain and filter droplets of micro-organisms expelled from the mouth and nasopharynx of theatre personnel during surgery, thereby providing protection for the patient [61]. Over the past decade several studies have challenged the accepted dogma of surgical facemask use. In 1981, Orr published the results of a study in which facemasks were abandoned in the OT of a British hospital for one month. There was no change in the postoperative wound infection rate so the study was extended to six months and included almost 1000 elective general surgical cases. Comparison of the wound infection rate with those of the same six-month periods in the previous four years revealed a 50% decrease in wound infections [62]. However, this study was seriously flawed. There was no adequate definition of a wound infection, the historical data were unreliable and the study was neither randomised nor controlled.

Very few randomised, controlled and blinded trials of facemask use have been published. In a Cochrane systematic review, Lipp and Edwards found only two studies that satisfied their stringent criteria as prospective, randomised clinical trials for inclusion [63]. Although one study failed to show that wearing or not wearing masks made any difference to wound infection rates in general surgery (orthopaedic, urological and cardiac cases were excluded) [64] **(Ib/A)**, the other study in gynaecology patients was abandoned in the early stages because of an unacceptable infection rate in the unmasked group [65] **(Ib/A)**.

Many other studies have produced sound scientific evidence of considerable benefits to patients and theatre staff. It has been reported that masks are 95% effective at filtering organisms but they become damp and transmit bacteria by a wick effect [18, 66] and they should be changed between cases. On the other hand Graf and Kersch reported that adaptable masks (green exterior) provided with multi-layered polyester filter pads proved to be the most suitable by their virtual impenetrability for bacteria. After several hours of use and heavy wetting of the filter's layers, no increase of bacterial transmission was observed [67]. Dineen also reported that prolonged use of masks and moistening of masks was not found to impair filtration efficiency [21]. Under certain conditions masks have been shown to reduce wound contamination seven-fold [39]. Berger *et al* studied the influence of surgical mask usage on bacterial contamination of the operative field during 30 procedures. The mask position was varied during each procedure according to a random table. The number of bacterial colonies recoverable when no mask was worn was significantly higher than that detected when a full mask was worn (p<0.002). Shedding of *Staphylococcus epidermidis* was greater when no mask was worn than with a full mask (p<0.004) [68] **(Ib/A)**. The AAORN Recommended Practices Committee has stated that "A mask should cover both mouth and nose and be secured in a manner that prevents venting" [50] **(IV/C)**.

In a study to assess the release of bacteria from theatre staff during normal conversation, Letts and Doermer used micro-spheres of human albumin sprayed on the face and in the nostrils under the facemask. They concluded that conversation contributes to airborne contamination in the OT but that contamination from this source can be lessened by wearing a facemask that extends underneath an overlapping hood [69] **(IIb/B)**.

In a randomised trial of the use of surgical masks in ophthalmic cataract surgery, Alwitry *et al* reported that

there were significantly fewer organisms cultured when the surgeon used a facemask (p=0.0006). The majority of organisms were *S. epidermidis*, *Bacillus spp*, and *Diphtheroid spp*; however, *S. aureus* and *Pseudomonas aeruginosa* were cultured on several occasions [70] **(Ib/A)**.

Skinner and Sutton produced a controversial paper in which they announced that, based on "published evidence", masks were abolished for the non-scrubbed staff in the OT in 1993 and that infection control monitoring showed no sign of an increase in the rate of postoperative infections [71]. However, in a letter to the editor of *Anaesthesia and Intensive Care*, Joffe and Lafferty pointed out that the infection control in that hospital was laboratory-based and that there had never been a study of the efficacy of facemasks [72]. They refuted that there was ever any "published evidence" to guide the decision to abandon the use of masks. They also pointed out that there were no prospective surgical site surveillance data before 1993 to compare with, so there was no way of knowing if there had been a change in the rate of postoperative wound infections. Joffe and Lafferty went on to say that "… in the absence of additional data … the hospital must abide by the Association of Operating Room Nurses and Operating Room Nurses Association of Canada recommended standards and practices which require the use of masks by anyone entering the surgical suite when open sterile items and equipment are present" [50, 72, 73] **(IV/C)**.

Masks are also promoted as protective barriers for the theatre staff. An experimental study by Weber *et al* tested eight different surgical masks for aerosol penetration through the filter media and through face-seal leaks. They concluded that the protection provided by surgical masks might be insufficient in environments containing potentially hazardous sub-micrometre-sized aerosols [74] **(IIb/B)**. However, Romney has cast doubt on whether this can be extrapolated to the clinical setting [75]. One multicentric study in the USA found that 24.2% of all "blood exposures" (patient's blood splashing onto theatre staff) occurred on the face and neck. Circulating staff accounted for 16.7% of blood exposures [76].

After reviewing the current literature and the evidence for the use of surgical facemasks, Romney

Chapter 1

concluded "Circulating personnel in the OT, including anaesthetists, should continue to wear surgical facemasks whenever open sterile items and equipment are present." "…most authorities now assert that masks also serve to protect the OT team as well as the patient" [75]. Romney also concluded that there is no evidence that the abandonment of masks is safe for patient or staff. Friberg has concurred, stating that at the present time there is no convincing evidence to support the abandonment of masks [60] **(IV/C)**.

The surgical scrub

Surgical hand scrubbing is recommended by numerous organisations including the ACDC [3] and the British Hospital Infection Society [77] (BHIS). However, recommended practices for scrubbing vary.

The surgical scrub with 4% chlorhexidine has been shown to reduce contamination by 80% and this is cumulative with successive washes [18]. In a study by Pereira et al, an initial scrub for three minutes and 30-second consecutive scrub was compared with a current standard regimen of a five-minute initial scrub and a three-minute consecutive scrub. They found that chlorhexidine gluconate was found to be responsible for lower numbers of colony-forming units of bacteria than povidone-iodine. The duration of the scrub had no significant effect on the numbers of bacteria when povidone-iodine was used. The optimal regimen was found to be the five-minute initial and three-minute consecutive scrubs with chlorhexidine gluconate [78] **(IIb/B)**. Since then, O'Shaugnessy has shown that no benefits accrue from scrubbing for more that two minutes [79]. Other authors have reported similar evidence [80-83]. No clinical trials have evaluated the impact of the antiseptic agent used for scrubbing on the risk of surgical wound infections [84-89].

The ACDC recommends the scrub is performed for at least two to five minutes using an appropriate antiseptic [3] **(IV/C)**. The BHIS recommends that a two-minute wash using aqueous disinfectants is required and alcoholic hand rubs are an acceptable alternative to repeated washing. The fingernails should be cleaned as part of the first scrub of the day and nailbrushes or nail sticks can be used to achieve this [3, 77] **(IV/C)**.

There is no set standard for the bacteriological quality of water used for scrubbing [19], although some institutions use sterile water for this purpose. Based on the results of studies in their hospital in which only environmental organisms were isolated from the water supply, Dharan and Pittet strongly believe that the use of sterile water for surgical hand disinfection is not necessary [19] **(III/B)**.

Jewellery and cosmetics

The results of a prospective, randomised study by Wynd et al provide statistically significant data that demonstrate that chipped fingernail polish or fingernail polish worn longer than four days fosters increased numbers of bacteria on the fingernails of OT nurses after surgical hand scrubs. Their data suggest OT nurses can wear fresh fingernail polish on healthy fingernails without risking increased bacterial counts [90] **(Ib/A)**. Despite these findings, the National Association of Theatre Nurses in Britain recommends that nail polish be removed. A number of authors have reported that long nails, either natural or synthetic may be associated with tears in surgical gloves [50, 91, 92] **(IV/C)**.

From a prospective study by Bartlett et al it was shown that finger rings, nose and ear piercings increased local surface bacterial counts when in situ, and especially after removal (p<0.0001) [93] **(IIb/B)**. Although these authors then stated that the effect of jewellery on skin disinfection needs further study before guidelines can be made concerning finger rings, it has been reported in two papers that the wearing of rings does not contribute significantly to contamination but there is a higher rate of glove perforation in staff who wear rings under surgical gloves [94, 95] **(IIb/B)**. In a Cochrane systematic review of the effect of wearing finger rings during scrubbing, the authors found no randomised controlled trials that compared the wearing of finger rings with the removal of finger rings [96]. Despite this the ACDC and the BHIS both recommend that theatre staff remove jewellery and also refrain from wearing artificial nails [3, 77] **(IV/C)**.

Gloves

A major source of wound contamination is from gloved hands that, initially, were sterile but become contaminated by the environment [12]. Therefore, it is logical to reduce the bacterial counts in the OT environment to a minimum by whatever means are necessary.

Various studies have shown that between 50% and 67% of gloves are perforated during joint replacement [97, 98]. Double gloving or wearing protective over-gloves of cotton can reduce this by three to nine times [94, 95] **(IIb/B)**.

In a Cochrane systematic review, Tanner and Parkinson analysed 18 controlled trials that measured glove perforations [99]. Nine trials compared single latex gloves versus double latex gloves. These found that the number of perforations to the double latex innermost glove was significantly reduced when two pairs of latex gloves were worn [94, 100-106]. One trial compared single latex orthopaedic gloves with double latex gloves. This showed that there was no difference in the number of perforations to the innermost gloves when wearing double latex gloves compared with a single pair of latex orthopaedic gloves [107] **(Ib/A)**. Three trials compared double latex gloves versus double latex indicator gloves. These trials showed similar numbers of perforations to both the innermost and the outermost gloves for both gloving groups. Perforations to the outermost gloves were detected more easily when double latex indicator gloves were worn. Wearing double latex indicator gloves did not increase the detection of perforations to the innermost gloves [108-110] **(Ib/A)**.

In the same Cochrane systematic review, two trials compared double latex gloves versus double latex gloves with liners. These trials showed a significant reduction in the number of perforations to the innermost glove when a glove liner was worn between two pairs of latex gloves [95, 111] **(Ib/A)**. Two trials compared double latex gloves versus latex inner with cloth outer gloves. These trials showed that wearing a cloth outer glove significantly reduced the number of perforations to the innermost latex glove [112, 113] **(Ib/A)**. The last study that was included in this review was one that compared double latex gloves versus latex inner with steel weave outer gloves and showed

that there was no reduction in the number of perforations to the innermost glove [114] **(Ib/A)**.

Drapes

The passage of bacteria through surgical drapes is a potential cause of wound infection. Previous studies have shown that liquids and human albumin penetrate certain types of drapes. Blom *et al* studied the passage of bacteria through seven different types of surgical drape and an operating tray and reported that bacteria easily penetrated all the woven re-usable fabrics within 30 minutes, but that the disposable non-woven drapes proved to be impermeable, as did the operating tray [115] **(IIb/B)**. Other authors have also reported that disposable drapes are more effective at reducing contamination than laundered cotton drapes [26, 97, 116] **(IIb/B)**. Verkkala *et al* assessed the effect of impervious clothing and surgical drapes on wound contamination in cardiac surgery and they reported that the contamination of the sternal wound was reduced by 46% and that of the leg wound by greater than 90% [116] **(IIb/B)**.

Sweating

Mills *et al* reported on a study in which ten surgeons each performed a mock total hip joint replacement operation under sterile conditions while not sweating and then repeated the operation while sweating. Settle plates were used to quantify the bacterial counts in the operative field in both phases. They found that for each subject a mean of 3.3cfu were present in the non-sweating phase and 6.9cfu were present in the sweating phase (p<0.05). The organisms that were grown were normal skin flora. They concluded that the sweating surgeon might be more likely to contaminate the surgical field than the non-sweating surgeon [117] **(IIb/B)**.

The patient

Sources of contamintion

A number of studies have shown that the patient's own skin flora are seldom implicated in postoperative wound infections. In the MRC controlled trial, only two infections were considered attributable to the patients' own bacteria [42] **(IIb/B)**.

Pre-operative preparation

Pre-operative showers for patients comparing 9% chlorhexidine, soap and controls showed that there was no significant difference in wound infection between any of the groups [79]. However, Garibaldi *et al* found that in a prospective, controlled clinical trial, that pre-operative showering and scrubbing with 4% chlorhexidine gluconate was more effective than povidone-iodine or triclocarban medicated soap in reducing skin colonisation at the site of surgical incision [118] **(IIa/B)**. Patients who showered twice with 4% chlorhexidine gluconate had lower mean colony counts of skin bacteria at the surgical incision site in the OT prior to the final scrub, than patients who showered twice with povidone-iodine solution or medicated bar soap. Patients in the chlorhexidine group had no growth on 43% of the incision site skin cultures compared with 16% in the povidone-iodine group and 6% in the soap and water group. Patients who showered and who were scrubbed with chlorhexidine also had lower rates of intra-operative wound contamination [118]. Other studies have corroborated this evidence [119, 120] **(IIa/B)**. Chlorhexidine gluconate is not inactivated by blood or serum proteins [121-124], whereas iodophors may be inactivated by them [122, 125].

The preparation of patients for surgery has traditionally included the routine removal of body hair from the intended surgical wound site, because its presence can interfere with the incision and the subsequent wound, the suturing of the incision and the application of adhesive drapes and wound dressings [126, 127]. Hair is also perceived to be associated with uncleanness and its removal is thought to reduce the risk of wound infections [128]. However, there are studies, that claim that pre-operative hair removal may have the opposite effect and should not be carried out [129-131] **(Ib/A)**.

Dry shaving excoriates the skin and produces a greater rate of infection than wet shaving, clipping or depilatory creams [132, 133]. Shaving the night before an operation is associated with a significantly higher risk of infection or damage to the skin than either depilatory creams or no shaving [134-136] **(IIb/B)**. In a prospective, randomised trial of shaving versus no shaving in patients undergoing appendicectomy, Rojanapirom and Danchaivijitr reported that their data showed no alteration in bacteria found on the skin or on the walls of the wound before closing [137] **(Ib/A)**.

The ACDC strongly recommends that hair should not be removed pre-operatively, unless the hair at or around the incision site will interfere with the operation [3] **(IV/C)**. The BHIS Working Party guidelines recommend that "only the area to be incised needs to be shaved" and that shaving should be avoided if possible [77] **(IV/C)**. Other research has suggested that hair removal should not take place in the OT, as loose hair may contaminate the sterile surgical field [138].

Skin preparation

Alcohol is readily available, inexpensive and remains the most effective and rapid-acting skin antiseptic [121]. Gilliam and Nelson have reported that skin preparation with 70% alcohol is as good as 2% aqueous chlorhexidine over five minutes [139] **(Ib/A)**. In another study reported by Geelhoed *et al*, they found in an analysis of a randomised study of pre-operative skin preparation techniques in thoracic and general surgical patients that the use of a one-minute alcohol cleansing and application of an antimicrobial film provided equivalent bactericidal activity to an iodophor scrub for five minutes and paint. The initial bacterial kill was greater with a one-minute alcohol cleansing than with a five-minute iodophor scrub. There were fewer patients with high bacterial counts at the time of closure in the groups treated with the antimicrobial film than in the traditional iodophor scrub group [140] **(Ib/A)**.

Conclusions

It is incumbent on all personnel who enter an OT suite to minimise the contamination of the environment by way of protecting patients from infections. The following recommendations are supported by scientific evidence.

Recommendations	Evidence level
◆ The number of personnel in an OT should be kept to a minimum, as should movements in and out of the OT.	IIb/B
◆ All personnel entering the OT suite should wear only theatre suite clothing (scrub suits) made of an approved material that minimises the passage of squames and bacteria.	Ib/A
◆ Clothing must not be reused without being laundered.	Ib/A
◆ Home laundering of OT apparel is not acceptable.	IV/C
◆ A cover gown may be used to pass from the OT suite but it must *completely* cover the theatre clothing underneath.	Ib/A
◆ Street clothing is unacceptable in the OT suite.	Ib/A
◆ A boiler suit covering street clothing is unacceptable.	IIa/B
◆ All personnel should wear footwear that is restricted for use only in the OT suite.	IIa/B
◆ Wellington (gum) boots are preferable to footwear with perforated or absorbent uppers.	IIa/B
◆ There is limited evidence that over shoes are not an acceptable alternative.	IIb/B
◆ Using OT suite footwear outside the OT suite is unacceptable.	IIa/B
◆ All personnel in the OT suite should have all hair covered and confined by a low-lint surgical hat.	IIa/B
◆ Skullcaps and bandanas that leave hair exposed are not acceptable.	IV/C
◆ All reusable theatre hats should be laundered at the end of each day by an approved laundry.	IV/C
◆ Home laundering of theatre hats is not acceptable.	IV/C
◆ The rate of wound infections is higher when OT staff don't wear face masks.	Ib/A
◆ All personnel in an OT, including anaesthetists and anaesthetic technicians should wear a surgical facemask whenever sterile items and equipment are exposed.	IV/C
◆ The mask should cover the mouth and nose.	IV/C
◆ The mask should be fitted tightly to the face to avoid venting.	IV/C
◆ Fingernails should be kept clean and, preferably, short.	IV/C
◆ Fresh nail polish is acceptable but old, chipped nail polish is unacceptable.	IIb/B
◆ Finger rings should be removed to avoid glove perforations.	IIa/B
◆ The surgical scrub should be carried out for between two and five minutes with an approved antiseptic soap substitute.	IIa/B
◆ Chlorhexidine gluconate is more effective at reducing contamination than povidone-iodine.	IIa/B
◆ No benefits accrue from scrubbing for more than two minutes.	Ib/A
◆ The reduction in contamination of the hands and forearms is cumulative with successive scrubs.	Ib/A
◆ Double gloves should be worn by the surgical team as a precaution against glove perforations.	Ib/A
◆ A single pair of orthopaedic gloves is an acceptable alternative.	Ib/A
◆ Patients should shower (preferably twice) with an antiseptic agent pre-operatively to reduce skin colony counts of bacteria and to reduce wound contamination.	IIa/B
◆ Do not remove hair from around the surgical site unless it will interfere with the operation.	Ib/A

References

1. Ayliffe G, Buckles A, Casewell M, Cookson B, Cox R, Duckworth G, *et al*. Revised guidelines for control of MRSA: applying appropriately-based recommendations. *Journal of Hospital Infection* 1999; 43(4): 315-6.

2. Ayliffe G, Buckles A, Casewell M, Cookson B, Cox R, Duckworth G, *et al*. Working Party Report. Revised guidelines for the control of methicillin-resistant *Staphylococcus aureus* infection in hospitals. Report of a combined working party of the British Society for Antimicrobial Chemotherapy, the Hospital Infection Society and the Infection Control Nurses Association. *Journal of Hospital Infection* 1998; 39(4): 253-90.

3. Mangram A, Horan T, Pearson M, Silver L, Jarvis W. Guideline for prevention of surgical site infection. *Infection Control & Hospital Epidemiology* 1999; 20(4): 247-78.

4. Boyce J, Potter-Bynoe G, Dziobek L. Hospital reimbursement patterns among patients with surgical wound infections following open heart surgery. *Infection Control & Hospital Epidemiology* 1990; 11(2): 89-93.

5. Poulsen K, Bremmelgaard A, Sorensen A, Raahave D, Petersen J. Estimated costs of postoperative wound infections. A case-control study of marginal hospital and social security costs. *Epidemiology & Infection* 1994; 113(2): 283-95.

6. Emmerson A, Enstone J, Griffin M, Kelsey M, Smyth E. The second national prevalence survey of infection in hospitals - overview of the results. *Journal of Hospital Infection* 1996; 32: 175-90.

7. Plowman R, Graves N, Griffin M. The socio-economic burden of hospital-acquired infection. London: Public Health Laboratory Service, 2000.

8. Wilson J. Infection control: surveying the risks (continuing education credit). *Nursing Standard* 1995; 9(15 Suppl Nu): 3-8.

9. Dreghorn C, Hamblin D. Revision arthroplasty: a high price to pay. *Br Med J* 1989; 298: 648-9.

10. Charnley J. A clean-air operating enclosure. *Br J Surg* 1964; 51: 202-5.

11. Lidgren L. Joint prosthetic infections: a success story. *Acta Orthop Scand* 2001; 72: 553-6.

12. Ritter M. Operating room environment. *Clin Orthop Relat Res* 1999; 369: 103-9.

13. Yin S, Xu S, Bo Y. Study of surgical instruments contamination by bacteria from air during the operation. *Chung-Hua Hu Li Tsa Chih Chinese Journal of Nursing* 1996; 31(12): 690-1.

14. Whyte W, Hambraeus A, Laurell G, Hoborn J. The relative importance of the routes and sources of wound contamination during general surgery. II. Airborne. *Journal of Hospital Infection* 1992; 22(1): 41-54.

15. Duhaime A, Bonner K, McGowan K, Schut L, Sutton L, Plotkin S. Distribution of bacteria in the operating room environment and its relation to ventricular shunt infections: a prospective study. *Childs Nervous System* 1991; 7(4): 211-4.

16. Lidwell O, Lowbury E, Whyte W, Blowers R, Stanley S, Lowe D. Airborne contamination of wounds in joint replacement operations: the relationship to sepsis rates. *Journal of Hospital Infection* 1983; 4(2): 111-31.

17. Lidwell O, Lowbury E, Whyte W, Blowers R, Stanley S, Lowe D. Bacteria isolated from deep joint sepsis after operation for total hip or knee replacement and the sources of the infections with *Staphylococcus aureus*. *Journal of Hospital Infection* 1983; 4(1): 19-29.

18. Bannister G. Prevention of infection in joint replacement. *Current Orthopaedics* 2002; 16: 426-33.

19. Dharan S, Pittet D. Environmental controls in operating theatres. *Journal of Hospital Infection* 2002; 51(2): 79-84.

20. Pawinska A, Dzierzanowska D. Bezpieczenstwo pacjentow i personelu na bloku operacyjnym. *Polski Merkuriusz Lekarski* 2002; 12(67): 7306.

21. Dineen P. Microbial filtration by surgical masks. *Surg Gynecol Obstetrics* 1971; 133(5): 812-4.

22. Hardin W, Nichols R. Aseptic technique in the operating room. In: *Surgical Infections*. Fry D, Ed. Boston: Little, Brown and Co, 1995: 109-18.

23. Smith R. What is the purpose of the scrub suit? *AORN Journal* 1980; 31(5): 769.

24. Dineen P. The role of impervious drapes and gowns preventing surgical infection. *Clin Orthop Relat Res* 1973; 96: 210-2.

25. Ha'eri G, Wiley A. The efficacy of standard surgical face masks: an investigation using 'tracer particles'. *Clin Orthop Relat Res* 1980; 148: 160-2.

26. Moylan JA, Fitzpatrick KT, Davenport KC. Reducing wound infections. Improved gown and drape barrier performance. *Arch Surg* 1987; 122: 152-7.

27. Moylan J, Balish E, Chan J. Intraoperative bacterial transmission. *Surgical Forum* 1974; 25: 29-30.

28. Lidwell O, Lowbury E, White W, Blowers R, Stanley S. Effect of ultraclean air in operating rooms on deep sepsis in the joint after total hip or knee replacement: a randomised study. *Br Med J* 1982; 285: 10-4.

29. Sheretz R, Reagan D, Hampton K, Robertson K, Streed S, Hoen H, *et al*. A cloud adult: the *Staphylococcus aureus*-virus interaction revisited. *Ann Int Med* 1996; 124(6): 539-47.

30. Schonholtz G. Maintenance of aseptic barriers in the conventional operating room: general principles. *J Bone Joint Surg Am* 1976; 58A(4): 439-45.

31. Duvlis Z, Drescher J. Untersuchungen uber den Luftkeimgehalt in konventionell klimatisierten Operationssalen. Zentralblatt fur Bakteriologie - 1 - Abt - Originale - B. *Hygiene, Krankenhaushygiene, Betriebshygiene, Praventive Medizin* 1980; 170(2): 185-98.

32. Chosky S, Modha D, Taylor G. Optimisation of ultraclean air. The role of instrument preparation. *J Bone Joint Surg Br* 1996; 78A(5): 835-7.

33. Pittet D, Ducel G. Infectious risk factors related to operating rooms. *Infection Control & Hospital Epidemiology* 1994; 15(7): 456-62.

34. Ayliffe G. Role of the environment of the operating suite in surgical wound infection. *Reviews of Infectious Diseases* 1991; 13 (Suppl 10): S800-4.

35. Fitzgerald R, Washington J. Contamination of the operative wound. *Orthop Clin N Am* 1975; 6(4): 1105-14.

36. Suzuki A, Namba Y, Matsuura M, Horisawa A. Airborne contamination in an operating suite: report of a five-year survey. *Journal of Hygiene* 1984; 93(3): 567-73.

37. Quraishi Z, Blais F, Sottile W, Adler L. Movement of personnel and wound contamination. *AORN Journal* 1983; 38(1): 146-7, 150-6.

38. Rudolph H. OP-Kleidung und Patientenabdeckung. Stand: 3. 7. 1992. *Unfallchirurg* 1993; 19(3): 186-9.

39. Whyte W, Bailey PV. Reduction of microbial dispersion by clothing. *J Parenter Sci Technol* 1985; 39: 51-60.

40. Scheibel J, Jensen I, Pedersen S. Bacterial contamination of air and surgical wounds during joint replacement operations. Comparison of two different types of staff clothing. *Journal of Hospital Infection* 1991; 19(3): 167-74.

41. Sanzen L. Occlusive clothing and ultraviolet radiation in hip surgery. *Acta Orthop Scand* 1989; 60(6): 664-7.

42. Lidwell O. Air, antibiotics and sepsis in replacement joints. *Journal of Hospital Infection* 1988; 11 (Supp C): 18-40.

43. Bergman B, Hoborn J, Nachemson A. Patient draping and staff clothing in the operating theatre: a microbiological study. *Scandinavian Journal of Infectious Diseases* 1985; 17(4): 421-6.

44. Andersen B, Solheim N. Occlusive scrub suits in operating theaters during cataract surgery: effect on airborne contamination. *Infection Control & Hospital Epidemiology* 2002; 23(4): 218-20.

45. Tammelin A, Hambraeus A, Stahle E. Routes and sources of *Staphylococcus aureus* transmitted to the surgical wound during cardiothoracic surgery: possibility of preventing wound contamination by use of special scrub suits. *Infection Control & Hospital Epidemiology* 2001; 22(6): 338-46.

46. Friberg B, Friberg S, Burman L. Inconsistent correlation between aerobic bacterial surface and air counts in operating rooms with ultra clean laminar air flows: proposal of a new bacteriological standard for surface contamination. *Journal of Hospital Infection* 1999; 42(4): 287-93.

47. Mitchell N, Evans D, Kerr A. Reduction of skin bacteria in theatre air with comfortable, non-woven disposable clothing for operating-theatre staff. *Br Med J* 1978; 1(6114): 696-8.

48. Whyte W, Vesley D, Hodgson R. Bacterial dispersion in relation to operating room clothing. *Journal of Hygiene* 1976; 76(3): 367-78.

49. Mailhot C, Slezak L, Copp G, Binger J. Cover gowns. Researching their effectiveness. *AORN Journal* 1987; 46(3): 482-90.

50. Association of Operating Rooms Nurses Recommended Practices Committee. Recommended practices for surgical attire. *AORN Journal* 1998; 68: 1048-52.

51. Belkin N. Home laundering of soiled surgical scrubs: surgical site infections and the home environment. *American Journal of Infection Control* 2001; 29(1): 58-64.

52. Brown A, Taylor G, Gregg P. Air contamination during skin preparation and draping in joint replacement surgery. *J Bone Joint Surg Br* 1996; 78B(1): 92-4.

53. Copp G, Mailhot C, Zalar M, Slezak L, Copp A. Covergowns and the control of operating room contamination. *Nursing Research* 1986; 35(5): 263-8.

54. Hambraeus A, Bengtsson S, Laurell G. Bacterial contamination in a modern operating suite. 3. Importance of floor contamination as a source of airborne bacteria. *Journal of Hygiene* 1978; 80(2): 169-74.

55. Humphreys H, Marshall RJ, Ricketts UE, Russell RJ, Reeves DG. Theatre overshoes do not reduce operating theatre floor bacterial counts. *Journal of Hospital Infection* 1991; 17: 117-23.

56. Hambraeus A, Malmborg A. The influence of different footwear on floor contamination. *Scandinavian Journal of Infectious Diseases* 1979; 11(3): 243-6.

57. Nagai I, Kadota M, Takechi M, Kumamoto R, Ueoka M, Matsuoka K, *et al.* Studies on the mode of bacterial contamination of an operating theatre corridor floor. *Journal of Hospital Infection* 1984; 5(1): 50-5.

58. Agarwal M, Hamilton-Stewart P, Dixon R. Contaminated operating room boots: the potential for infection. *American Journal of Infection Control* 2002; 30(3): 179-83.

59. Garner B, editor. *Infection control.* 10th ed. St Louis: Mosby-Year Book Inc, 1995.

60. Friberg B, Friberg S, Ostensson R, Burman L. Surgical area contamination - comparable bacterial counts using disposable head and mask and helmet aspirator system, but dramatic increase upon omission of head-gear: an experimental study in horizontal laminar air-flow. *Journal of Hospital Infection* 2001; 47(2): 110-5.

61. Mikulicz J. Das Operieren in sterilisierten Zwirnhandschuhen und mit Mundbinde. *Zentralbl Chirurg* 1897; 26: 714.

62. Orr N. Is a mask necessary in the operating theatre? *Ann R Coll Surg Engl* 1981; 63(6): 390-2.

63. Lipp A, Edwards P. Disposable surgical face masks for preventing surgical wound infection in clean surgery. *Cochrane Database of Systematic Reviews* 2002; 4.

64. Tunevall T. Postoperative wound infections and surgical face masks: a controlled study. *World J Surg* 1991; 15(3): 383-7.

65. Chamberlain G, Houang E. Trial of the use of masks in the gynaecological operating theatre. *Ann R Coll Surg Engl* 1984; 66(6): 432-3.

66. Rogers K. An investigation into the efficiency of disposable face masks. *Journal of Clinical Pathology* 1980; 33(11): 1086-91.

67. Graf W, Kersch D. Bakteriologische Bewertung chirurgischer Gesichtsmasken. *Zentralblatt fur Bakteriologie, Mikrobiologie und Hygiene - 1 - Abt - Originale B, Hygiene* 1980; 171(2-3): 142-57.

68. Berger S, Kramer M, Nagar H, Finkelstein A, Frimmerman A. Effect of surgical mask position on bacterial contamination of the operative field. *Journal of Hospital Infection* 1993; 23(1): 51-4.

69. Letts R, Doermer E. Conversation in the operating theater as a cause of airborne bacterial contamination. *J Bone Joint Surg Am* 1983; 65A(3): 357-62.

70. Alwitry A, Jackson E, Chen H, Holden R. The use of surgical facemasks during cataract surgery: is it necessary? *British Journal of Ophthalmology* 2002; 86(9): 975-7.

71. Skinner M, Sutton B. Do anaesthetists need to wear surgical masks in the operating theatre? A literature review with evidence-based recommendations. *Anaesthesia and Intensive Care* 2001; 29(4): 331-8.

72. Joffe A, Lafferty S. Do anaesthetists need to wear surgical face masks in the operating theatre? *Anaesthesia and Intensive Care* 2002; 30: 530-3.

73. Operating Room Nurses Association of Canada. Recommended practices for perioperative nursing practice, 4th ed. ORNAC, 1998.

74. Weber A, Willeke K, Marchioni R, Myojo T, McKay R, Donnelly J, *et al*. Aerosol penetration and leakage characteristics of masks used in the health care industry. *American Journal of Infection Control* 1993; 21(4): 167-73.

75. Romney M. Surgical face masks in the operating theatre: re-examining the evidence. *Journal of Hospital Infection* 2001; 47(4): 251-6.

76. White M, Lynch P. Blood contact and exposures among operating room personnel: a multicenter study. *American Journal of Infection Control* 1993; 21(5): 243-8.

77. Woodhead K, Taylor E, Bannister G, Chesworth T, Hoffman P, Humphreys H. Behaviours and rituals in the operating theatre: a report from the Hospital Infection Society Working Group in Infection Control in the Operating Room 2001. Hospital Infection Society, 2001.

78. Pereira L, Lee G, Wade K. The effect of surgical handwashing routines on the microbial counts of operating room nurses. *American Journal of Infection Control* 1990; 18(6): 354-64.

79. O'Shaugnessy M, O'Malley VP, Corbett G, Given HF. Optimum duration of surgical scrub time. *Br J Surg* 1991; 78: 685-6.

80. Hingst V, Juditzki I, Heeg P, Sonntag H. Evaluation of the efficacy of surgical hand disinfection following a reduced application time of 3 instead of 5 min. *Journal of Hospital Infection* 1992; 20(2): 79-86.

81. Wheelock S, Lookinland S. Effect of surgical hand scrub time on subsequent bacterial growth. *AORN Journal* 1997; 65(6): 1087-92.

82. Deshmukh N, Kramer J, Kjellberg S. A comparison of 5-minute povidone-iodine scrub and 1-minute povidone-iodine scrub followed by alcohol foam. *Military Medicine* 1998; 163(3): 145-7.

83. Masterton B. Cleansing the surgeon's hands. *Scientific American Surgeon* 1996; 2: 3-9.

84. Rubio P. Septisol antiseptic foam: a sensible alternative to the conventional surgical scrub. *International Surgery* 1987; 72(4): 243-6.

85. Babb J, Davies J, Ayliffe G. A test procedure for evaluating surgical hand disinfection. *Journal of Hospital Infection* 1991; 18 (Suppl B): 41-9.

86. Holloway P, Platt J, Reybrouck G, Lilly H, Mehtar S, Drabu Y. A multi-centre evaluation of two chlorhexidine-containing formulations for surgical hand disinfection. *Journal of Hospital Infection* 1990; 16(2): 151-9.

87. Kobayashi H. Evaluation of surgical scrubbing. *Journal of Hospital Infection* 1991; 18 (Suppl B): 29-34.

88. Nicoletti G, Boghossian V, Borland R. Hygienic hand disinfection: a comparative study with chlorhexidine detergents and soap. *Journal of Hospital Infection* 1990; 15(4): 323-37.

89. Rotter M, Koller W. Surgical hand disinfection: effect of sequential use of two chlorhexidine preparations. *Journal of Hospital Infection* 1990; 16(2): 161-6.

90. Wynd C, Samstag D, Lapp A. Bacterial carriage on the fingernails of OR nurses. *AORN Journal* 1994; 60(5): 796, 799-805.

91. Hardin W, Nichols R. Hand washing and patient skin preparation. In: *Critical Issues in Operating Room Management*. Malangoni M, editor. Philadelphia: Lippincott-Raven, 1997: 133-49.

92. Committee on Control of Surgical Infections of the Committee on Pre- and Postoperative Care. In: *Manual on Control of Infection in Surgical Patients*. American College of Surgeons, editor. Philadelphia: J.B. Lippincott & Co, 1984.

93. Bartlett GE, Pollard TCB, Bowker KE, Bannister GC. Effects of jewellery on surface bacterial counts of operating theatres. *Journal of Hospital Infection* 2002; 52(1): 68-70.

94. Doyle P, Alvi S, Johanson R. The effectiveness of double gloving in obstetrics and gynaecology. *British Journal of Obstetrics and Gynaecology* 1992; 992: 83-4.

95. Sebold E, Jordan L. Intraoperative glove perforation: a comparative analysis. *Clin Orthop Relat Res* 1993; 297: 242-4.

96. Arrowsmith V, Maunder J, Sargent R, Taylor R. Removal of nail polish and finger rings to prevent surgical infection. *Cochrane Database of Systematic Reviews* 2002; 4.

97. Lankester BJA, Bartlett GE, Garneti N, Blom AW, Bowker KE, Bannister GC. Direct measurement of bacterial penetration through surgical gowns: a new method. *Journal of Hospital Infection* 2002; 50: 281-5.

98. Nicola P, Adam CM, Alien PW. Increased awareness of glove perforation in major joint replacements. *J Bone Joint Surg Br* 1997; 79B: 371-3.

99. Tanner J, Parkinson H. Double gloving to reduce surgical cross-infection. *Cochrane Database of Systematic Reviews* 2003; 3.

100. Avery C, Gallacher P, Birnbaum W. Double gloving and a glove perforation indication system during the dental treatment of HIV positive patients: are they really necessary? *British Dental Journal* 1999; 186(1): 27-9.

101. Berridge D, Starkey G, Jones N, Chamberlain J. A randomised controlled trial of double versus single gloving in vascular surgery. *J Roy Coll Surg Edin* 1998; 43: 9-10.

102. Jensen S, Kristensen B, Fabrin K. Double gloving as self-protection in abdominal surgery. *Eur J Surg* 1997; 163(3): 163-7.

103. Kovavasich E, Vanitchanon P. Perforation in single and double gloving methods for cesarian section. *International Journal of Gynaecology and Obstetrics* 1999; 67(3): 157-61.

104. Marin Bertolin M, Gonzale Martinez R, Gimenez C, Marquina Vila P, Amorrortu Veleyos J. Does double gloving protect surgical staff from skin contamination during plastic surgery? *Plastic and Reconstructive Surgery* 1997; 99(4): 956-60.

105. Naver L, Gottrup F. Incidence of glove perforations in gastrointestinal surgery and the protective effect of double gloves: a prospective randomised controlled study. *Eur J Surg* 2000; 166: 293-5.

Chapter 1

106. Thomas S, Agarwal M, Mehta G. Intraoperative glove perforation - single versus double gloving in protection against skin contamination. *Postgraduate Medical Journal* 2001; 77(909): 458-60.

107. Turnquest M, How H, Allen S, Voss D, Spinnato J. Perforation rate using a single pair of orthopaedic gloves vs. a double pair of gloves in obstetric cases. *Journal of Maternal-Fetal Medicine* 1996; 5(6): 362-5.

108. Avery C, Taylor J, Johnson P. Double gloving and a system for identifying glove perforations in maxillofacial trauma surgery. *British Journal of Oral and Maxillofacial Surgery* 1999; 4: 316-9.

109. Duron J, Keilani K, Elian N. Efficacy of double gloving with a coloured inner pair for immediate detection of operative glove perforations. *Eur J Surg* 1996; 162: 941-4.

110. Nicolai P, Aldam C, Allen P. Increased awareness of glove perforation in major joint replacement. *J Bone Joint Surg Br* 1997; 79B: 371-3.

111. Sutton P, Greene T, Howell F. The protective effect of a cut-resistant glove liner. *J Bone Joint Surg Br* 1998; 80B: 411-3.

112. Sanders R, Fortin P, Ross E, Helfet D. Outer gloves in orthopaedic procedures. *J Bone Joint Surg Am* 1990; 72A: 914-7.

113. Underwood M, Weerasena N, Graham T, Hosie K, Dunning J, Bailey J, *et al*. Prevalence and prevention of glove perforation during cardiac operations. *J Thorac Cardiovasc Surg* 1993; 1066(2): 375-7.

114. Louis S, Steinberg E, Gruen O, Bartlett C, Helfet D. Outer gloves in orthopaedic procedures: a polyester stainless steel wire weave glove liner compared with latex. *J Orthop Trauma* 1998; 12(2): 101-5.

115. Blom A, Estela C, Bowker K, MacGowan A, Hardy JR. The passage of bacteria through surgical drapes. *Ann R Coll Surg Engl* 2000; 82(6): 405-7.

116. Verkkala K, Eklund A, Ojajarvi J, Tiittanen L, Hoborn J, Makela P. The conventionally ventilated operating theatre and air contamination control during cardiac surgery - bacteriological and particulate matter control garment options for low level contamination. *Eur J Cardio-Thorac Surg* 1998; 14(2): 206-10.

117. Mills S, Holland D, Hardy A. Operative field contamination by the sweating surgeon. *ANZ J Surg* 2000; 70(12): 837-9.

118. Garibaldi R. Prevention of intraoperative wound contamination with chlorhexidine shower and scrub. *Journal of Hospital Infection* 1988; 11 (Suppl B): 5-9.

119. Paulson D. Efficacy evaluation of a 4% chlorhexidine gluconate as a full-body shower wash. *American Journal of Infection Control* 1993; 21(4): 205-9.

120. Hayek L, Emerson J, Gardner A. A placebo-controlled trial of the effect of two preoperative baths or showers with chlorhexidine detergent on postoperative wound infection rates. *Journal of Hospital Infection* 1987; 10(2): 165-72.

121. Larson E. Guideline for use of topical antimicrobial agents. *American Journal of Infection Control* 1991; 16(6): 253-66.

122. Mayhall C. Surgical infections including burns. In: *Prevention and Control of Nosocomial Infections*. 2nd ed. Wenzel R, Ed. Baltimore: Williams and Wilkins, 1993: 614-64.

123. Brown T, Ehrlich C, Stehman F, Golichowski A, Madura J, Eitzen H. A clinical evaluation of chlorhexidine gluconate spray as compared with iodophor scrub for preoperative skin preparation. *Surg Gynecol Obstet* 1984; 158: 363-6.

124. Lowbury E. The effect of blood on disinfection of surgeons' hands. *Br J Surg* 1974; 61: 19-21.

125. Ritter M. The antimicrobial effectiveness of operative-site preparative agents: a microbiological and clinical study. *J Bone Joint Surg Am* 1980; 62A(5): 826-8.

126. Millar J, Webster P, Patel S, Ramey J. Intracranial surgery: to shave or not to shave. *Otology and Neurology* 2001; 22: 908-11.

127. Hallstrom R, Beck S. Implementation of the AORN skin shaving standard. *AORN Journal* 1993; 58(3): 498-506.

128. Kumar K, Thomas J, Chan C. Cosmesis in neurosurgery: is the bald head necessary to avoid postoperative infection. *Annals of Academic Medicine of Singapore* 2002; 31: 150-4.

129. Alexander J, Fischer J, Boyajian M, Palmquist J, Morris M. The influence of hair removal methods on wound infections. *Arch Surg* 1983; 11: 347-52.

130. Court-Brown C. Pre-operative skin depilation and its effect on postoperative wound infections. *J Roy Coll Surg Edin* 1981; 26: 238-41.

131. Horgan M, Piatt J. Shaving of the scalp may increase the rate of infection in CSF shunt surgery. *Paediatric Neurosurgery* 1997; 26: 180-4.

132. Cruse PJ, Foord R. A five-year prospective study of 23,649 surgical wounds. *Arch Surg* 1973; 107: 206-16.

133. Serodian R, Reynolds BM. Wound infections after preoperative depilatory versus razor preparation. *Am J Surg* 1971; 121: 251-4.

134. Cruse P, Foord R. The epidemiology of wound infection. A 10-year prospective study of 62,939 wounds. *Surg Clin N Am* 1980; 60(1): 27-40.

135. Mishriki S, Law D, Jeffery P. Factors affecting the incidence of postoperative wound infection. *Journal of Hospital Infection* 1990; 16(3): 223-30.

136. Hamilton H, Hamilton K, Lone F. Preoperative hair removal. *Can J Surg* 1977; 20(3): 269-71.

137. Rojanapirom S, Danchaivijitr S. Pre-operative shaving and wound infection in appendectomy. *Journal of the Medical Association of Thailand* 1992; 75 (Suppl 2): 20-3.

138. Mews P. *Patient care during operative and invasive procedures*. Philadelphia: WB Saunders & Co, 2000.

139. Gilliam D, Nelson C. Comparison of one-step idorphor skin preparation versus traditional preparation in total joint surgery. *Clin Orthop Relat Res* 1990; 250: 258-60.

140. Geelhoed G, Sharpe K, Simon G. A comparative study of surgical skin preparation methods. *Surg Gynecol Obstet* 1983; 157(3): 265-8.

Chapter 2

The investigation of skeletal malignancy

Simon Carter FRCS

Consultant Orthopaedic Oncologist

ROYAL ORTHOPAEDIC HOSPITAL, BIRMINGHAM, UK

Introduction

The commonest malignancies affecting the skeleton are metastases. A half of all primary tumours produce bony metastases. Only the liver and lungs are more frequent sites of metastatic disease [1]. The commonest tumours resulting in bone metastases are: prostate (32%), breast (22%) and kidney (16%) with lung and thyroid as the next commonest [2]. The commonest sites of disease in order of frequency are the spine, pelvis, ribs, skull and proximal long bones [3]. In the USA, 1.2 million cases of cancer are diagnosed annually; thus, there is the potential for 600,000 cases of bony metastases developing [4] **(IV/C)**; 20% of these will develop clinically relevant bony metastases during their lifetime; another 50% will have metastases identified at autopsy [5] **(IV/C)**. The diagnosis and management may not follow any particular protocol, as the diagnosis depends on the past history of malignancy, the stage of that disease and treatments received. In the case of a suspected malignancy in the absence of a past history of cancer, the lesion should be considered a sarcoma until proven otherwise, although it may eventually be diagnosed as a skeletal metastasis of unknown origin, as is the situation in 3%-4% of all skeletal metastases [6] **(IV/C)**. Over the same period of one year in the USA, only 8,000 cases of sarcoma will be diagnosed.

Methodology

The literature search strategy used was via the Medline database to obtain consensus articles on the management of musculoskeletal malignancy and to obtain the available data on denominator numbers.

Features of skeletal malignancy

It has been demonstrated that patients with solitary metastases can have a longer survival with the avoidance of pathological fractures and an improved quality of life if the metastatic lesion is resected [7] **(IIa/B)**; the main exception to this being metastases from bronchogenic carcinoma, which presents with late and aggressive bone metastases. These patients have a short life expectancy and surgery should be avoided.

Primary sarcomas are tumours arising from structures derived from embryonal mesodermal tissues, unlike carcinomas which arise from endodermal or ectodermal tissues. Sarcomas are malignant, with the features of malignancy of local invasion and metastatic potential, but there are differences in behaviour when compared to carcinomas. Sarcomas tend to metastasise via the blood stream with the majority of

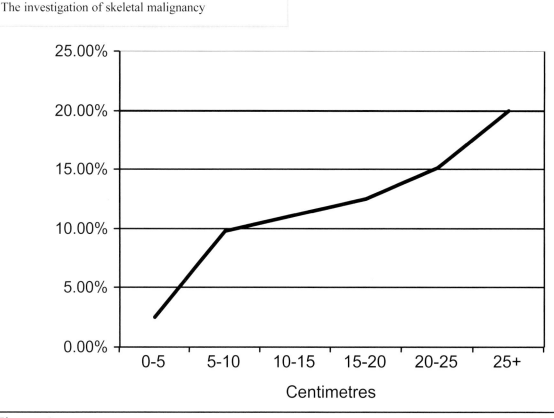

Figure 1. Incidence of metastases at diagnosis.

metastases appearing in the lungs (85%) or bone. Lymph node and hepatic metastases are rare.

Primary bone sarcomas, as sarcomas in general, are rare. The commonest, osteosarcoma, occurs with a frequency of about three cases per million of the population a year. Soft tissue sarcomas present with a frequency of 10-15 cases per million per year.

All primary bone sarcomas present in similar ways; with symptoms of pain and or swelling and occasionally as a pathological fracture. The nature of the pain is that it is a constant, non-mechanical pain often noticed at night and, as the majority of these tumours arise in childhood, the pain is ascribed to growing pains. The duration of symptoms can often be surprisingly long, the average duration of symptoms at presentation of an osteosarcoma being 13 weeks. The pain may be localised to the site of the tumour but referred pain is often a presenting symptom in pelvic tumours. The incidence of presentation of a primary bone tumour as a pathological fracture is 6-10%; careful history taking can, however, elicit symptoms which predated the fracture.

The delay in the presentation of tumours has, over the last 15 years, not altered. The mean delay to diagnosis from the onset of symptoms was for osteosarcoma 16 weeks in 1986 and the same in 2000; similarly, Ewing's sarcoma remained at 40 weeks and chondrosarcoma, 54 weeks. In both reviews of patient presentation, 25% of patients had the tumour missed on initial radiographs. The delay in presentation results in large tumour sizes. It is well recognised that large tumours have a worse prognosis than smaller lesions. Larger tumours have a greater likelihood of metastatic disease at presentation (Figure 1).

When a patient presents with a history and features suggestive of a primary bone sarcoma, what investigations should be performed? The differential diagnosis of a primary bone sarcoma is infection; therefore, an infection screen should be performed. A raised ESR, however, does not exclude sarcoma, as in Ewing's sarcoma, a raised ESR is recognised as a poor prognostic factor, especially when combined with systemic symptoms, for example, night sweats and fever.

Radiographs of the affected part are by far the most important diagnostic tool, often showing features of bone destruction, neoplastic bone formation, soft tissue swelling and periosteal reaction. The role of bone scanning and MRI in diagnosis is limited but both are vital parts of the tumour work-up to identify the site, extent and relationship of the tumour to adjacent structures in order to plan management.

Having identified a possible primary bone sarcoma, what should be the next step in the management of the patient? Ideally, the patient should be referred to a specialised treatment centre for biopsy, staging and treatment [8] **(IIa/B)**. The investigations performed are: chest CT scanning and a whole body bone scan, to identify the presence of metastatic disease, and an MRI of the tumour to assess its anatomical relationships. Staging studies can be performed at the presenting institution if there is no delay to the referral. At the referring centre, after the staging studies have been completed, a biopsy will be performed. The purpose of staging the patient's tumour is to plan treatment and to allow for comparison of treatment results between centres.

The diagnostic factors suggesting malignancy in a soft tissue lesion are (see Table 1 for corresponding risk of malignancy): 1) size greater than 5cm; 2) increasing size of the lesion; 3) a mass deep to the deep fascia; and 4) a painful mass.

Table 1. Diagnostic features suggesting malignancy.

Features	Risk of malignancy
None	Nil
1	16%
2	43%
3	65%
4	86%

If these risk factors are combined then the possibility of the lesion being sarcomatous can be assessed. A recurrent lump, irrespective of the previous histology, should also be considered malignant until proven otherwise.

The overall management of the patient depends on the diagnosis of the tumour and the presence or otherwise of metastatic disease. All patients are staged before biopsy and the biopsy should be performed with an awareness of the eventual surgical treatment.

Staging studies

Irrespective of the diagnosis (as it is not known at this stage) all patients should undergo investigations prior to biopsy to assess the extent of the disease. The investigations needed are MRI scanning of the affected part, bone scanning and a chest CT.

MRI scanning of the affected part

The MRI should show the entire bone and adjacent joints (Figure 2). Osteosarcoma and Ewing's sarcoma can have multiple foci of tumour within the affected

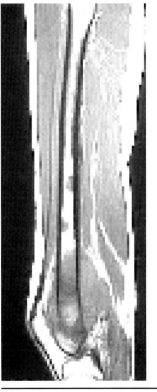

Figure 2. MRI scan of a distal femur showing the presence of skip metastases, soft tissue swelling and absence of joint involvement, but with a swelling beneath the synovium of the suprapatella pouch.

Chapter 2

bone; the skip lesions have the same prognostic significance as metastatic disease. The involvement of an adjacent joint or bone may limit the surgical options available. MRI after biopsy may alter the appearance of size of the tumour as a result of oedema or haemorrhage.

Bone scanning

The scan should be of the entire body. Many bone scan departments, for reasons of economy, do not routinely produce images distal to the knee or elbow; 60% of osteosarcoma occur around the knee and a significant proportion may, therefore, be missed.

The bone scan may identify the extent of bone involvement, the presence of skip lesions or other bone metastases and may occasionally identify ossifying lung metastases. The renal images may be useful, as an abnormal image may suggest a renal primary tumour with the bone lesion being a metastatic renal cell malignancy. The bone scan must be performed before the biopsy as the biopsy itself will produce a 'hot spot'. The investigation of a possible bone tumour requires an idea of the activity of the lesion; a quiescent lesion would appear, therefore, to be active on bone scan after biopsy.

Chest CT

Eighty-five percent of all metastases from primary bone sarcomas are to the chest as a result of haematogenous spread. A chest radiograph will identify lesions of about 1cm in diameter, whereas a CT will pick up lesions of 1-2mm in size. It is not the size of the metastasis that is prognostically important but the presence or otherwise of metastases. There is no role for abdominal CT, angiography or ultrasound in the staging of primary bone sarcomas.

Once the staging studies have been performed, with the possible exception of the chest CT, a biopsy should be the next investigation. The biopsy should be performed following review of the imaging studies of the tumour.

Sarcomas are often heterogeneous with areas of viable tissue and areas of necrosis. Review of the

MRI will identify those areas where there is a greater likelihood of obtaining representative viable tissue; an example of this is when biopsying a chondroid tumour arising in conjunction with a pre-existing enchondroma. Care should be taken to avoid any area of persisting enchondroma but tissue should be taken from sites of tumour activity at areas of endosteal scalloping. The biopsy tract will, of course, be contaminated by tumour and care should be taken to avoid spreading the tumour into previously uncontaminated compartments. The site of the biopsy should allow for the tract to be excised with the tumour at the time of resection and should, therefore, be in line with the incision of the definitive procedure. The biopsy should be performed at the centre performing the definitive treatment. Such centres should have pathologists experienced in the diagnosis of primary bone tumours, which is well recognised as being a particularly difficult area of pathology.

The quantity of tissue required for diagnosis should be determined by the requirements of the pathologist. In many centres, needle biopsies are usually considered adequate but there must be sufficient tissue for histopathological studies and for further immunohistopathology and cytogenetic studies, microbiology, and tissue for further studies including research. The pathological diagnosis of musculoskeletal malignancies is difficult and, therefore, specimens should be sent to experienced pathology departments, which are usually only available at tumour centres.

It is therefore apparent that to perform a biopsy there must be co-operation of the clinical staff, radiologists and pathologists, all forming part of a multidisciplinary team. There is no place for a biopsy of a suspected sarcoma to be performed outside a specialist centre.

A review of 597 biopsies of musculoskeletal malignancies revealed that only 315 were performed at a musculoskeletal tumour centre. The risk of a major error in diagnosis was twice as high if the biopsy was performed at the referring centre, and the errors, complications, changes in course and outcome were between two to 12 times greater when performed outside specialist centres [9] **(IIa/B)**.

Pathological fracture as the initial presentation does cause some problems during the staging studies, as the haemorrhage associated with the fracture may give the appearance that the tumour is of a larger size. Also, the fracture haematoma may result in the spread of tumour cells into adjacent compartments or perhaps the dissemination of micrometastases. The presence of a fracture may result in a delay in presentation, as it may not be apparent initially that the fracture occurred at the site of a primary bone sarcoma and may be subjected to inappropriate surgery.

In soft tissue sarcomas, an excisional biopsy may be performed if the lesion is less than 2-3cm.

At the completion of the staging studies and biopsy, the results should be combined to stage the tumour and plan management. It is vital that such discussions are conducted within a multidisciplinary setting. It is the presence of such a team that is associated with a better long-term result for the patient.

Conclusions

Urgent referral to a centre specialising in the investigation and treatment of these conditions is strongly recommended, as inappropriate delays and investigations may prejudice the eventual outcome for the patient.

Recommendations	Evidence level
As musculoskeletal malignancy can present in a variety of ways in any anatomical site and may be one of literally hundreds of differing pathological entities, there are no randomised trials concerned with the investigation of musculoskeletal malignancy. The following recommendations are the result of consensus opinions derived by bodies concerned with these malignancies.	
◆ Do not biopsy a malignant musculoskeletal tumour if it is a solitary lesion or is a suspected sarcoma with or without fracture; refer to a musculoskeletal tumour centre.	IIa/B
◆ During the presentation of a patient with suspected metastatic disease, perform the following investigations: local plain films, chest radiograph, laboratory tests. If suspicious, then proceed to a bone scan, if the lesion is: o monostotic - CT/MR imaging, biopsy (ideally at musculoskeletal tumour centre); o polyostotic, no impending fracture - biopsy most accessible lesion; impending fracture - biopsy and stabilise/resect.	IIa/B
◆ In a patient with suspected sarcoma (bone or soft tissue), refer to a musculoskeletal tumour centre.	IIa/B
◆ Should there be any concern about the care of a patient with musculoskeletal malignancy, the local treatment centre should be contacted for advice.	IV/C

Chapter 2

References

1. Hage AD, Aboulafia AJ, Aboulafia DM. Incidence, location and diagnostic evaluation of metastatic disease. *Orthop Clin North Am* 2000; 31: 515-28.

2. Clain A. Secondary malignant disease of bone. *Br J Cancer* 1965; 19: 15-29.

3. Silverberg E. Cancer statistics 1986. *Ca Cancer J Clin* 1986; 36: 9-25.

4. Cancer facts and figures, Atlanta, GA. American Cancer Society, 1999; 1-36.

5. Mirra JM. Bone Tumours. In: *Bone Tumours*. Malvern, PA: Lea and Febiger 1989: 1498.

6. Holmes FF, Fouts TL. Metastatic cancer of unknown primary site. *Cancer* 1970; 26: 816-20.

7. Capanna R, Campanacci DA. The treatment of metastases in the appendicular skeleton. *J Bone Joint Surg* 2001; 83-B: 471-81.

8. Springfield DS, Rosenberg A. Biopsy: complicated and risky. *J Bone Joint Surg* 1996; 78-A,5: 639-43.

9. Mankin HJ, Mankin CJ, Simon MA. The hazards of biopsy revisited. *J Bone Joint Surg* 1996; 78-A,5: 656-63.

Chapter 3

The management of paediatric long bone fractures

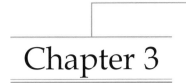

Paul J Harwood MRCS
Specialist Registrar, Orthopaedic Surgery
Peter A Templeton FRCS (Orth)
Consultant in Orthopaedic Surgery

THE GENERAL INFIRMARY AT LEEDS, LEEDS, UK

Introduction

Due primarily to advances in the treatment of infective disease, paediatric illness and mortality have fallen significantly over the past three decades. Traumatic injury is now the most common cause of hospital attendance and mortality in paediatric patients over one year of age [1-4]. An overall fracture rate of 36.1/1000 per year within the paediatric population of the UK has been reported [2]. Amongst childhood injuries, long bone fractures account for up to 35% of admissions [5]. Fractures in childhood deserve special consideration for several reasons, all related intimately to age, the adolescent patient behaving in an increasingly adult manner with respect to responses to injury.

A child's bone has different biomechanical properties from that of an adult. Paediatric bone is not only more elastic than adult bone, but also suffers a higher degree of plastic deformation prior to ultimate failure [6]. The periosteum forms a much more substantial layer than that of an adult, contributing significantly to the overall strength of the bone. This periosteum is seldom completely divided during fracture, altering the way in which paediatric fractures

displace and sometimes hindering or aiding reduction. The growing bone has a propensity to remodel, allowing a greater degree of fracture displacement to be accepted, and heals rapidly after fracture. The presence of an open epiphysis, however, also raises the prospect of physeal injury and subsequent growth disturbance.

The overall needs of younger patients must also be considered in contrast to those of adults. Children respond differently to injury, both physiologically and psychologically. Their reaction to pain and hospitalisation requires special consideration leading to different methods of analgesia and anaesthetic. A high index of suspicion must always be maintained for the possibility of non-accidental injury.

Patterns of injury change with the patient's age, influenced both by environmental factors and by the development of the child. A bimodal distribution of trauma-related mortality is reported with peaks at the beginning and end of childhood [2]. Rates of fracture increase with age; in older children an increasing proportion occur in males, to match the strong male preponderance of traumatic injury observed in the adult population [7]. In general, long bone fracture rates are seen to increase with age, although this increase is greater in males, whilst femoral fractures actually become less common with age in females [7].

Methodology

An electronic database search was undertaken using the Cochrane library, Pubmed and Embase. Combinations of the terms 'humerus', 'radius OR ulna OR forearm', 'femur', 'tibia', 'child OR paediatric' and 'shaft OR diaphyseal' were used to identify potentially relevant papers. Abstracts were retrieved and reviewed, pertinent papers were selected with priority given to well designed clinical trials with stronger levels of evidence. Only papers published in the last ten years were considered, with precedence given to more recent publications. Information was supplemented with further literature searches on specific topics as appropriate. This chapter is intended to offer an update on current evidence rather than a comprehensive systematic literature review.

Femur

Femoral shaft fracture is encountered relatively frequently and has recently been reported as the commonest cause of paediatric orthopaedic inpatient treatment, accounting for almost 22% of a series detailing more than 80,000 patients from the USA [8]. The peak incidence in this series occurred at two years of age with a male preponderance of 3:1 [8]. As in adult patients, femoral fracture is commonly seen in patients with multiple injuries [9]. Typically, femoral shaft fracture, particularly in younger patients, has been associated with a high risk of non-accidental injury, with rates of 60%-80% reported in some series [10, 11]. However, Schwend et al, by examining 139 cases from their institution, emphasise that other factors in the patient's presentation are more important than the fracture distribution in determining the likelihood of child abuse. Indeed, whilst a 42% risk of non-accidental injury was reported in children who have not started walking, this risk fell to 2.6% in patients who have. The need for vigilance is clear, although the risk of damage to the family unit by overzealous pursuit of these cases is highlighted.

Femoral shaft fractures in children are seldom complicated by delayed or non-union, reported problems generally arising due to the deformity associated with malunion or overgrowth [12]. Traditionally, paediatric patients with femoral shaft fracture have been treated non-operatively with good results, either by traction or cast immobilisation in a hip spica. Although these methods are still advocated [13], new innovations have offered the opportunity to facilitate rapid mobilisation. Several studies have highlighted the potential for early discharge and cost saving by adopting early operative management protocols rather than traction **(IIa/B)** [14, 15]. Firm indications for operative management include concomitant multiple, ipsilateral tibial ('floating knee') [16] or head injury, local soft tissue damage and pathological fractures. Relative indications include the age and size of the child, social and economic factors; in older patients with a diminished potential for remodelling, more accurate reduction becomes increasingly important [17]. A survey of current practice amongst American paediatric orthopaedic surgeons, carried out in 1998, showed an increasing trend towards operative management with increasing patient age [18]. A consensus statement describing the care most frequently recommended for each age group and fracture pattern is summarised in Table 1. Treatment options were early spica, traction then cast, Pavlik harness, flexible nail, external fixator, plate and screws and reamed intramedullary nail (IMN). Simple fractures were divided into spiral and transverse patterns; there were few differences between the responses for these two groups except for the six to nine-year-olds and those older than nine years where external fixation was also recommended by 29% and 28% of respondents for spiral, but not transverse fractures. It is clear from this data that considerable difference of opinion still remains regarding the different treatment options available, which is likely in part, to be due to the relative lack of data from properly controlled clinical trials. The protocol for a Cochrane systematic review has been published in the Cochrane library but this is as yet incomplete [19].

Table 1. Summary of questionnaire responses from paediatric orthopaedic surgeons regarding treatment of femoral fracture (adapted from Sanders *et al* [18]). Where the second most common response was 75% as frequently given as the first, multiple results are given. Numbers in parentheses show the percentage of respondents giving that answer.

Age group	Simple	Multi-fragmentary	Polytrauma
<1 year	Early spica (80%)	Early spica (82%)	Early spica (49%)
1-6 years	Early spica (70%)	Early spica (44%) Traction then cast (36%)	Ex-fix (49%)
6-9 years	Traction then cast (38%) Ex-fix (29%)	Ex-fix (44%) Traction then cast (42%)	Ex-fix (49%)
>9 years	Reamed IMN (30%) Flexible nail (30%)	Ex-fix (46%)	Ex-fix (39%) Reamed IMN (34%)

Traction

Although there has been a progressive shift away from traction as definitive management of femoral shaft fractures for economic and social reasons, it still has a role to play (Figure 1). It is frequently used as a temporising method whilst the patient is prepared for theatre or for a period prior to spica casting to allow easier control of the fracture position during application. Other than the economic data supporting a move away from definitive traction, little recent literature is available on the subject. A case series from the Middle East described comparable results in their practice with conservative and operative treatment from a series of more than 300 patients, 45% and 22% of whom were treated by balanced skin or skeletal traction, respectively [13]. A further case series from Eastern Europe reported good results in a series of 209 patients treated by gallows or balanced skin traction dependent on their age **(III/B)** [20].

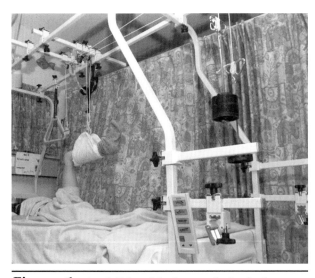

Figure 1. A child with femoral shaft fracture treated by balanced skeletal traction.

Spica

Hip spica application offers a non-invasive method of femoral stabilisation, with a cast applied from chest to toes immobilising the hip and knee at approximately 90°. Although traditionally applied following a period of traction, to achieve some prior stability of the fracture site, this has been increasingly advocated as an early primary treatment option [21, 22]. However, the cast is only suitable for younger, smaller patients, is extremely cumbersome and treatment can be complicated by pressure sores [23]. Various case series document successful use of this method in patients less than ten years of age, with union rates of 100% reported. Loss of position, particularly in terms of length, is problematic with rates of cast reapplication reported at 9% to 20% [21, 22]. This was particularly problematic in patients older than seven years, and some authors have recommended its use in patients only aged six or less **(III/B)** [22]. It has been shown that the position achieved at seven to ten days correlates well with final position at union [21].

In a recent well designed, prospective randomised trial, Wright *et al* compared early spica immobilisation with operative management in the form of external fixation. This study included 108 patients aged four to ten years, assessed two years post-injury [24]. Eleven percent of patients treated by spica casting required conversion to other forms of fixation, due to unacceptable loss of position, with a further 3.5% requiring re-manipulation and spica application. Similarly, 11% of patients treated by external fixation required adjustment of the fixator under anaesthetic and two patients (4%) re-fractured after removal of the device, both successfully treated by open reduction and plate fixation. The mean treatment duration was significantly longer in the external fixation group (77 vs. 58 days). Twenty patients in the external fixation group received a course of oral antibiotics for pin-site infection but none required hospitalisation and there were no cases of deep infection. Rates of malunion, defined as 2cm of leg length discrepancy, 15° AP angulation or 10° varus / valgus angulation, were significantly higher in the spica group (45% vs. 16%, relative risk 2.86, number needed to treat 3.4). Therefore, one malunion was avoided for approximately every four patients treated by external fixation rather than spica cast **(Ib/A)**. Grouping the patients by age did not alter this. Although the long-term effects of malunion in these patients are unknown, the authors conclude that at two years follow-up, the majority of remodelling will already have occurred and this deformity is likely to be permanent. A further randomised trial examining gait patterns in 31 patients also treated by external fixation or spica immobilisation found persisting gait abnormalities in the patients treated by spica not present in the external fixation group **(Ib/A)** [25]. It is concluded that spica immobilisation should be employed with care and possibly reserved for patients less than three years of age.

External fixation

External fixation has offered an attractive method of treatment for children with femoral fracture, as it is relatively quick and easy to perform and spares the growth plate (Figure 2). However, pin-site care can be problematic and the fixator is often seen as a focus of anxiety for the parents and the child. It is therefore of interest that in Wright's study, patient and parent treatment satisfaction scores were not significantly different from those treated by casting, suggesting that the problem may be less significant than is generally supposed [24]. Another major concern limiting

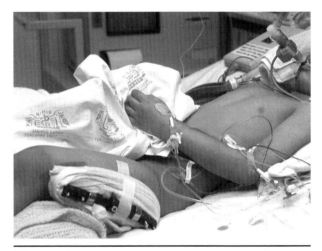

Figure 2. A multiply injured child with femoral shaft fracture treated by external fixation.

application of this technique has been the high frequency of re-fracture following removal of the fixator, with rates of up to 22% reported [26]. Again this concern may well be unfounded, with a re-fracture rate of 4% in Wright's study and no serious infections **(Ib/A)**. Similarly, several case series document good overall results following external fixation. Hedin *et al* reported 86% of fractures within 10° of neutral angulation at union, with the remaining fractures remodelling to acceptable positions within one year; this was unaffected by the patient's age **(III/B)** [27]. Infection was common in this series, occurring in 37% of cases, but all were superficial and treated by pin-site cleaning or antibiotics alone (50% each). In another series of 192 patients treated by a combination of traction with conversion to a spica cast or external fixation, reviewed at a mean of six years, no significant difference in re-fracture rate was recorded (0% vs. 1.8%) However, a higher rate of 20% was observed in a further group treated by open reduction and external fixation **(III/B)** [28]. Domb *et al* reported a 2% re-fracture rate, a 21% rate of infection (2% serious) and a 4% mal-reduction rate, requiring adjustment of the fixator **(III/B)**. In this series, 53 patients were randomised to dynamisation of their fixators when early callus formation was observed. No significant difference between the groups was observed in terms of time to union, fixator removal or full weight-bearing, with the conclusion that axial dynamisation offers no advantage over static external fixation **(Ib/A)**. Overall therefore, it would appear that external fixation offers a safe and effective treatment method with good rates of union, low rates of malunion and lower than expected rates of re-fracture.

In a study of patients treated by external fixation, a mean overgrowth of 0.3cm at one year and 0.5cm at two years was observed. Overgrowth was significantly more pronounced in the youngest group of patients (three to four years old). There was no observed effect on overgrowth by angulation or displacement of the fracture, the degree of shortening, the type or location of the fracture or the sex of the patient **(IIb/B)** [27].

Open reduction and internal fixation (compression plating)

Open plating of femoral fractures offers the advantages of operative treatment in terms of early mobilisation and discharge, as well as rigid, anatomic fixation, with better control of fractures located towards the bone ends. However, the large exposure with consequent scarring and blood loss, alongside the potential requirements for implant removal, must be considered. Caird *et al* reported their experience with 60 patients, with a mean age of eight years, treated via a lateral approach using 3.5mm or 4.5mm dynamic compression plates as appropriate to the child's size **(III/B)** [29]. Two patients required blood transfusion. The mean time to clinical and radiological union was eight weeks and the hardware was removed in all patients at a mean of 11 months (3-24). One patient (1.6%) suffered early hardware failure

and two (3.2%) re-fractured; all patients went on to eventual union with other treatments. Although two patients had significant leg length discrepancy, there were no instances of hip avascular necrosis, premature physeal closure, infection or neurovascular injury and all patients had returned to their pre-injury level of activity at the end of follow-up. Eren *et al* reported a series of 46 similarly treated patients, with a mean age of eight years (four to ten years), followed-up for a mean of six years, 28 of whom underwent hardware removal at a mean of 18 months **(III/B)** [30]. Fracture healing was observed in all at ten weeks; there was one case of osteomyelitis (2.1%) successfully treated by debridement and early plate removal at five months without subsequent problems. A mean of 1.2cm leg length discrepancy was observed due to overgrowth, occurring in 15 patients, none of whom had subjective problems or gait abnormality. Interestingly, only 20% of the patients with retained metalwork had a leg length discrepancy, compared with 50% of those in whom the plate was removed. No patients with retained plates reported local symptoms. Successful bridge plating of closed, multi-fragmentary fractures using a percutaneous technique has also been described **(III/B)** [31]. In a series of 14 patients there were no incidences of metalwork failure, and the mean time to union was 12 weeks. At a mean of 48 months follow-up all patients had achieved a full range of motion in the hip and knee and there were no clinically relevant leg length discrepancies.

Interlocked intramedullary nailing

Intramedullary nailing offers stable femoral fixation and reamed, locked antegrade nailing is the treatment of choice for femoral shaft fracture in adults [32]. In children, concerns over damage to the greater trochanteric apophysis and the blood supply to the femoral head, alongside good results achieved through other methods, have meant that this method has not been widely employed in this group. Although avascular necrosis is a relatively rare complication, its consequences are devastating for this young group of patients [33, 34]. In adolescents, however, controversies remain [18]. Momberger *et al* have described their experience with a series of 50 patients, aged from ten to 16 years (mean 13.2) treated by standard reamed, locked, antegrade nailing, with the nail entry point posterior and lateral to the piriformis fossa **(III/B)** [35]. There were no infections or non-unions and at a mean of 16 months follow-up there were no patients with clinical or radiological evidence of femoral head osteonecrosis. Average hospital stay in patients without other injuries was 3.2 days. One patient required transfusion. Articulo-trochanteric distance was observed to be reduced to an average of 4.5mm compared with the non-operated side. However, no patients had a symptomatic gait disturbance or an observed leg length discrepancy of over 10mm. The benefits of choosing an entry point lateral to the piriformis fossa and avoiding use of the awl are highlighted in avoiding damage to the retinacular vessels. Whilst these results are impressive, it should be noted that in general, reamed antegrade intramedullary nailing is not recommended in the skeletally immature **(IV/C)**.

Titanium elastic nailing

A relatively recent addition to available treatment options, titanium elastic nails have renewed the interest in intramedullary fixation of paediatric fractures. Their flexibility allows insertion through a small incision without injury to the physis, by a relatively straightforward technique. Various case series have demonstrated that this method can be used successfully with good union rates and a very low rate of fracture displacement [36-38]. In addition, patients have reported satisfaction with the treatment and outcome [38], but several authors have reported relatively high rates of adverse events. Luhmann et al reported a 49% complication rate in 49 patients, including one case of septic arthritis on nail removal, one case of delayed union and one atrophic non-union [39]. In one patient, in whom nail insertion caused significant comminution at the fracture site, the procedure was abandoned and the fracture successfully treated by open reduction and plate fixation. Twenty-nine percent reported significant pain at the nail insertion site and 9% suffered nail erosion though the skin; each of these problems was associated with protrusion of the nail end from the insertion point by more than 40mm with an optimum length of 25mm recommended. Similarly, Narayanan et al reported a 53% rate of local symptoms along with rates of 10% for malunion and 2.5% for

both re-fracture and superficial infection [40]. By logistic regression analysis it was determined that prominence of the nail ends greater than 10mm from the cortex measured in the transverse plane was associated with an increased risk of local problems (adjusted odds ratio [OR] 4.5). By similar methods, malunion and significant loss of position was strongly associated with mismatched nail diameters (OR 19.4), as well as fracture comminution (OR 5.3) and multiple injuries (OR 4.4). Interestingly, in a group of 25 patients who were asymptomatic at six months post-op and therefore did not have their nails removed, none had become symptomatic by final follow-up (mean 3.6 years).

A biomechanical analysis, examined different nail configurations utilising a model of a six-year-old child's femur. The constructs examined were a pair of C-shaped nails, a pair of straight nails (inserted retrograde from medial and lateral sides in both cases), and one S-shaped and one C-shaped nail (inserted antegrade through the lateral cortex). The study identified no difference in the mechanical properties of these different patterns, suggesting that any of these configurations could be used, as preferred, in each case [41]. A similar study from Gwyn et al investigated the torsional stability of transverse, oblique, spiral, butterfly, and comminuted femoral fractures stabilised using titanium elastic nails. Whilst the oblique and spiral fractures exhibited the highest stability in internal and external rotation respectively, all constructs were found to be at least as stable as in simple transverse fractures. It was concluded that in this respect, flexible nailing was a suitable treatment for all fracture types [42].

Tibia

Tibial fractures are relatively uncommon in children compared to the population as a whole; however, their incidence rises sharply through adolescence with peak occurrence in 20 to 30-year-olds [5, 43]. Despite this, tibial fracture remains the second most common fracture requiring inpatient care in a paediatric population, accounting for 21.5% of orthopaedic trauma admissions [8]. Non-operative treatment methods are employed in more than 90% of cases with good results [44, 45]. Indications for operative management include failure of conservative methods, multi-level, open or comminuted fractures and polytrauma [46]. External fixation and intra-medullary devices have both been successfully employed; however, only limited evidence was identified comparing different methods of fixation, probably due to the relative infrequency of operative management in these patients.

Non-operative management

The mainstay of treatment in paediatric tibial fractures remains closed reduction and plaster-cast immobilisation. Gicquel *et al* have described their experience with conservative methods in a series of 102 patients treated by closed reduction and long-leg casting, with conversion to a Sarmiento patellar tendon weight-bearing cast at a mean of 26 days **(III/B)** [46]. The mean total immobilisation time was 64 days. All fractures united, although one patient suffered re-fracture at the same level five months later following a significant injury.

Intact fibula

From the above series, eight patients (7.8%) united with more than 5° of angular deformity. The presence of an intact fibula was associated with a persistent varus deformity, occurring in 76% of 21 patients, although the deformity was greater than 5° in only three patients. This is consistent with findings from another series of 95 children with isolated tibial fractures and an intact fibula. Whilst 76 patients initially had a varus or posterior angular deformity, 32 (42%) had recurrence of this deformity following closed reduction, all occurring within 21 days of injury [47]. Although 15 (47%) required cast wedging, none required operative intervention and it is concluded that conservative management is still appropriate in these cases, with serial X-rays for three weeks to monitor for loss of position. In a series reported by Wessel *et al*, isolated tibial fracture was significantly associated with increased risk of leg length discrepancy, as was repeated manipulation and age less than ten years at the time of fracture. This group recommended operative management of older children **(IIb/B)** [48].

Operative management

Intramedullary nailing

Flexible nails offer similar advantages in tibial fractures as in femoral fractures. Good results have been described using pairs of matched, C-shaped antegrade nails inserted using an entry point 1.5-2cm distal to the physis, with the nail tips left 1 cm proud to allow removal [38, 49, 50]. In a series of 16 patients treated in such a manner following failure of closed manipulation, 100% union rates were achieved at a mean of nine weeks, despite the fact that 14 (88%) were high energy injuries and three (19%) were open fractures. At union, no patients had angular deformity of greater than 10° in the sagittal or 5° in the coronal plane and there were no tibial length inequalities of greater than 7mm. All nails were removed without complication **(III/B)** [44]. It has been observed that the eccentric placement of the tibia within its soft tissue envelope coupled with its triangular cross-sectional shape mean that with standard nail placement, there will be a tendency for the tibia to drift into recurvatum. It is therefore recommended that the nail tips are turned dorsally to counteract this deforming force [51].

Court-Brown *et al* have published a series of 36 adolescent (13 to 16 years old) but skeletally immature patients, treated by reamed, locked, antegrade nailing for closed diaphyseal tibial fractures. Nails were placed using an entry point just above the tibial tubercle, slightly lower than usual, to reduce the risk of injury to the proximal tibial growth plate. No patients suffered problems related to premature physeal closure and all patients united (mean 11.5 weeks). There was a relatively high rate of compartment syndrome (8%) but no other significant complications **(III/B)** [52].

External fixation

The feasibility of external fixation for stabilisation of paediatric tibial fractures has been demonstrated in several case series [53-56]. Gordon *et al* describe a series of 46 tibial fractures treated by mono-lateral (29) or circular, fine wire (16) fixators. It was found that in patients aged more than 12 years, loss of reduction was relatively common in those with mono-lateral frames but did not occur with circular fixators **(IIb/B)** [57].

In the only identified comparative study for paediatric tibial fractures, Kubiak *et al* recently reported results comparing 31 skeletally immature patients treated by external fixation (15) or elastic nailing (16) for tibial shaft fractures **(IIb/B)** [58]. Fifty-three percent and 32%, respectively, of these fractures were open injuries. The mean time to union was significantly shorter in the nailing group (seven vs. 18 weeks, p<0.01) and significantly better functional outcome, as estimated using the Paediatric Outcomes Data Collection Instrument, was also recorded. Although the rates of open fracture were not significantly different between the groups in this series due to the sample size, given the impact of soft tissue injury in these patients, it would be interesting to evaluate these results further using a larger sample or randomisation of treatment method.

Open tibial fractures

Several series reported experience treating open tibial fractures in children [59-64]. Soft tissue injuries are treated using the same principles as in adults, with early debridement and subsequent soft-tissue cover where required. In contrast to adults with open tibial fractures, however, most of the patients in these series had their fractures stabilised using casts (45%-83%); the majority of the remainder were treated by external fixation or intramedullary nailing with plate fixation used in a few cases (Figure 3). Overall, results were good, with 92%-98% of fractures uniting without further intervention. Union was achieved in an average of 9-14 weeks for patients treated in plaster and 15-20 weeks for those treated using an external fixator. In general it was observed that union occurred significantly faster in patients with grade I/II injuries compared to those with grade III injuries. Infection rates were low, with superficial infections in 5%-8% and deep infections reported in 0%-10% of cases. Complication rates in younger patients were lower than observed in adults, suggesting that less aggressive treatment might be appropriate; however, in patients older than 11 years the clinical course parallels that in adults **(III/B)** [53, 60, 62-64].

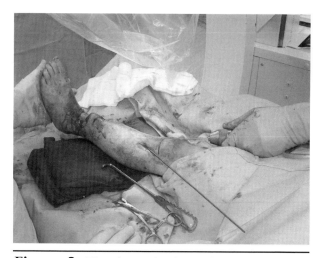

Figure 3. Titanium elastic nailing of an open tibial fracture.

Levy *et al* assessed the social impact of open tibial fractures in a series of 40 patients, 40% of whom had suffered grade I, 25% grade II and 35% grade III injuries. It was found that on average children missed four months of school and 33% needed to repeat the year. Twenty-five percent reported nightmares relating to the accident and 30% reported chronic pain, despite solid union at the fracture site **(IIb/B)** [65].

Humerus

Paediatric humeral shaft fracture is relatively uncommon, although varying rates have been reported, with the injury accounting for between 2% and 8% of admissions for fracture in children [5, 8, 66]. The majority of these injuries can be treated conservatively as, due to the potential for remodelling, anatomic reduction is not required **(IV/C)** [67]. Indeed, traditional practice in proximal humeral fractures has shown that children under five can tolerate 70° of angulation and complete displacement and even children aged more than 12 years can tolerate 40° of angulation with 50% displacement [68]. In mid-shaft fractures, 20-30° varus angulation, and 20° of anterior bowing have been found to be tolerable. Shortening of 1-2cm is also acceptable, as overgrowth is often observed and this deformity is well tolerated even when residual [69]. Due to the muscle bulk of the upper arm, clinical appearance is often more important than radiographic measurements, with varus angulation less well tolerated and deformity being more obvious in more distal humeral fractures. Non-operative treatment options include slings, hanging casts and functional bracing for three to six weeks, depending on the child's age. Indications for operative management include failure of conservative treatment, open fractures, pathological fracture [70] and multiple injuries. Due to the popularity and success of conservative measures, little recent literature specifically regarding the management of paediatric humeral shaft injuries is available. As with other long bone fractures, several papers have recently highlighted the fact that although a high level of vigilance must be maintained for non-accidental injury, rates are probably much lower than previously suggested and factors other than fracture site and pattern are more important in predicting such cases [71, 72]. These include inconsistent history, delayed presentation, children who have not started walking and previous fracture.

Operative management

Successful, retrograde, elastic intramedullary nailing of paediatric humeral shaft fractures has been reported by several groups, although no comparative studies are available (III/B) [38, 49, 50, 73, 74]. Good outcome from these limited series is reported, with similar potential problems to those encountered in nailing of other long bone fractures. Retrograde insertion using two nails from the lateral side is recommended to avoid damage to the ulnar nerve [51]. Open reduction and internal fixation has also been described. A small series reports good results from internal fixation of simultaneous humeral shaft and forearm fractures [75]. Another small series reports good results from external fixation of humeral shaft fractures with few complications in patients with multiple injuries and open fractures (III/B) [76]. Opinion on early exploration of primary and secondary radial nerve injuries remains divided, with the majority of the literature pertaining to adult patients alone or mixed adult and paediatric populations. Several groups state that early exploration in either case is advisable and leads to better outcome [77, 78]. Ring et al reported in a series of adult patients that transection of the nerve is almost universally associated with open injury and that

the results of early reconstruction are poor, most likely because of the extent of the injuries. Palsies in the context of closed humeral fracture almost always recovered spontaneously in this series, although the mean time to signs of recovery was seven weeks [79]. This is concordant with findings from other groups who report spontaneous recovery rates of greater than 80% in radial nerve palsy associated with simple, closed humeral fracture [80, 81]. In general, exploration of post-manipulation radial nerve injuries has been recommended to identify those nerves trapped in the fracture site. Lim et al reported 100% spontaneous recovery rates in their series of patients with radial nerve palsy following open reduction and internal fixation, recommending an expectant approach [81].

Forearm

Diaphyseal fractures of the forearm bones are relatively common in childhood, accounting for up to 15% of paediatric orthopaedic trauma admissions [16]. Although non-operative management has formed the mainstay of treatment, and some groups recommend this approach [82], others have reported relatively poor results, particularly with more proximal injuries [83-85] and increasing rates of operative management have been reported in more recent years (IV/C) [5]. The main functional impairment resulting from these deformities is a loss of forearm rotation [86]. Open reduction and internal fixation of mid-shaft forearm fractures has been used successfully in adult patients for many years. However, the extensive surgical exposure required and subsequent scarring makes this approach less attractive in children. Percutaneous nailing therefore represents an appealing alternative in younger patients [87]. Indications for operative management include angulation of greater than 10°, unstable fracture patterns, comminution, failure of reduction, failure of non-operative management and open fractures [88, 89]. External fixation has also been recommended for open and grossly comminuted injuries.

Closed reduction and casting

Despite changes in the available treatment methodologies, closed reduction and stabilisation in a well moulded plaster remains the mainstay of treatment for most children's forearm fractures. Indeed, various groups have called for caution in the adoption of more aggressive treatment regimes, citing the good results of non-operative management with low complication rates [82, 84]. Jones *et al* reported a retrospective series of more than 730 consecutive patients with closed forearm fractures treated in their unit [82]. Four hundred of these patients had suffered diaphyseal fractures. In these patients the indications for manipulation were angulation of more than 10° in those aged less than nine years and more than 8° in older children. Up to 1cm of shortening was also accepted in the younger patients. Post reduction X-rays were taken twice in the first three weeks with the same indications for re-manipulation. If a satisfactory position was achieved, the patient was returned to a long-arm cast, if not, the cast was supplemented with K-wires placed percutaneously into the thumb metacarpal and distal ulna to aid traction. These wires were then included in the plaster cast. Overall, 41% of patients required closed manipulation. Unfortunately it is unclear from the manuscript what proportion had suffered diaphyseal fractures. Of these patients, only 7% required re-manipulation and in just over half of these, supplemental K-wires were used. One hundred percent union rates are reported with no cases of malunion. Two of the 12 patients treated with supplemental wires suffered wound infection treated with oral antibiotics and two had restriction of forearm pronation and supination. These results are contrasted with the rates of complications reported in series employing various methods of internal fixation. Although the method of operative management employed is somewhat unusual, with most groups now using internal fixation or intramedullary nailing, this series highlights the high rates of success with non-operative treatment, which was used in 96.5% of patients.

Younger *et al* investigated factors affecting quality of reduction by multiple logistic regression analysis in a series of 369 patients with forearm fractures treated by closed manipulation and plaster application. Amongst the influential factors, loss of position in the cast at clinic review and the quality of initial reduction were the only significant predictors of position at cast removal **(IIb/B)**. Other factors under consideration

were age, fracture site, sex, number of bones fractured, side of fracture and use of an above or below-elbow cast. However, diaphyseal fractures were treated exclusively in above-elbow casts [90]. In a series of 109 patients with distal 1/3 radial fractures randomised to immobilisation in pronation, neutral rotation or supination, Boyer *et al* found that this had no significant effect on the position of the fracture at cast removal **(Ib/A)** [91]. In this series only fracture type significantly predicted final position, with greater angulation observed in displaced fractures compared with greenstick type.

Johari *et al* reported in a prospective observational study, that distal radial remodelling in patients with diaphyseal fractures only occurred in those aged ten years or less. This was not the case in distal radial fractures with significant remodelling occurring up to the age of 15 **(IIb/B)**. It was observed that malalignment in the radio-ulnar plane was least likely to remodel and most likely to cause loss of motion. All patients were treated by closed reduction and plaster immobilisation and the median follow-up time was three years. In a similar study of 100 patients, Qairul *et al* found all fractures united at three to six weeks and that remodelling occurred at a rate of 1.5° per month in the mid-shaft and 2.5° per month in proximal and distal 1/3 fractures [92].

Although general anaesthesia is used to facilitate closed reduction of forearm fractures in children, certainly in UK practice, several series have reported the success of intravenous regional anaesthesia for this purpose. Bratt *et al* have published a randomised, double blind trial of high and low-dose intravenous lidocaine (1.5mg/kg vs. 3.0mg/kg), including 283 children aged from three and a half to 16 years old **(Ib/A)** [93]. It was found that 96% of patients reported satisfactory anaesthesia in the higher-dose group. Lower rates were reported in patients with more displaced fractures (93%) and in this group of patients significantly less patients reported satisfaction when the low-dose anaesthesia was used (67%). There were no complications of anaesthesia. Other studies have also reported successful use of regional anaesthesia for upper limb surgery in children.

Operative treatment

Operative fixation of paediatric forearm fractures is indicated in cases where closed reduction either cannot be achieved or maintained. Open reduction and fixation using plates and screws as in adult fractures has been employed with union rates approaching 100% and relatively few complications in some series **(III/B)** [94, 95] (Figure 4). This is in contrast to reports of corrective osteotomy for malunited forearm fracture with relatively poor results and high complication rates **(III/B)** [96]. The comparison focuses on the need for accurate reduction and reliable immobilisation using operative intervention if indicated, but not ignoring the potential risk of complication as reported in other series [97]. Although all but one fracture united, Smith *et al* reported complication rates of 33% and 44% for internal fixation by open reduction and internal fixation, and intramedullary fixation, respectively, compared with 5% in patients immobilised in plaster [97]. In a series of 20 patients treated by intramedullary fixation with rush pins or Kirschner wires for diaphyseal forearm fractures, Cullen *et al* highlighted the relatively high complication rates seen with the technique in their patients [98]. Although union was achieved in all patients and 19 patients reported excellent or good clinical results, ten patients suffered complications. These included five cases of hardware migration, four infections (one osteomyelitis in a grade II open fracture), loss of reduction in two cases, three nerve injuries, one re-fracture, one malunion and one synostosis. Four patients required re-operation. Similar results are reported in various other series, although rates of adverse events vary [99]. It is concluded that although good results can be achieved, complications of the technique are to be expected. Limited reports of external fixation in paediatric forearm fractures for open fractures or multiple injuries are also available, with good results reported [76].

Van der Reis *et al* compared the results of these methods in a series of patients with displaced, diaphyseal both bone forearm fracture [100]. Of 434 patients admitted with forearm fracture, 91 met the inclusion criteria for fracture type. Fifty of these were treated by closed reduction and casting, leaving 41 treated by internal fixation. Twenty-one were treated by

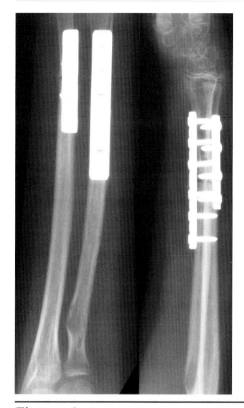

Figure 4. A forearm fracture treated by open reduction and internal fixation.

intramedullary rush-pin fixation, the ulnar wire placed antegrade, crossing the apophysis, the radial wire placed antegrade from the radial styloid, and 18 by traditional plate and screw fixation using AO / ASIF (Association for the Study of Internal Fixation) techniques. There were no significant differences between the groups, with 78% in each achieving 'excellent' and 22% 'poor' clinical results. Complications were relatively common. In the plate and screws group, there were two non-unions, one osteomyelitis, one nerve injury, one hardware failure and one case of complex-regional pain syndrome. In the intramedullary pin group, there was one delayed union, two cases of rotational malunion, and one compartment syndrome; again, there were no significant differences between the groups. The nailing procedures were significantly shorter both for the primary procedure and removal of the metal-work which was performed in all cases. Although it would appear that these techniques are equally applicable, this study is non-randomised and it is unclear how the treatments were allocated. Furthermore it is likely that the study is insufficiently powered to detect differences in complication rates or outcome between the groups **(IIa/B)**.

Flexible nailing

Elastic nailing has also been employed in paediatric forearm fractures, with union rates of 96%-100% reported and normal range of motion achieved in 90%-99% of patients **(III/B)** [38, 101-103] (Figure 5). Complication rates in these series were in the region of 10%-12% and include skin irritation and breakdown, superficial and deep infection, osteomyelitis and nerve injury. Serious complications were reported in very small numbers of patients. Various techniques are described including retrograde radial wiring, antegrade and retrograde ulnar wiring, the use of straight nails or convex bend to the medial side in the ulna and lateral bend in the radius [103]. The intention is to maintain the bow of the radius in relation to the ulna, stretching the interosseous membrane. Mann *et al* reported results from 54 patients treated by this technique, of which 7% required open reduction prior to nailing [63]. All fractures united, seven patients suffered superficial infections and there were three transient nerve palsies. One patient suffered a reduced range of motion due to exuberant callus formation but all others achieved full mobility. In a group of 34 children treated in different institutions by K-wire or elastic titanium nail intramedullary fixation, Calder *et al* reported no difference in outcome **(IIa/B)** [104]. All fractures united and no patients reported subjective disability, although a measurable loss of forearm rotation was observed in 11% treated with K-wires and 9% treated by elastic nailing; axial malunion greater than 10° was observed in 8% of the K-wire patients. Complication rates were similar. The cost saving by the use of K-wires is highlighted, with the hardware costing between 2% and 5% of that used in elastic nailing. Furthermore, only 50% of patients with K-wires required a second general anaesthetic to facilitate removal. It is acknowledged by the authors that the elastic nails do offer theoretical advantages. The study design and power may mean that real differences in outcome are not found.

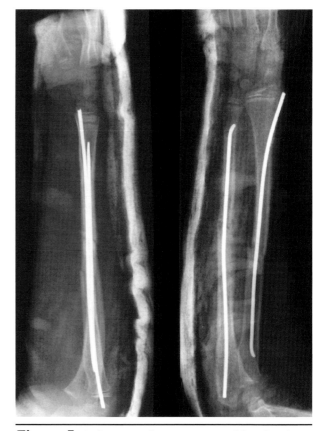

Figure 5. A forearm fracture treated by titanium elastic nailing.

Single or both bone fixation?

In a retrospective analysis of 32 children with unstable both bone forearm fracture, Bhaskar *et al* found no difference in radiological or functional outcome in patients treated by single bone or conventional both bone fixation. There were significantly more complications in the both bone fixation group, both at fixation and at subsequent plate removal. Their practice was to begin with fixation of the ulna and if an acceptable reduction of the radius was simultaneously achieved (<10° angulation), then the radius would not be addressed. They concluded that this was safe practice and may avoid complications **(IIb/B)** [105]. Flynn *et al* reported a similar series of 17 patients with both bones diaphyseal forearm fracture [106]. In cases where closed reduction was possible but could not be maintained, the ulna was fixed preferentially by intramedullary K-wiring, using an antegrade technique crossing the ulnar apophysis (nine patients). Where radial reduction was impossible, an open reduction was performed, with soft tissue interposition being found in all cases. For these patients, internal fixation of the radius was performed using a plate and screws. If this resulted in a stable ulnar reduction, second bone plating was not performed. In all cases, a long-arm cast was applied. All fractures healed and all but two patients, who lost 5° of pronation, achieved a full range of motion. It should be recognised that both these series represent a highly selected group of patients. In a further series from Lee *et al*, 32% of 22 fractures treated by single bone ulnar fixation lost position, despite supplemental cast immobilisation [107]. No fractures treated by both bones or isolated radial fixation lost position, although there were only three patients in the latter group. Similarly, Shoemaker *et al* found single bone fixation to be associated with loss of position requiring re-operation [108]. Although single-bone fixation has been employed successfully it should be used with caution and only be applied if stable reduction of the unfixed bone is clearly achieved.

Conclusions

We have attempted to summarise the recent literature regarding contemporary management of long bone fractures in paediatric patients. Although evidence-based practice is increasing, a variety of treatment methods are still applicable and wide variation in protocol is evident. Conservative management remains appropriate for the majority of patients and fractures, although the application of operative methods is increasing. It is therefore imperative that surgeons are aware of relevant indications and potential complications. More and larger randomised, controlled trials of the different operative interventions are required before meaningful evidence-based treatment guidelines can be produced. Due to the relative rarity of operative intervention in many cases, a multicentre approach to this would be advantageous.

Chapter 3

Recommendations	Evidence level
Femoral fracture	
◆ A 42% risk of non-accidental injury is reported in children with femoral fractures who do not walk, falling to <3% in those who do.	IIb/B
◆ Early operative management has been shown to reduce costs.	IIa/B
◆ Traction is still a safe method of treatment and can be used to gain temporary control of the fracture.	IIa/B
◆ Compared with external fixation, spica cast immobilisation in patients aged over three years is associated with increase rates of malunion and persisting gait abnormalities.	Ib/A
◆ Regarding external fixation, high rates of re-fracture are not observed in randomised trials and fixator dynamisation offers little advantage. Higher rates of re-fracture have been observed following open reduction.	Ib/A, III/B
◆ Both titanium elastic nailing and plate fixation have been shown to be safe, although no randomised or comparative studies were identified.	III/B

Recommendations	Evidence level

Tibial fracture

- The mainstay of treatment for tibial fracture is closed reduction and cast immobilisation, with good results reported. — III/B
- The presence of an intact fibula is associated with loss of position, although successful non-operative management is reported. Some groups recommend operative treatment in older children (>ten years). — IIb/B, IV/C
- Where operative treatment is used, elastic stable intramedullary nailing has been shown to result in more rapid union and superior functional outcome compared with external fixation. — IIa/B
- Successful treatment of open fractures is reported using similar techniques to those employed in adults. Younger children (<12 years) appear to have more favourable outcome. — III/B
- The significant psychological and social impact of these injuries has been reported, with patients missing four months of school on average and a third needing to repeat the year. — IIb/B

Humeral fracture

- Due to the potential for remodelling and the fact that moderate malunion is generally well tolerated, non-operative management is recommended for the majority of paediatric humeral shaft fractures. — III/B
- Successful elastic nailing, internal and external fixation have been reported. — III/B
- Opinion is divided on early exploration of radial nerve injuries. High rates of spontaneous recovery are reported, particularly in closed fractures and following internal fixation. — III/B

Forearm fracture

- Malunion of forearm fractures is associated with poor functional outcome, particularly with more proximal injury in older patients. — III/B
- Coronal malalignment is least well tolerated. — IIb/B
- Significant remodelling following diaphyseal forearm fractures is only observed in patients aged less than 11 years. — IIb/B
- Rates of 1.5° per month are reported. — III/B
- Quality of initial reduction and loss of position in the cast are the only significant predictors of position at cast removal. — III/B
- The position of the immobilisation with regard to forearm rotation has no effect in patients with distal 1/3 forearm fractures. — Ia/A
- Regional anaesthesia can be successfully employed in paediatric patients. — Ib/A
- Fixation of forearm fractures by a range of methods in children has been associated with varying results; high complication rates are reported in some series, occurring in up to 44% of patients. — III/B
- Several case series report superior results with elastic nailing. — III/B
- In a small non-randomised comparative study, no difference could be shown between elastic nailing and the use of less expensive intramedullary K-wires. — IIb/B
- Single bone fixation has been shown to be effective in patients if the second bone is stable and reduced following fixation of the first. — III/B

References

1. WISQARSTM (Web-based Injury Statistics Query and Reporting System), 2002.

2. Dowd MD, Keenan HT, Bratton SL. Epidemiology and prevention of childhood injuries. *Crit Care Med* 2002; 30(11 Suppl): S385-92.

3. Mallon B, Cullen A, Keenan P, *et al*. A profile of attenders at the A&E Department of the Children's Hospital, Temple Street, Dublin. *Ir Med J* 1997; 90(7): 266-7.

4. Ziv A, Boulet JR, Slap GB. Emergency department utilization by adolescents in the United States. *Pediatrics* 1998; 101(6): 987-94.

5. Cheng JC, Ng BK, Ying SY, Lam PK. A 10-year study of the changes in the pattern and treatment of 6,493 fractures. *J Pediatr Orthop* 1999; 19(3): 344-50.

6. Currey JD, Butler G. The mechanical properties of bone tissue in children. *J Bone Joint Surg Am* 1975; 57(6): 810-4.

7. Lyons RA, Delahunty AM, Kraus D, *et al*. Children's fractures: a population-based study. *Inj Prev* 1999; 5(2): 129-32.

8. Galano GJ, Vitale MA, Kessler MW, *et al*. The most frequent traumatic orthopaedic injuries from a national pediatric inpatient population. *J Pediatr Orthop* 2005; 25(1): 39-44.

9. Winthrop AL, Brasel KJ, Stahovic L, *et al*. Quality of life and functional outcome after pediatric trauma. *J Trauma* 2005; 58(3): 468-73; discussion 73-4.

10. Anderson WA. The significance of femoral fractures in children. *Ann Emerg Med* 1982; 11(4): 174-7.

11. Thomas SA, Rosenfield NS, Leventhal JM, Markowitz RI. Long-bone fractures in young children: distinguishing accidental injuries from child abuse. *Pediatrics* 1991; 88(3): 471-6.

12. Shapiro F. Fractures of the femoral shaft in children. The overgrowth phenomenon. *Acta Orthop Scand* 1981; 52(6): 649-55.

13. Al-Habdan I. Diaphyseal femoral fractures in children: should we change the present mode of treatment? *Int Surg* 2004; 89(4): 236-9.

14. Clinkscales CM, Peterson HA. Isolated closed diaphyseal fractures of the femur in children: comparison of effectiveness and cost of several treatment methods. *Orthopedics* 1997; 20(12): 1131-6.

15. Nork SE, Hoffinger SA. Skeletal traction versus external fixation for pediatric femoral shaft fractures: a comparison of hospital costs and charges. *J Orthop Trauma* 1998; 12(8): 563-8.

16. Yue JJ, Churchill RS, Cooperman DR, *et al*. The floating knee in the pediatric patient. Non-operative versus operative stabilization. *Clin Orthop Relat Res* 2000; 376: 124-36.

17. Kissel EU, Miller ME. Closed Ender nailing of femur fractures in older children. *J Trauma* 1989; 29(11): 1585-8.

18. Sanders JO, Browne RH, Mooney JF, *et al*. Treatment of femoral fractures in children by pediatric orthopedists: results of a 1998 survey. *J Pediatr Orthop* 2001; 21(4): 436-41.

19. Morton L, Bridgman S, Dwyer J, Theis J. Interventions for treating femoral shaft fractures in children and adolescents. (Protocol). *The Cochrane Database of Systematic Reviews* 2001; 4: Art. No CD003473. DOI: 10.1002/14651858. CD003473.

20. Rybka D, Trc T, Mrzena V. Conservative treatment of femoral fractures in children in data from the Orthopedic Clinic of the 2nd Medical Faculty of Charles University. *Acta Chir Orthop Traumatol Cech* 2003; 70(3): 170-6.

21. Ferguson J, Nicol RO. Early spica treatment of pediatric femoral shaft fractures. *J Pediatr Orthop* 2000; 20(2): 189-92.

22. Illgen R, 2nd, Rodgers WB, Hresko MT, *et al*. Femur fractures in children: treatment with early sitting spica casting. *J Pediatr Orthop* 1998; 18(4): 481-7.

23. Hughes BF, Sponseller PD, Thompson JD. Pediatric femur fractures: effects of spica cast treatment on family and community. *J Pediatr Orthop* 1995; 15(4): 457-60.

24. Wright JG, Wang EE, Owen JL, *et al*. Treatments for paediatric femoral fractures: a randomised trial. *Lancet* 2005; 365(9465): 1153-8.

25. Wong J, Boyd R, Keenan NW, *et al*. Gait patterns after fracture of the femoral shaft in children, managed by external fixation or early hip spica cast. *J Pediatr Orthop* 2004; 24(5): 463-71.

26. Miner T, Carroll KL. Outcomes of external fixation of pediatric femoral shaft fractures. *J Pediatr Orthop* 2000; 20(3): 405-10.

27. Hedin H, Hjorth K, Larsson S, Nilsson S. Radiological outcome after external fixation of 97 femoral shaft fractures in children. *Injury* 2003; 34(4): 287-92.

28. Kesemenli CC, Subasi M, Arslan H, *et al*. Is external fixation in pediatric femoral fractures a risk factor for refracture? *J Pediatr Orthop* 2004; 24(1): 17-20.

29. Caird MS, Mueller KA, Puryear A, Farley FA. Compression plating of pediatric femoral shaft fractures. *J Pediatr Orthop* 2003; 23(4): 448-52.

30. Eren OT, Kucukkaya M, Kockesen C, *et al*. Open reduction and plate fixation of femoral shaft fractures in children aged 4 to 10. *J Pediatr Orthop* 2003; 23(2): 190-3.

31. Agus H, Kalenderer O, Eryanilmaz G, Omeroglu H. Biological internal fixation of comminuted femur shaft fractures by bridge plating in children. *J Pediatr Orthop* 2003; 23(2): 184-9.

32. Forster MC, Aster AS, Ahmed S. Reaming during antegrade femoral nailing: is it worth it? *Injury* 2005; 36(3): 445-9.

33. Buckaloo JM, Iwinski HJ, Bertrand SL. Avascular necrosis of the femoral head after intramedullary nailing of a femoral shaft fracture in a male adolescent. *J South Orthop Assoc* 1997; 6(2): 97-100.

34. Thometz JG, Lamdan R. Osteonecrosis of the femoral head after intramedullary nailing of a fracture of the femoral shaft in an adolescent. A case report. *J Bone Joint Surg Am* 1995; 77(9): 1423-6.

35. Momberger N, Stevens P, Smith J, *et al*. Intramedullary nailing of femoral fractures in adolescents. *J Pediatr Orthop* 2000; 20(4): 482-4.

36. Flynn JM, Hresko T, Reynolds RA, *et al*. Titanium elastic nails for pediatric femur fractures: a multicenter study of early results with analysis of complications. *J Pediatr Orthop* 2001; 21(1): 4-8.

Chapter 3

37. Linhart WE, Roposch A. Elastic stable intramedullary nailing for unstable femoral fractures in children: preliminary results of a new method. *J Trauma* 1999; 47(2): 372-8.

38. Till H, Huttl B, Knorr P, Dietz HG. Elastic stable intramedullary nailing (ESIN) provides good long-term results in pediatric long-bone fractures. *Eur J Pediatr Surg* 2000; 10(5): 319-22.

39. Luhmann SJ, Schootman M, Schoenecker PL, *et al.* Complications of titanium elastic nails for pediatric femoral shaft fractures. *J Pediatr Orthop* 2003; 23(4): 443-7.

40. Narayanan UG, Hyman JE, Wainwright AM, *et al.* Complications of elastic stable intramedullary nail fixation of pediatric femoral fractures, and how to avoid them. *J Pediatr Orthop* 2004; 24(4): 363-9.

41. Kiely N. Mechanical properties of different combinations of flexible nails in a model of a pediatric femoral fracture. *J Pediatr Orthop* 2002; 22(4): 424-7.

42. Gwyn DT, Olney BW, Dart BR, Czuwala PJ. Rotational control of various pediatric femur fractures stabilized with titanium elastic intramedullary nails. *J Pediatr Orthop* 2004; 24(2): 172-7.

43. Grutter R, Cordey J, Buhler M, *et al.* The epidemiology of diaphyseal fractures of the tibia. *Injury* 2000; 31 Suppl 3: C64-7.

44. O'Brien T, Weisman DS, Ronchetti P, *et al.* Flexible titanium nailing for the treatment of the unstable pediatric tibial fracture. *J Pediatr Orthop* 2004; 24(6): 601-9.

45. Shannak AO. Tibial fractures in children: follow-up study. *J Pediatr Orthop* 1988; 8(3): 306-10.

46. Gicquel P, Giacomelli MC, Basic B, *et al.* Problems of operative and non-operative treatment and healing in tibial fractures. *Injury* 2005; 36 Suppl 1: A44-50.

47. Yang JP, Letts RM. Isolated fractures of the tibia with intact fibula in children: a review of 95 patients. *J Pediatr Orthop* 1997; 17(3): 347-51.

48. Wessel L, Seyfriedt CS, Hock S, Waag KL. Pediatric tibial fractures: is conservative therapy still currently appropriate? *Unfallchirurg* 1997; 100(1): 8-12.

49. Bartl V, Melichar I, Gal P. Personal experience with elastic stable intramedullary osteosynthesis in children. *Rozhl Chir* 1996; 75(10): 486-8.

50. Jubel A, Andermahr J, Isenberg J, *et al.* Experience with elastic stable intramedullary nailing (ESIN) of shaft fractures in children. *Orthopade* 2004; 33(8): 928-35.

51. Slongo TF. Complications and failures of the ESIN technique. *Injury* 2005; 36 Suppl 1: A78-85.

52. Court-Brown CM, Byrnes T, McLaughlin G. Intramedullary nailing of tibial diaphyseal fractures in adolescents with open physes. *Injury* 2003; 34(10): 781-5.

53. Blasier RD, Barnes CL. Age as a prognostic factor in open tibial fractures in children. *Clin Orthop Relat Res* 1996; 331: 261-4.

54. Hull JB, Sanderson PL, Rickman M, *et al.* External fixation of children's fractures: use of the Orthofix Dynamic Axial Fixator. *J Pediatr Orthop B* 1997; 6(3): 203-6.

55. Platz A, Kach K. Management of unstable shaft fractures of the lower extremity in children using the external fixator. *Swiss Surg* 1996; 2(6): 284-9.

56. Siegmeth A, Wruhs O, Vecsei V. External fixation of lower limb fractures in children. *Eur J Pediatr Surg* 1998; 8(1): 35-41.

57. Gordon JE, Schoenecker PL, Oda JE, *et al.* A comparison of monolateral and circular external fixation of unstable diaphyseal tibial fractures in children. *J Pediatr Orthop B* 2003; 12(5): 338-45.

58. Kubiak EN, Egol KA, Scher D, *et al.* Operative treatment of tibial fractures in children: are elastic stable intramedullary nails an improvement over external fixation? *J Bone Joint Surg Am* 2005; 87(8): 1761-8.

59. Cullen MC, Roy DR, Crawford AH, *et al.* Open fracture of the tibia in children. *J Bone Joint Surg Am* 1996; 78(7): 1039-47.

60. Grimard G, Naudie D, Laberge LC, Hamdy RC. Open fractures of the tibia in children. *Clin Orthop Relat Res* 1996; 332: 62-70.

61. Irwin A, Gibson P, Ashcroft P. Open fractures of the tibia in children. *Injury* 1995; 26(1): 21-4.

62. Jones BG, Duncan RD. Open tibial fractures in children under 13 years of age - 10 years experience. *Injury* 2003; 34(10): 776-80.

63. Robertson P, Karol LA, Rab GT. Open fractures of the tibia and femur in children. *J Pediatr Orthop* 1996; 16(5): 621-6.

64. Song KM, Sangeorzan B, Benirschke S, Browne R. Open fractures of the tibia in children. *J Pediatr Orthop* 1996; 16(5): 635-9.

65. Levy AS, Wetzler M, Lewars M, *et al.* The orthopedic and social outcome of open tibia fractures in children. *Orthopedics* 1997; 20(7): 593-8.

66. Landin LA. Epidemiology of children's fractures. *J Pediatr Orthop B* 1997; 6(2): 79-83.

67. Machan FG, Vinz H. Humeral shaft fracture in childhood. *Unfallchirurg* 1993; 19(3): 166-74.

68. Beaty JH. Fractures of the proximal humerus and shaft in children. *Instr Course Lect* 1992; 41: 369-72.

69. Wilkins KE. Principles of fracture remodeling in children. *Injury* 2005; 36 Suppl 1: A3-11.

70. Knorr P, Schmittenbecher PP, Dietz HG. Treatment of pathological fractures of long tubular bones in childhood using elastic stable intramedullary nailing. *Unfallchirurg* 1996; 99(6): 410-4.

71. Shaw BA, Murphy KM, Shaw A, *et al.* Humerus shaft fractures in young children: accident or abuse? *J Pediatr Orthop* 1997; 17(3): 293-7.

72. Taitz J, Moran K, O'Meara M. Long bone fractures in children under 3 years of age: is abuse being missed in Emergency Department presentations? *J Paediatr Child Health* 2004; 40(4): 170-4.

73. Oestern HJ, Rieger G, Jansen T. The internal fixation of fractures in children. *Unfallchirurg* 2000; 103(1): 2-11.

74. Shah MH, Heffernan G, McGuinness AJ. Early experience with titanium elastic nails in a trauma unit. *Ir Med J* 2003; 96(7): 213-4.

75. Kayali C, Agus H, Sanli C. Simultaneous ipsilateral humerus and forearm fractures in children. *Acta Orthop Traumatol Turc* 2002; 36(2): 117-23.

76. Bennek J. The use of upper limb external fixation in paediatric trauma. *Injury* 2000; 31 Suppl 1: 21-6.

Chapter 3

77. Alnot J, Osman N, Masmejean E, Wodecki P. Lesions of the radial nerve in fractures of the humeral diaphysis. Apropos of 62 cases. *Rev Chir Orthop Reparatrice Appar Mot* 2000; 86(2): 143-50.

78. Brug E, Joist A, Meffert R. Postoperative radial paralysis. Fate or negligence, conservative wait or revision? *Unfallchirurg* 2002; 105(1): 82-5.

79. Ring D, Chin K, Jupiter JB. Radial nerve palsy associated with high-energy humeral shaft fractures. *J Hand Surg Am* 2004; 29(1): 144-7.

80. Larsen LB, Barfred T. Radial nerve palsy after simple fracture of the humerus. *Scand J Plast Reconstr Surg Hand Surg* 2000; 34(4): 363-6.

81. Lim KE, Yap CK, Ong SC, Aminuddin. Plate osteosynthesis of the humerus shaft fracture and its association with radial nerve injury - a retrospective study in Melaka General Hospital. *Med J Malaysia* 2001; 56 Suppl C: 8-12.

82. Jones K, Weiner DS. The management of forearm fractures in children: a plea for conservatism. *J Pediatr Orthop* 1999; 19(6): 811-5.

83. Czerny F, Linhart W, Rueger JM, *et al.* Forearm fractures in children. *Unfallchirurg* 1994; 20(4): 203-10.

84. Ostermann PA, Richter D, Mecklenburg K, *et al.* Pediatric forearm fractures: indications, technique, and limits of conservative management. *Unfallchirurg* 1999; 102(10): 784-90.

85. Wurfel AM, Voigt A, Linke F, Hofmann von Kap-herr S. New aspects in the treatment of complete and isolated diaphyseal fracture of the forearm in childhood. *Unfallchirurg* 1995; 21(2): 70-6.

86. McHenry TP, Pierce WA, Lais RL, Schacherer TG. Effect of displacement of ulna-shaft fractures on forearm rotation: a cadaveric model. *Am J Orthop* 2002; 31(7): 420-4.

87. Lascombes P, Prevot J, Ligier JN, *et al.* Elastic stable intramedullary nailing in forearm shaft fractures in children: 85 cases. *J Pediatr Orthop* 1990; 10(2): 167-71.

88. Greenbaum B, Zionts LE, Ebramzadeh E. Open fractures of the forearm in children. *J Orthop Trauma* 2001; 15(2): 111-8.

89. Schmittenbecher PP. State-of-the-art treatment of forearm shaft fractures. *Injury* 2005; 36 Suppl 1: A25-34.

90. Younger AS, Tredwell SJ, Mackenzie WG. Factors affecting fracture position at cast removal after pediatric forearm fracture. *J Pediatr Orthop* 1997; 17(3): 332-6.

91. Boyer BA, Overton B, Schrader W, *et al.* Position of immobilization for pediatric forearm fractures. *J Pediatr Orthop* 2002; 22(2): 185-7.

92. Qairul IH, Kareem BA, Tan AB, Harwant S. Early remodeling in children's forearm fractures. *Med J Malaysia* 2001; 56 Suppl D: 34-7.

93. Bratt HD, Eyres RL, Cole WG. Randomized double-blind trial of low- and moderate-dose lidocaine regional anesthesia for forearm fractures in childhood. *J Pediatr Orthop* 1996; 16(5): 660-3.

94. Ortega R, Loder RT, Louis DS. Open reduction and internal fixation of forearm fractures in children. *J Pediatr Orthop* 1996; 16(5): 651-4.

95. Wyrsch B, Mencio GA, Green NE. Open reduction and internal fixation of pediatric forearm fractures. *J Pediatr Orthop* 1996; 16(5): 644-50.

96. Trousdale RT, Linscheid RL. Operative treatment of malunited fractures of the forearm. *J Bone Joint Surg Am* 1995; 77(6): 894-902.

97. Smith VA, Goodman HJ, Strongwater A, Smith B. Treatment of pediatric both-bone forearm fractures: a comparison of operative techniques. *J Pediatr Orthop* 2005; 25(3): 309-13.

98. Cullen MC, Roy DR, Giza E, Crawford AH. Complications of intramedullary fixation of pediatric forearm fractures. *J Pediatr Orthop* 1998; 18(1): 14-21.

99. Luhmann SJ, Gordon JE, Schoenecker PL. Intramedullary fixation of unstable both-bone forearm fractures in children. *J Pediatr Orthop* 1998; 18(4): 451-6.

100. Van der Reis WL, Otsuka NY, Moroz P, Mah J. Intramedullary nailing versus plate fixation for unstable forearm fractures in children. *J Pediatr Orthop* 1998; 18(1): 9-13.

101. Griffet J, el Hayek T, Baby M. Intramedullary nailing of forearm fractures in children. *J Pediatr Orthop B* 1999; 8(2): 88-9.

102. Mann D, Schnabel M, Baacke M, Gotzen L. Results of elastic stable intramedullary nailing (ESIN) in forearm fractures in childhood. *Unfallchirurg* 2003; 106(2): 102-9.

103. Richter D, Ostermann PA, Ekkernkamp A, *et al.* Elastic intramedullary nailing: a minimally invasive concept in the treatment of unstable forearm fractures in children. *J Pediatr Orthop* 1998; 18(4): 457-61.

104. Calder PR, Achan P, Barry M. Diaphyseal forearm fractures in children treated with intramedullary fixation: outcome of K-wire versus elastic stable intramedullary nail. *Injury* 2003; 34(4): 278-82.

105. Bhaskar AR, Roberts JA. Treatment of unstable fractures of the forearm in children. Is plating of a single bone adequate? *J Bone Joint Surg Br* 2001; 83(2): 253-8.

106. Flynn JM, Waters PM. Single-bone fixation of both-bone forearm fractures. *J Pediatr Orthop* 1996; 16(5): 655-9.

107. Lee S, Nicol RO, Stott NS. Intramedullary fixation for pediatric unstable forearm fractures. *Clin Orthop Relat Res* 2002; 402: 245-50.

108. Shoemaker SD, Comstock CP, Mubarak SJ, *et al.* Intramedullary Kirschner wire fixation of open or unstable forearm fractures in children. *J Pediatr Orthop* 1999; 19(3): 329-37.

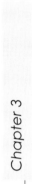

Chapter 3

Chapter 4

Congenital talipes equinovarus

James S Huntley MA (Hons) DPhil MB BChir MRCS
Lecturer and Honorary Specialist Registrar
Malcolm F Macnicol MB ChB BSc (Hons) FRCS MCh FRCSEd (Orth)
Consultant Orthopaedic Surgeon

ROYAL HOSPITAL FOR SICK CHILDREN, EDINBURGH, SCOTLAND

Introduction

Incidence and epidemiology

Congenital talipes equinovarus (CTEV) is a musculoskeletal condition characterised by rigid (non-reducible) ankle equinus, with hindfoot varus and forefoot adductus. It is a challenging condition, recognised since ancient times [1], with a marked variation in incidence according to geography and race [2]. In Caucasian populations the incidence is held to be 1.2 per 1000 live-births [2], although slightly lower rates have been documented recently for Scotland (0.89/1000) [3] and the USA (0.6/1000) [4]. The rate is higher for South Pacific populations (6 to 7 per 1000 live births), and lower in Japan (0.5 per 1000 live births) [5]. There is a male to female ratio of (2 to 2.5):1, and about 50% of cases are bilateral [2, 6]. Left and right feet are equally affected [7]. Most cases of CTEV are 'isolated' (i.e. occur in a child without other identifiable abnormalities). However, a minority are 'syndromic', occurring in conjunction with other anomalies (Table 1).

Table 1. Associations of 'syndromic' CTEV.

- Foetal-alcohol syndrome
- Spina bifida/myelomeningocoele
- Arthrogryposis
- Down's syndrome
- Constriction band syndrome
- Freedman-Sheldon syndrome
- Sacral agenesis
- Diastrophic dwarfism

Aetiology

Many aetiological theories have been advanced, including intra-uterine moulding, developmental defects, and anomalies of other systems (neurogenic, myogenic, vascular) [8, 9]. Both genetic and environmental factors have been implicated [10]. Almost one quarter of patients with CTEV has a positive family history for the condition [6]. Furthermore, if a twin has CTEV, there is a marked increase in CTEV risk for the sibling if the twins are monozygotic, as opposed to dizygotic [11]. Thus, there appears to be a strong basis for a genetic component [10]. However, there is also a seasonal variation in CTEV presentation [3, 12].

There are multiple tissue abnormalities in clubfeet, including:

- a large increase in the type I:II muscle fibre ratio, type IIB fibre deficiency, and abnormal fibre grouping [13];
- bone and joint deformities, e.g. of the talus and calcaneocuboid joint [14-16];
- vascular hypoplasia [17] (also, parents of children with CTEV were much less likely to have a dorsalis pedis pulse [18]);
- anomalous musculature [7];
- increased vimentin and myofibroblastic characteristics [19].

However, it is difficult to discern which of these might be primary (cause), and which secondary (effect).

Intra-uterine factors may be important. For instance, an association has been documented with early (<11 weeks) amniocentesis, especially if there was an amniotic fluid leak [20]. Swart [21] reported delayed closure of the neural canal at L4/5, the level of peronei innervation.

Anatomy

An understanding of the morbid anatomy is paramount. Most authorities suggest that the primary bony deformity in CTEV occurs in the talus - with the neck being short, angled medially and flexed plantarwards [2, 22]. The navicular is subluxed medially, and the calcaneus shortened and widened. Continued talar head growth medially causes the calcaneus to become adducted (and varised). The cavus results from Hick's 'pronation-twist': a relatively greater flexion of the first metatarsal in relation to the hindfoot. This is the key to Ponseti's argument that the cavus deformity must be corrected by supination of the forefoot, before any attempts at correction of the other components of the deformity [23].

Classification systems

Many classification systems have been proposed for CTEV. For a system to be of value it should be easy to apply, have good inter- and intra-observer reliability, have relevance prognostically and particularly as a guide to treatment [24]. Wainwright et al [25] noted that CTEV classification is awkward: the deformity is complex, three-dimensional and partly dynamic. They assessed the inter-observer reliabilities of the following classification systems:

- Ponseti and Smoley [26]. On the basis of measurements of ankle dorsiflexion, hindfoot varus, forefoot supination and tibial torsion, the CTEV foot can be designated good, acceptable or poor.
- Harrold and Walker [27]. On the basis of the degree of passive correctability of the equinovarus deformity, a grade of 1-3 can be allotted.
- Catterall [28]. On the basis of several clinical observations, the CTEV foot can be allotted to one of four 'patterns': 'resolving', 'tendon contracture', 'joint contracture', and 'false correction'.
- Dimeglio et al [29]. On the basis of four indices (equinus in the sagittal plane, varus deviation in the frontal plane, derotation of the calcaneo-forefoot block around the talus, adduction of the forefoot on the hindfoot in the frontal plane), and four supplementary observations (medial crease, posterior crease, cavus, deficient calf musculature), a score of between 4 and 20 is summated, allowing the CTEV foot to be assigned to one of four groups:

  o I benign <5;
  o II moderate 5-10;
  o III severe 11-15;
  o IV very severe 16-20.

Although complex, the Dimeglio et al classification gave the best inter-observer agreement for the CTEV foot. In addition, in the case series of Souchet et al [30] (see below), for functional physical therapy, the pretreatment Dimeglio et al classification correlated to outcome. Both the Dimeglio system and the Pirani system (see below) have been assessed in another study as having good inter-observer reliability [31].

The Pirani system [32, 33] is also being used at many centres. It grades the deformity by considering six different components: posterior crease, empty heel, and rigid equinus (hindfoot group), and medial crease, lateral border curvature, and position of the talar head (midfoot group). Each component is given a score of 0, 0.5, or 1. Thus, the scale ranges from 0-6, with higher numbers representing increasingly severe deformity.

Attitudes to management

Recently, there has been a trend to conservative (as opposed to surgical) modes of treatment [24]. Whilst the case series evidence for the Ponseti technique is encouraging, the need for ancillary surgery is variable, but sometimes frequent. Conversely, some long-term results for surgically treated clubfeet have been disappointing [34]. Heterogeneous aetiology, marked variation in severity, inadequate and multiple grading systems, multiple surgical options and dilemmas, as well as differences in outcome/rating assessments make the design of prospective comparative long-term studies awkward [9], and for certain questions some might argue unethical. These factors are reflected in the paucity of the evidence base.

Methodology

Medline (Pubmed) and the Cochrane Library were searched ('club foot' OR 'clubfoot'). No systematic reviews were identified. In total, 2518 references were retrieved of which most were excluded on the basis of screening the title and abstract. Those not excluded were assessed further. Five recent substantive non-systematic reviews were identified [2, 9, 35-37]. Supplemental references were obtained from the review articles, and also from expert knowledge of the literature. The remainder of this chapter considers aspects of the management of CTEV in four sections outlining conservative treatments, surgical treatments, the evidence (key studies), and conclusions with recommendations (and levels of evidence).

Conservative treatments

Conservative treatments involve stretching, manipulation, strapping, plasters, and percutaneous tenotomies. Manipulative treatment has had many advocates since Hippocrates.

Kite's method

In the 1930s, Kite [38, 39] advocated serial correction of the CTEV deformities using gentle manipulative treatment and below-knee casting in sequence from distal to proximal in strict order, only progressing when the previous step had been accomplished i.e. varus forefoot first, inverted hindfoot second, and subsequently, ankle and subtalar deformities.

Ponseti's method

In the 1940s, Ponseti developed a technique similarly involving manipulation and serial casting [40]. However, the cavus is reduced first by supinating the forefoot to align it properly with the hindfoot. Thereafter, the hindfoot varus, inversion and adduction deformities are corrected simultaneously, by simultaneous lateral shift of the navicular, cuboid and calcaneus; this is performed by abducting the foot against counter-pressure exerted at the lateral talar head (avoiding pressure at the calcaneocuboid joint against a stabilised heel - a malfeasance termed Kite's error by Ponseti [41]). Cast application is a skilled process: after manipulation, a below-knee cast is applied and moulded appropriately; the cast is then extended above the thigh, maintaining hyperabduction of the foot. In most cases, a correction can be obtained after five casts. The Achilles tendon may require percutaneous lengthening before application of the last cast (which is left on three weeks), as long as the heel varus has been corrected. A foot-abduction brace is a critical adjunct to the manipulation and casting protocol [4]. It consists of a bar (length equal to child's shoulder width) with shoes at both ends. These are rotated externally 40° (normal side) and 70° (CTEV). The brace should be worn full time for two to three months and then at night and naptimes (at least ten hours per day) for three to four years.

The functional method

The other major conservative mode of treatment to have been developed is the 'functional method' [30, 42, 43], also termed the 'French method' [44]. This starts as soon as possible in the neonatal period. Initially, the manipulations (c. 30 minutes per foot) are done each day but after two weeks, they are progressively decreased to two sessions per week (usual time to correction six to eight weeks). A flexible below-knee splint is worn between manipulations, allowing some spontaneous movement but maintaining the reduction obtained. The method consists of five 'stages':

- correction of mid-tarsal deformities, in particular reduction of the talonavicular articulation together with correction of forefoot adduction;
- correction of hindfoot varus and partial correction of calcaneal equinus;
- increasing reduction of the talus in the ankle mortise;
- lateral derotation of the calcaneo-forefoot unit; and
- correction of hindfoot equinus.

Continuous passive movement machines have been incorporated into this regime at certain centres [44].

Botulinum toxin as an adjunct

Alvarez *et al* [45] reported on an uncontrolled, non-randomised cohort of 73 CTEV feet from 51 patients, using Botulinum toxin A to defunction triceps surae instead of a tenotomy during a Ponseti-type protocol. Mean follow-up post-Botulinum was only nine months for children in whom treatment was initiated at less than 30 days, and only 15 months in those presenting between one and eight months of age. Outcome (surgical rate, Pirani score, ankle dorsiflexion and recurrences) at this very early stage yielded only one failure requiring surgery, meaning this technique compares favourably with tenotomy. However, this treatment can only be regarded as experimental at the current time.

Surgical treatments

Assessment

Clinical

Assessment of the components of the deformity is pivotal; if all components are maintained, despite conservative treatment, then a full posteromedial and plantar lateral release is likely to be required. However, if the midfoot yields a straight lateral border and a flexible border then confining the operation to a posterior release may be sufficient [36].

Radiological

Plain films are generally taken in anteroposterior and lateral planes, allowing definition of the talocalcaneal angles/index, cavus and degrees of subluxation at the calcaneocuboid and talonavicular joints. Simons [46] assessed the CTEV deformity radiologically, in terms of the longitudinal axes of the talus and calcaneus on anteroposterior (normally 20°-40°; less than 20° in CTEV) and lateral views. Addition of these angles gives the talocalcaneal index, (TCI - normally 51°-77°). Correction of the CTEV should give a TCI >50°. However, it is difficult to take standard planar radiographic views of this complex three-dimensional deformity; radiographic assessment is further complicated because much of the deformity is of cartilage anlages rather than bone [9].

Optimum timing of surgery

There are no published prospective randomised trials concerning the timing of surgery for CTEV [9]. Some authorities have advocated surgery in the neonatal phase [47, 48]. In contrast, Turco favoured surgery between one and two years of age; in his follow-up [49] he found a markedly higher failure rate in the group operated on at less than one year. Advocates of operating early reason that the younger the skeleton, the more capacity there is for correction and remodelling. However, there is also an increased anaesthetic risk and surgical risk given that the smaller operative field decreases the margin for error.

In a retrospective notes review with subsequent follow-up, Porat et al [50] compared outcomes of 37 CTEV feet (26 children) treated surgically at either <3 months (mean follow-up age 3.5 years) or late (mean age at operation three years seven months, and age at follow-up nine years two months). 'Satisfactory' results were obtained in 82% and 23%, respectively; however, initial severities were not clear. Furthermore, the nature of the surgery varied, and the heterogeneous follow-up times do not make easy comparison. Tibrewal et al [51] reported a high re-operation rate (39%) due to under-correction in patients operated on with subtalar realignment at six weeks of age.

Depuy and Drennan (1989) [52] reported on a small series of 30 patients (44 feet) which they divided into three groups based on average age of operation (4.4 months, 9.1 months, and 16.1 months). Initial severities and modes of operation were similar. The best results in both radiographic and clinical terms were on those patients operated on earliest. However, Ghali et al [53] found no significant difference between early and later soft tissue releases. There seems to be consensus that primary surgery should be done in the first year of life if possible, because of the greater capacity for remodelling [2] (IV/C).

Approaches

Here we outline the historical development of salient surgical approaches to the club foot. Rather than adopting a one operation fits all approach, surgery should be tailored to the particular patient - the 'a la carte' approach as advocated by Bensahel [54], with recognition that under-correction may allow relapse/recurrence, whilst over-correction may lead to a valgus heel and stiff/painful foot [9] (IV/C).

Posterior

Attenborough [55] confined his operative approach to cases in which a good correction was not obtained quickly by manipulation and casting. Nevertheless, the preferred age for operation was 'early', between two and four months. His rationale was that the fundamental deformity in severe CTEV is fixed plantar flexion of the talus. Therefore, when manipulating/ casting, he concentrated on the equinus and forefoot varus deformities, and ignored inversion. The operation involves a vertical incision halfway between the Achilles tendon and the medial border of the tibia, allowing the tendons and neurovascular bundle to be identified. Initially, the Achilles is z-lengthened (later sutured). Tibialis posterior and flexor digitorum longus are divided. The posterior aspect of the ankle joint can then be exposed, and divided, both horizontally and vertically, to release the strong talofibular ligament. Finally, flexor hallucis longus is divided. Attenborough reported 22 CTEV feet in 14 children with follow-up ranging from six months to four years, finding mobile corrected feet and apparently normal tendon function within a few months of surgical treatment.

Posteromedial

In response to dissatisfaction with the surgical results of CTEV correction at that time, Turco [7] developed the 'one-stage posteromedial release with internal fixation' with an initial report of 58 feet from 41 patients with 'severe recalcitrant' CTEV treated over the course of 7.5 years (31 feet from 23 patients over two to seven years). He described three groups of contractures in CTEV:

- posterior (posterior capsule of ankle and subtalar joints, Achilles tendon, and posterior talofibular and calcaneofibular ligaments);
- medial (deltoid and spring ligaments, talonavicular joint capsule, tendons of tibialis posterior, flexor digitorum longus, and flexor hallucis longus); and
- subtalar (including the subtalar interosseous and Y-bifurcated ligament).

He emphasised the importance of adequate surgical exposure to all meticulous sharp dissection without damage to articular cartilage. The operation involves an 8-9cm incision from the base of the first metatarsal running posterior, just under the medial malleolus to the Achilles tendon. Taking care to protect the neurovascular bundle, tibialis posterior, flexor digitorum longus, flexor hallucis longus, and the distal 2-3cm of the Achilles tendon are identified and freed from their sheaths. The knot of Henry is divided to free flexor hallucis longus and flexor digitorum longus.

Chapter 4

Thereafter, Turco describes three steps:

- posterior release (Achilles tendon, posterior capsulotomy of ankle joint, posterior capsulotomy of subtalar joint and calcaneofibular ligament, posterior insertion of deltoid ligament on calcaneus);
- medial release (much fibrotic tissue is to be excised from this region, tibialis posterior tendon is divided just above the medial malleolus, deltoid ligament is excised from the talonavicular joint, the spring ligament is incised and detached from the sustentaculum tali, and the navicular mobilised); and
- subtalar release (this is important to allow mobilisation of the anterior calcaneus; the talocalcaneal ligament above the sustentaculum tali is divided, and then the navicular mobilised by cutting the Y-ligament). Talonavicular fixation is secured with a K-wire, and the Achilles tendon is sutured in its lengthened position. (Authors' note: it is vital to leave the tibiotalar component of the deltoid ligament intact - otherwise, fixed valgus of the hindfoot may result.)

Turco [49] published medium-term follow-up (2-15 years) of 149 feet, with excellent/good results in 83.8%.

Lateral-posteromedial

McKay [56, 57] emphasised the patho-anatomy of the calcaneocuboid joint and described a surgical procedure allowing more derotation of the calcaneus after release of the lateral structures, together with recession of the flexor sheaths in an attempt to cause less scarring around the tendons.

'Hanging foot'

Simons [58, 59] described the 'extensive complete subtalar release'. This consists of a standard posteromedial release supplemented by release of lateral parts of the talonavicular joint, subtalar joint, interosseous talocalcaneal ligament and calcaneofibular ligament, to allow a more complete derotation of the calcaneus. He further described augmentation procedures such as calcaneal/calcaneocuboid osteotomies and plantar release, and recommended the Cincinnati incision [60] for this procedure. Simons [59] evaluated his results from two historical cohort groups (group 1 - posteromedial release/lateral release; group 2 - complete subtalar release) with at least two years follow-up by clinical evaluation and radiography. He found a higher percentage (72% v. 50%) of satisfactory results in the complete subtalar release group.

Secondary surgery

There is a risk of approximately 25% that a relapse (or over-correction) will occur post-surgery, of such a degree that secondary surgery is required [2]. After clinical and roentgenographic assessment, a number of procedures may be contemplated - an algorithm for guidance has been developed [61]. The Ilizarov method has been applied [62] after relapse in children who had originally undergone conventional surgery. Bradish and Noor reported a series of 17 relapsed feet (12 children) treated with gradual distraction in an 'unconstrained' frame. Follow-up at three years post-surgery showed a maintained correction with good/excellent results in 13. Additional tendon transfers were performed in five (all good/excellent).

Evidence - key studies

Outcomes after treatment

Laaveg and Ponseti [63] reported long-term results of the Ponseti protocol in treatment of CTEV in 104 feet of 70 patients. Inclusion criteria were:

- no other congenital abnormality;
- the patient was less than six months old when first seen; and
- either there had been no previous treatment except splinting or fewer than three casts had been applied. Outcomes were evaluated at ten to 27 years using a 100-point functional rating system (Table 2). This system has a subjective

Table 2. Functional rating system for measuring outcome after treatment for club foot. Adapted from [63].
Reproduced with permission from the Journal of Bone and Joint Surgery, Inc.

Category	Points
Subjective (ex 70)	
Pain (ex 30)	
My clubfoot:	
a) is never painful	30
b) occasionally causes mild pain during strenuous activities	24
c) usually is painful after strenuous activities only	18
d) is occasionally painful during routine activities	12
e) is painful during walking	6
Function (ex 20)	
In my daily living, my clubfoot:	
a) does not limit my activities	20
b) occasionally limits my strenuous activities	16
c) usually limits me in strenuous activities	12
d) limits me occasionally in routine activities	8
e) limits me in walking	4
Satisfaction (ex 20)	
I am:	
a) very satisfied with the end result	20
b) satisfied with the end result	16
c) neither satisfied nor unsatisfied with the end result	12
d) unsatisfied with the end result	8
e) very unsatisfied with the end result	4
Objective (ex 30)	
Heel position (standing) (ex 10)	
Heel neutral, 0° or some valgus	10
Heel varus, 1-5°	5
Heel varus, 6-10°	3
Heel varus, >10°	0
Passive movement (ex 10)	
Dorsiflexion	1 point per 5° (up to 5)
Total varus-valgus heel	1 point per 10° (up to 3)
Total anterior inversion-eversion foot	1 point per 25° (up to 2)
Gait (ex 10)	
Normal	6
Can toe-walk	2
Can heel-walk	2
Limp	-2
No heel-strike	-2
Abnormal toe-off	-2
TOTAL	ex 100

Chapter 4

component (satisfaction, function and pain) and an objective component (position of heel, passive range of motion, and gait). The functional rating system has been adopted by several later studies allowing some comparison of outcomes.

Results are classified according to score: excellent (90-100), good (80-89), fair (70-79), poor (<70).

Of 104 feet, 13 required manipulation and casting only, 42 required Achilles tendon lengthening (93% of these were performed percutaneously under local anaesthesia), 48 required tibialis anterior transfer to the third cuneiform (of these 48, only two had tibialis anterior transfer alone, 29 also had an Achilles lengthening and 17 had a variety of other surgical procedures), one required a tibialis posterior transfer. A 'relapse' was defined as a club foot having a recurrent deformity that required further treatment: 55 (53%) clubfeet had no relapse; 49 had one relapse (mean age 39 months), 25 a second relapse (mean age 53 months), ten a third relapse (mean age 63 months), three a fourth relapse (mean age 77 months). The final mean score for all feet was 87.5 (standard deviation 11.7, range 50-100), and 74% were rated excellent/good. However, in most patients, foot and ankle movement was limited and radiographic angles were not fully corrected.

Cooper and Dietz [64] reported a 30-year follow-up of 45 patients (71 clubfeet), of whom 29 were from the original series [63]. Using pain and functional limitation as the outcome criteria, 78% had an excellent/good outcome compared with 85% of matched controls. Conversely, Hutchins et al [65] reported excellent/good results, on the Laaveg and Ponseti rating scale, in 57% of patients treated with early surgical release.

A retrospective cohort study by Haasbeek and Wright [66] compared the functional outcomes of two groups of surgically treated patients (<two years age):

* posterior release (1963-1971); and
* comprehensive release (1973 onwards).

The posterior release involved open Achilles lengthening, usually with a subtalar and posterior ankle release. The comprehensive release involved both medial and posterolateral approaches, and included lengthening of the Achilles tendon, flexor digitorum longus, flexor hallucis longus, and tibialis posterior, together with release of the talonavicular, calcaneocuboid, posterior ankle and subtalar joints [67]. Functional outcome assessed on the Laaveg and Ponseti scale gave mean scores of 81 for the posterior release group (at mean 28-year follow-up) and 86 for the comprehensive release group (at mean 16-year follow-up); these were not significantly different. Although the ankle range of movement was similar, the posterior release group had a significantly higher re-operation rate, and a higher percentage of patients with subtalar stiffness.

Herzenberg et al [68] conducted a retrospective cohort study comparing two groups of CTEV patients (treatment initiated within first three months of life) treated with Ponseti or 'traditional' methods of casting, with comparison of need for posteromedial release within the first year - 3% in the Ponseti group, and 94% in the 'traditional' group. In the Ponseti group, 91% of patients had a percutaneous Achilles tenotomy at the age of two to three months. There was significantly better range of movement in the Ponseti-treated group.

A retrospective cohort review by Ippolito et al [69] compared long-term outcomes in CTEV patients treated by two different protocols (starting in first three weeks of life), involving serial manipulation/casting followed by surgery. Entry into each group was dependent on historical time of presentation (i.e. 1973-1977, group 1; 1979-1984, group 2). The first group was treated by Marino-Zuco manipulation (which unfortunately involved forefoot pronation as its first manipulative step) followed by posteromedial release [49] in resistant cases. The second group was treated by Ponseti manipulation [26] followed by heel-cord z-lengthening and posterior capsulectomy of the ankle. Subsequent bracing procedures were similar for each group. The system of Laaveg and Ponseti [63] was used to assess outcomes at 25 and 19 years respectively. These long-term results were better in patients treated by the second protocol; 43% of group 1 feet and 78% of group 2 feet were classed as good or excellent. Group 2 mean score and percentage excellent/good results were similar for patients reported earlier [63]. The authors felt that the results of posteromedial release were disappointing, but these may reflect rather on the manipulative method that preceded surgery. CT analysis of the same groups showed that whilst equinus was well corrected in both groups, the cavus, supination and adduction deformities were better corrected in the second group.

Recently, Morcuende et al [4] published a consecutive case series for CTEV (157 patients; 256 clubfeet; January 1991 to December 2001). These data were held to describe a radical reduction in the rate of extensive corrective surgery in patients treated by the Ponseti method. Outcome measurements were initial correction of the deformity, rate of extensive surgery and relapse rate. Although no patient was lost to follow-up, the average age at 'last follow-up' was reported as 26 months (range six months to eight years). Correction was obtained in 98% feet, but we suggest this is far too early to assess. A percutaneous tenotomy was performed in 86% cases. A complication of cast treatment occurred in 8% of patients, attributed to a deficiency in casting technique. Only 2.5% (four) patients required extensive corrective surgery (one posteromedial release and three posterior releases with Achilles tenotomy). There were 17 (10%) relapses which were associated with non-compliance with the foot-abduction brace. The authors attributed these encouraging early results to improved technique, in particular the degree of hyper-abduction obtained in the long leg cast, and increased compliance in the foot-abduction brace. However, it may be premature to make any judgements concerning relapse and the need for extensive surgery, as the average age at last follow-up in this study was only 26 months; the mean age of first relapse in the long-term study of Laaveg and Ponseti was 39 months. We await the longer-term results of this series with interest.

Souchet et al [30] reported on 350 CTEV feet (234 patients) treated by the 'functional method' described earlier. Average time of final follow-up was 14 years (range 11-18 years), but outcomes were also recorded at the age of six years with good results in 77%. Initial classification was 'at birth' [29], allowing categorisation of CTEV into one of four groups (as above - see Classification systems). The outcome evaluation was that recommended by the International Club Foot Study Group (ICFSG) [70] (Table 3). Initially, group A (mild) contained four feet (1%), group B (moderate) 109 feet (31%), group C (severe) 178 feet (51%), and group D (very severe) 59 feet (17%). Over the course of functional treatment, all groups improved. Feet requiring surgery were operated on at an average of one year of age. They found that feet that improved progressively over the course of three months treatment would have a good result, i.e. the prognosis of conservative treatment can be assessed in the first months. Table 4 shows the heterogeneous array of studies that report outcomes from conservative treatment, with good results (by different outcome assessments) ranging from 25% to 77%.

Predicting need for tenotomy during the Ponseti protocol

Scher et al [33] rated 50 CTEV feet (35 patients) using both the Dimeglio and Pirani systems. The tenotomy rate during the Ponseti protocol was 72%. Initial severity correlated to the likelihood of requiring a tenotomy; indeed, CTEV with an initial score >4 on the Pirani system, or Dimeglio Grade IV are very likely to require a tenotomy **(IIb/B)**.

Predicting likelihood of relapse after Ponseti treatment

Dobbs et al [71] performed a retrospective study on 51 consecutive CTEV patients (86 feet) treated using the Ponseti method; the major risk factor for risk of recurrence was non-compliance with the foot-abduction orthosis (odds ratio 183). Parental educational level was also found to be a significant risk factor **(III/B)**.

Table 3. ICFSG rating system for outcome evaluation for treatment of clubfeet [70]. *Reproduced with permission from Lippincott Williams & Wilkins.*

Morphology

		Score	
A Hindfoot			
1. Varus or valgus	0	1 (10°)	2 (>10°)
2. Equinus or calcaneus	0	1 (10°)	2 (>10°)
B Midfoot			
1. Supination or pronation	0	1 (10°)	2 (>10°)
2. Adduction or abduction	0	1 (10°)	2 (>10°)
C Global alignment of the foot			
1. Rotation: medial or lateral (thigh-knee foot angle)	0	1 (10°)	2 (>10°)
2. Pes cavus or flat foot	0	1 (10°)	2 (>10°)
Maximum		12	

Functional evaluation

		Score	
A Passive motion			
1. Ankle			
i Dorsiflexion	0	1 (0°)	2 (negative)
ii Plantar flexion	0	1 (10°)	2 (0 or negative)
2. Subtalar varus-valgus	Flexible/stiff	0	1
3. Midtarsal joint motion: pronation-supination	Flexible/stiff	0	1
B Muscle function	*Normal*	*Moderate*	*Severe*
Jones' classification	(5,4)	(3)	(2,1,0)
1. Triceps surae	0	1	2
2. Toe flexors	0	1	2
3. Extensors	0	1	2
4. Anterior tibia tendon	0	1	2
5. Extensor hallicis longus	0	1	2
6. Posterior tibia tendon	0	1	2
7. Peroneal tendon	0	1	2
8. Flexor hallicis longus	0	1	2
C Dynamic function			
1. Gait	*None*	*Positive*	
i Intoeing (medial rotation)	0	1 (10°)	2 (>10°)
ii Calcaneus	0	1 (10°)	2 (>10°)
iii Equinus	0	1 (10°)	2 (>10°)
iv Dynamic supination	0	1 (10°)	2 (>10°)
v Limping	0	1	
vi Ability to run	1	0	
vii Ability to jump	1	0	
2. Shoe wear	Normal 0		Abnormal 1
3. Heel walking or toe walking	Yes 0		No 1
D Pain			
1. No pain	0		
2. Pain with activity	1		
3. Pain with sports	2		
4. Constant	3		
Maximum		36	

Table 3. *Continued:*

Radiologic evaluation

	Score	
	Normal	*Abnormal*
A Standing anteroposterior views (in weight-bearing position)		
1. Talocalcaneal angle	0	1
2. Cuboid-calcaneo alignment	0	1
3. Cubo-M5 axis	0	1
4. Talo-M1 angle	0	1
5. Talonavicular position	0	1
B Standing lateral views (foot in weight-bearing position)		
1. Talocalcaneal angle	0	1
2. Tibiocalcaneal angle	0	1
3. Talonavicular position	0	1
4. Talo-M1 axis	0	1
5. Calcaneo-M5 axis	0	1
6. Flat top talus	0	1
C Ankle anteroposterior standing	0	1
(Posterior border of medial and lateral malleoli lined up at same plane when taking radiograph)		
Maximum		12

Scores are from 0 for a perfect result to 60 for the worst result (0-5=excellent, 6-15=good, 16-30=fair, >30=poor).

Table 4. Outcome evaluation - good results from conservative treatment [30, 72-81].

Study	Cases (n)	Pre-treatment classification	Good results conservative treatment	Follow-up (years)	Outcome evaluation
Dimeglio *et al*, 1996	171	Birth	76 (44%)	ND	ND
Lefort *et al*, 1994	260	2 groups	47 (18%)	7	100 points
Harrold & Walker, 1983	129	3 groups	48%	ND	ND
Karski & Woski, 1989	435	ND	217 (50%)	ND	ND
Laaveg & Ponseti, 1980	104	ND	12.5% (conservative alone) 40% (with PAT)	18	100 points
Morcuende *et al*, 1994	ND	ND	89% (with PAT)	34	ND
Cooper & Dietz, 1995	71	ND	5 (conservative alone) 27 (with PAT)	34	ND
Napiontek, 1996	49	ND	Radiographic assessment	8.3	ND
Seringe & Atia, 1990	269	3 groups	130 (48%)	6	5 groups
Yamamoto *et al*, 1990, 1998	113	3 groups	72 (63%)	12	McKay
Bensahel *et al*, 1980	600	ND	48%	10-15	ND
Bensahel *et al*, 1990	338	ND	48%	10-14	ND
Campenhout *et al*, 2001	100	Dimeglio	25%	3.2	Campenhout
Souchet *et al*, 2004	350	Dimeglio	77%	11-18	60 points, ICFSG
Richards *et al*, 2005	142	Dimeglio	42% (conservative alone) 9% (with PAT)	3	Richards

ND = no data; PAT = percutaneous Achilles tenotomy; ICFSG = International Clubfoot Study Group

Chapter 4

Conclusions

The paucity of the evidence base emphasises the importance of prospectively grading cohorts of patients receiving interventions (or not), before objective outcomes are assessed. Although difficult to perform rigorously, in certain areas randomisation to treatment arms in controlled trials might allow better identification of indications for particular treatment modalities. Despite the current trend towards conservative management, the skills required to operate on later 'failed' cases mandates the maintenance of operative centres for tertiary referral.

Recommendations	Evidence level
◆ All treatment should initially be conservative, involving one of the modern regimens.	III/B
Conservative treatment	
◆ Should be started as soon as possible after birth.	IV/C
◆ At birth, grading of CTEV predicts outcome of conservative treatment (functional method).	IIb/B
◆ At birth, grading of CTEV predicts requirement for tenotomy.	IIb/B
◆ Ponseti/Functional/French protocols show improved results over earlier methods.	III/B
◆ Non-compliance with the foot-abduction bar is an important cause of failure in the Ponseti method.	IIa/B
◆ Forced manipulation and casting may lead to oedema and later fibrosis, making later surgery more difficult.	IV/C
Surgical treament	
◆ Pre-treatment classification predicts requirement for later surgery.	IIb/B
◆ Is optimally timed before 12 months of age.	IV/C
◆ 'A la carte' surgery is justified in resistant CTEV.	IV/C

References

1. Fixsen JA. Children's orthopaedic surgery. In: *The evolution of orthopaedic surgery*. Klenerman L, Ed. London: Royal Society of Medicine, 2002; chapter 10: 149-58.
2. Roye DP, Roye BD. Idiopathic congenital talipes equinovarus. *J Am Acad Orthop Surg* 2002; 10: 239-48.
3. Barker SL, Macnicol MF. Seasonal distribution of idiopathic congenital talipes equinovarus in Scotland. *J Pediatr Orthop B* 2002; 11: 129-33.
4. Morcuende JA, Dolan LA, Dietz FR, Ponseti IV. Radical reduction in the rate of extensive corrective surgery for clubfoot using the Ponseti method. *Pediatrics* 2004; 113: 376-80.
5. Chapman C, Stott NS, Port RV, Nicol RO. Genetics of clubfoot in Maori and Pacific people. *J Med Genet* 2000; 37: 680-3.
6. Lochmiller C, Johnston D, Scott A, Risman M, Hecht JT. Genetic epidemiology study of idiopathic talipes equinovarus. *Am J Med Genet* 1998; 79: 90-6.
7. Turco VJ. Surgical correction of the resistant club foot: one-stage posteromedial release with internal fixation: a preliminary report. *J Bone Joint Surg* 1971; 53A: 477-97.
8. Macnicol MF, Nadeen MF. Evaluation of the deformity in club foot by somatosensory evoked potentials. *J Bone Joint Surg* 2000; 82B: 731-5.
9. Ballantyne JA, Macnicol MF. Congenital talipes equinovarus (clubfoot): an overview of the aetiology and treatment. *Curr Orthop* 2002; 16: 85-95.

10. Wynne-Davies R. Genetic and environmental factors in the etiology of talipes equinovarus. *Clin Orthop* 1972; 84: 9-13.

11. Idelberger K. Die ergebnisse der zwillingsforschung beim angeborenen Klumpfuss. *Verhandlungen der Deutschen Orthopadischen Gesellschaft* 1939; 33: 272-6.

12. Robertson WWJr, Corbett D. Congenital clubfoot. Month of conception. *Clin Orthop* 1997; 338: 14-8.

13. Handelsman JE, Glasser R. Muscle pathology in clubfoot and lower motor neuron lesions. In: *The clubfoot: the present and a view of the future.* New York: Springer-Verlag, 1994: 21-31.

14. Simons GW. Calcaneocuboid joint deformity in talipes equinovarus: an overview and update. *J Pediatr Orthop B* 1995; 4: 25-35.

15. Thometz JG, Simons GW. Deformity of the calcaneocuboid joint in patients who have talipes equinovarus. *J Bone Joint Surg* 1993; 75A: 190-5.

16. Ippolito E. Update on pathological anatomy of clubfoot. *J Pediatr Orthop B* 1995; 4: 17-24.

17. Sodre H, Bruschini S, Mestriner LA, Miranda F Jr, Levinsohn EM, Packard DS Jr, Crider RJ Jr, Schwartz R, Hootnick DR. Arterial abnormalities in talipes equinovarus as assessed by angiography and the Doppler technique. *J Pediatr Orthop* 1990; 10: 101-4.

18. Muir L, Laliotis N, Kutty S, Klenerman L. Absence of the dorsalis pedis pulse in the parents of children with club foot. *J Bone Joint Surg* 1995; 77B: 114-6.

19. Sano H, Uhtoff HK, Jarvis JG, Mansingh A, Wenckebach GF. Pathogenesis of soft tissue contracture in club foot. *J Bone Joint Surg* 1998; 80B: 641-4.

20. Farrell SA, Summers AM, Dallaire L, Singer J, Johnson JA, Wilson RD. Club foot, an adverse outcome of early amniocentesis: disruption or deformation? CEMAT. Canadian Early and Mid-Trimester Amniocentesis Trial. *J Med Genet* 1999; 36: 843-6.

21. Swart JJ. Clubfoot: a histological study. *SA Bone Joint Surg* 1993; 3: 17-23.

22. Ippolito E, Ponseti IV. Congenital club foot in the human fetus: a histological study. *J Bone Joint Surg* 1980; 62A: 8-22.

23. Ponseti IV. Treatment of congenital club foot. *J Bone Joint Surg* 1992; 74A: 448-454.

24. Macnicol MF. The management of club foot: issues for debate. *J Bone Joint Surg* 2003; 85B: 167-70.

25. Wainwright AM, Auld T, Benson MK, Theologis TN. The classification of congenital talipes equinovarus. *J Bone Joint Surg* 2002; 84B: 1020-4.

26. Ponseti IV, Smoley EN. Congenital club foot: the results of treatment. *J Bone Joint Surg* 1963; 45A: 261-75.

27. Harrold AJ, Walker CJ. Treatment and prognosis in congenital club foot. *J Bone Joint Surg* 1983; 65B: 8-11.

28. Catterall A. A method of assessment of the clubfoot deformity. *Clin Orthop* 1991; 264: 48-53.

29. Dimeglio A, Bensahel H, Souchet P, Mazeau P, Bonnet F. Classification of clubfoot. *J Pediatr Orthop B* 1995; 4: 129-36.

30. Souchet P, Bensahel H, Themar-Noel C, Pennecot G, Csukonyi Z. Functional treatment of clubfoot: a new series of 350 idiopathic clubfeet with long-term follow-up. *J Pediatr Orthop B* 2004; 13: 189-96.

31. Flynn JM, Donohoe M, Mackenzie WG. An independent assessment of two clubfoot-classifications systems. *J Pediatr Orthop* 1998; 18: 323-7.

32. Pirani S, Outerbridge H, Moran M, Sawatsky BJ. A method of evaluating the virgin clubfoot with substantial interobserver reliability. Pediatric Orthopedic Society of North America 1995 meeting, Miami, Florida, May 1995.

33. Scher DM, Feldman DS, van Bosse HJP, Sala DA, Lehman WB. Predicting the need for tenotomy in the Ponseti method for correction of clubfeet. *J Pediatr Orthop* 2004; 24: 349-52.

34. Ippolito E, Fraracci L, Farsetti P, Di Mario M, Caterini R. The influence of treatment on the pathology of club foot: CT study at maturity. *J Bone Joint Surg* 2004; 85B: 574-80.

35. Macnicol MF. The surgical mangement of congenital talipes equinovarus (club foot). *Curr Orthop* 1994; 8: 72-82.

36. Cummings RJ, Davidson RS, Armstrong PF, Lehman WB. Congenital clubfoot. *J Bone Joint Surg* 2002; 84A: 290-308.

37. Noonan KJ, Richards BS. Non-surgical management of idiopathic clubfoot *J Am Acad Orthop Surg* 2003; 11: 392-402.

38. Kite JH. The treatment of congenital clubfoot. *JAMA* 1932; 99: 1156.

39. Kite JH. Principles involved in the treatment of congenital club-foot. *J Bone Joint Surg* 1939; 21: 595-606.

40. Ponseti IV. *Congenital club foot. Fundamentals for treatment.* Oxford: Oxford University Press, 1996.

41. Ponseti IV. The Ponseti technique for correction of congenital clubfoot. *J Bone Joint Surg* 2002; 84A: 1889-91.

42. Bensahel H, Degrippes Y, Billot C. Comments about 600 club feet. *Chir Pediatr* 1980; 21: 335-42.

43. Bensahel H, Dimeglio A, Souchet P. Final evaluation of clubfoot. *J Pediatr Orthop B* 1995; 4: 137-41.

44. Richards BS, Johnston CE, Wilson H. Non-operative clubfoot treatment using the French physical therapy method. *J Pediatr Orthop* 2005; 25: 98-102.

45. Alvarez CM, Tredwell SJ, Keenan SP, Beauchamp RD, Choit RL, Sawazky BJ, De Vera MA. Treatment of idiopathic clubfoot utilizing botulinum A toxin. *J Pediatr Orthop* 2005; 25: 229-35.

46. Simons GW. Analytical radiography of club feet. *J Bone Joint Surg* 1977; 59B: 485-9.

47. Ryoppy S, Sairanen H. Neonatal operative treatment of club foot: a preliminary report. *J Bone Joint Surg* 1983; 65B: 320-5.

48. Pous JG, Dimeglio A. Neonatal surgery in club foot. *Orthop Clin North Am* 1978; 9: 233-40.

49. Turco VJ. Resistant congenital club foot: one-stage posteromedial release with internal fixation. A follow-up report of a fifteen-year experience. *J Bone Joint Surg* 1979; 61A: 805-14.

50. Porat S, Milgrom C, Bentley G. The history of treatment of congenital clubfoot in the Royal Liverpool Children's Hospital: improvement of results by early extensive posteromedial release. *J Pediatr Orthop* 1984; 4: 331-8.

51. Tibrewal SB, Benson MK, Howard C, Fuller DJ. The Oxford club foot programme. *J Bone Joint Surg* 1992; 74A: 528-33.

Chapter 4

52. DePuy J, Drennan JC. Correction of idiopathic clubfoot: a comparison of results of early versus delayed posteromedial release. *J Pediatr Orthop* 1989; 9: 44-8.

53. Ghali NN, Smith RB, Clayden AD, Silk FF. The results of pantalar reduction in the management of congenital talipes equinovarus. *J Bone Joint Surg* 1983; 65B: 1-7.

54. Bensahel H, Csukonyi Z, Desgrippes Y, Chaumien JP. Surgery in residual clubfoot: one-stage medioposterior release 'a La Carte'. *J Pediatr Orthop* 1987; 7: 145-8.

55. Attenborough CG. Severe congenital talipes equinovarus. *J Bone Joint Surg* 1966; 48B: 31-9.

56. McKay DW. New concept of and approach to clubfoot treatment: II. Correction of the clubfoot. *J Pediatr Orthop* 1983a; 3: 10-21.

57. McKay DW. New concept of and approach to club foot treatment: III. Evaluation and results. *J Pediatr Orthop* 1983b; 3: 141-8.

58. Simons GW. Complete subtalar release in club feet. I: a preliminary report. *J Bone Joint Surg* 1985a; 67A: 1044-55.

59. Simons GW. Complete subtalar release in club feet. II: comparison with less extensive procedures. *J Bone Joint Surg* 1985b; 67A: 1056-65.

60. Crawford AH, Marxen JL, Osterfeld DL. The Cincinnati incision: a comprehensive approach for surgical procedures of the foot and ankle in childhood. *J Bone Joint Surg* 1982; 64A: 1355-8.

61. Lehman WB, Atar D, Grant AD, Strongwater AM. Re-do clubfoot: surgical approach and long-term results. *Bull NY Acad Med* 1990; 66: 601-17.

62. Bradish CF, Noor S. The Ilizarov method in the management of relapsed club feet. *J Bone Joint Surg* 2000; 82B: 387-91.

63. Laaveg SJ, Ponseti IV. Long-term results of treatment of congenital club foot. *J Bone Joint Surg* 1980; 62A: 23-31.

64. Cooper DM, Dietz FR. Treatment of idiopathic clubfoot. A thirty-year follow-up. *J Bone Joint Surg* 1995; 77A: 1477-89.

65. Hutchins PM, Foster BK, Paterson DC, Cole EA. Long-term results of early surgical release in club feet. *J Bone Joint Surg* 1980; 62A: 23-31.

66. Haasbeek JF, Wright JG. A comparison of the long-term results of posterior and comprehensive release in the treatment of clubfoot. *J Pediatr Orthop* 1997; 17: 29-35.

67. Carroll NC. Congenital clubfoot: pathoanatomy and treatment. *Instr Course Lect* 1987; 36: 117-21.

68. Herzenberg JE, Radler C, Bor N. Ponseti versus traditional methods of casting for idiopathic clubfoot. *J Pediatr Orthop* 2002; 22: 517-21.

69. Ippolito E, Farsetti P, Caterini R, Tudisco C. Long-term comparative results in patients with congenital clubfoot treated with two different protocols. *J Bone Joint Surg* 2003; 85A: 1286-94.

70. Bensahel H, Kuo K, Duhaime M, the ICFSG. The outcome evaluation of clubfoot. *J Pediatr Orthop B* 2003; 12: 269-71.

71. Dobbs MB, Rudzki JR, Purcell DB, Walton T, Porter KR, Gurnett CA. Factors predictive of outcome after use of the Ponseti method for the treatment of idiopathic clubfeet. *J Bone Joint Surg* 2004; 86A: 22-7.

72. Dimeglio A, Bonnet F, Mazeau P, De Rosa V. Orthopaedic treatment and passive motion machine: consequences for the surgical treatment of clubfoot. *J Pediatr Orthop B* 1996; 5: 173-80.

73. Lefort G, Sleiman M, Lefebvre P, Dooud S. Congenital clubfoot. Analysis of 260 cases followed from birth. *Rev Chir Orthop Reparatrice Appar Mot* 1994; 80: 246-51.

74. Karski T, Wosko I. Experience in the conservative management of congenital clubfoot in newborns and infants. *J Pediatr Orthop* 1989; 9: 134-6.

75. Napiontek M. Clinical and radiographic appearance of congenital talipes equinovarus after successful non-operative treatment. *J Pediatr Orthop* 1996; 16: 67-72.

76. Seringe R, Atia R. Idiopathic congenital club foot: results of functional treatment (269 feet). *Rev Chir Orthop Reparatrice Appar Mot* 1990; 76: 490-501.

77. Yamamoto H, Furuya K. Treatment of congenital club foot with a modified Denis Browne splint. *J Bone Joint Surg* 1990; 72B: 460-3.

78. Yamamoto H, Muneta T, Morita S. Nonsurgical treatment of congenital clubfoot with manipulation, cast, and mofied Denis Browne splint. *J Pediatr Orthop* 1998; 18: 538-42.

79. Bensahel H, Catterall A, Dimeglio A. Practical applications in idiopathic clubfoot: a retrospective multicentric study in EPOS. *J Pediatr Orthop* 1990; 10: 186-8.

80. Bensahel H, Guillaume A, Csukonyi Z Degrippes Y. Results of physical therapy for idiopathic clubfoot: a long-term follow-up study. *J Pediatr Orthop* 1990; 10: 189-90.

81. Campenhout A, Molenaers G, Moens P, Fabry G. Does functional treatment of idiopathic clubfoot reduce the indication for surgery? Call for a widely accepted rating system. *J Pediatr Orthop B* 2001; 10: 315-8.

Chapter 5

Acute management of the patient with spinal cord injury

Jan Borremans Neurosurgeon (GMC)
Specialist Registrar in Spinal Injuries
Brian Gardner BM BCH MA (Oxon) FRCS FRCP (Lond & Edin)
Consultant Surgeon in Spinal Injuries
Patrick Kluger Surgeon for Trauma and Orthopaedics (GMC)
Consultant in Spinal Injuries

NATIONAL SPINAL INJURIES CENTRE, STOKE MANDEVILLE HOSPITAL, AYLESBURY, UK

Introduction

Every system of the body is affected in the case of a spinal cord injury (SCI). The effective management of all aspects from the early stages onwards, influences the successful care of the SCI patient and avoids unnecessary morbidity or mortality.

Before 1940, most SCI patients died from complications within months to years after their injury. If they survived, they often were doomed to destitute institutional lives [1].

Sir Ludwig Guttmann established the first centre of comprehensive care in the world at Stoke Mandeville soon after World War II. He introduced radical changes by proving that fragmentation of care resulted in poor outcome. Through application of a comprehensive approach to care he was able to dramatically alter the five-year survival prognosis for tetraplegic patients from 5% to 90% [2, 3].

Initially in the UK and later in the Commonwealth, Continental Europe, USA, Japan and more recently in China and India, comprehensive systems of care were developed according to Guttmann's principles.

In one-roof systems, the same centre deals with all aspects of medical care following the Accident and Emergency phase. In two-roof systems, the acute care is carried out in one hospital followed by sub-acute and chronic care elsewhere. The latter have some disadvantages compared with the one-roof systems, but both have improved outcomes compared with those where care is either fragmented or carried out by those lacking the required knowledge and experience [3].

Methodology

An electronic database search of Pubmed and Ovid Medline was executed using the search term 'spinal cord injury(ies)', limited to abstracts in core clinical journals and combined with the words 'acute, diagnosis', 'epidemiology', 'management', 'methylprednisolone', 'pathophysiology', 'rehabilitation', 'surgery' and 'traumatic'. Additional manual searching was performed, using reference lists from recent publications and from the National Spinal Injuries Centre Guidelines and Protocols. In total, 158 relevant publications were identified and are cited in this chapter.

Classification

The two most commonly used classification systems are those of Frankel [4] and the American Spinal Injury Association [5] (ASIA) (Table 1).

They both define a SCI as complete if there is no motor or sensory function below the level of injury. There is paraplegia when the arms are spared and a tetraplegia when they are involved. If there is any residual neurological function below the level of injury, the injury is incomplete (Frankel) or has a zone of partial preservation (ASIA). In the ASIA classification, some sacral sensation must be present to have an incomplete lesion.

The potential for any functional neurological recovery within 18 months after an acute SCI (ASCI) in a patient with a complete lesion is estimated at less than 5% [6].

According to the pattern of the neurological deficits after a SCI, some clinical syndromes may be distinguished: central cord syndrome, Brown Sequard syndrome, anterior cord syndrome, posterior cord syndrome, conus medullaris syndrome and cauda equina syndrome.

Epidemiology and demographics

Incidence and prevalence

The annual incidence of acute traumatic SCI varies between series and countries, but is usually in the range of 10 to 50 per million population [3, 7, 8]. Typically only one in 40 polytrauma victims admitted to a major trauma centre has suffered an acute SCI [9]. Most published reports on ASCI do not consider pre-admission deaths. Early indications from an ongoing audit of new admissions into Accident and Emergency Departments in the South of England suggest an annual incidence of spinal trauma with spinal cord at risk, of 16 per million and an incidence of actual spinal cord damage of 12 per million per year [3]. The prevalence in ASCI is defined as all persons with an SCI in a specified population at a particular point of time. Prevalence rates quoted in the literature vary between 130 and 1124 per million population [10-14].

Despite the low incidence, the mortality of these injuries at the scene of injury, or before hospital admission, is estimated between 48% and 79% [15]. Deaths after hospital admission for ASCI vary from 4% to 17% [16]. Respiratory complications are the leading

Table 1. The Frankel classification and American Spinal Injury Association (ASIA) impairment.

Frankel classification

A = Complete	Complete motor and sensory lesion below the level of the lesion
B = Sensory only	No motor function, but some sensation present below the level of the lesion
C = Motor useless	Some motor power present below the lesion, but of no practical use
D = Motor useful	Useful motor power present below the lesion
E = Recovery	Free of neurological symptoms, but abnormal reflexes may be present

ASIA impairment scale

A = Complete	No sensory or motor function is preserved in the sacral segments S4-S5
B = Incomplete	Sensory but no motor function is preserved below the neurological level and includes the sacral segments S4-S5
C = Incomplete	Motor function is preserved below the neurological level and more than half of key muscles below the neurological level have a muscle grade less than 3 (grades 0-2)
D = Incomplete	Motor function is preserved below the neurological level and at least half of key muscles below the neurological level have a muscle grade greater than or equal to 3
E = Normal	Sensory and motor function are normal

cause of death, followed by heart disease, septicaemia and pulmonary emboli. Urological complications no longer seem to be a prominent cause [17].

Causes and prognostic factors

The commonest causes of SCI in frequency of occurrence are road traffic accidents (motor vehicle, bicycle, pedestrian) (40%-50%), falls (20%), sports and recreation (10%-25%), accidents at work (10%-25%), and violence (10%) [10]. The causes of injury vary between countries and age groups. Some recent trends have been observed: in developed countries, sports and leisure causes have increased and work-related causes have decreased. Alarming increases are reported in the violence-related group. Falls tend to affect the older population, whereas high velocity-high impact accidents are predominantly observed in the younger age groups [9, 18, 19].

The most important prognostic factors for survival after ASCI are age, level of injury and neurological grade. The mortality rate for patients with lesions at levels C1-C3, C4-C5 and C6-C8 is respectively 6.6, 2.5 and 1.5 times higher than for patients with paraplegia [20, 21].

Level of injury and neurological deficit

Approximately 55% of ASCI occur at the cervical levels (C1 to C7/T1) and about 15% occur in each of the following levels: thoracic (T1 to T11), thoracolumbar (T11/12 to L1/2) and lumbosacral levels (L2 to S5) [10].

Whereas three to four decades ago, 66% of ASCI were complete, more recently, a shift has been observed: 45% are complete, 15% ASIA B, 10% ASIA C and 30% ASIA D. This reflects an improvement in pre-hospital care, initial hospital care and an awareness of the importance of immobilisation [22-26].

Age and sex

The majority of ASCIs occur in young male patients, aged between 20 and 40. The male to female ratio is between 3:1 and 4:1. The mean age of an individual

with SCI is 35 years. Two thirds of new SCI occur in patients less than 30 years of age [10, 15, 26, 27].

Associated injuries

Isolated SCI occurs in only 20% of cases. In ASCI, 20% to 57% of the cases have a significant associated brain or thoracic injury and 10% to 15% have another spinal lesion below the level of injury [9, 28-31].

A neurological deficit is observed in 10% of those with vertebral fractures. The types of vertebral column injuries associated with ASCI are fracture dislocations (40%), burst fractures (30%), minor fractures (10%), dislocations (5%), SCI without obvious radiographic abnormality or without obvious radiographic evidence of trauma (15%) [10, 18]. Approximately 10% of unstable spinal fractures are still missed in the UK [3, 32].

Prevention

Experience from preventative programmes indicate that behaviour is more likely to be changed by laws with sanctions than by voluntary good sense and sound education [3]. For example, RTAs are less likely to result in spinal cord injury when speed limits are observed and when rear and front seat belts, side impact support systems and front and side airbags are in place. Sports injuries are more reduced by adherence to rules, proper training and expert supervision, than by good education and encouragement.

Pathophysiology

Primary traumatic SCI is due to a combination of the initial impact with or without subsequent persisting spinal cord compression, usually resulting in transection, laceration, contusion or concussion [33].

It is now generally accepted that ASCI is a two-step process. The primary mechanism involves the initial mechanical injury due to the local deformation and energy transformation, whereas the secondary mechanism encompasses a cascade of biochemical and cellular processes that are initiated by the primary impact and may cause ongoing cellular damage and even cell death [34, 35].

The secondary cascade includes:

◆ vascular and microvascular changes consisting of ischaemia, impaired autoregulation, haemorrhage, vasospasm and thrombosis [35-37];

◆ ionic derangement with increased intracellular calcium and extracellular potassium and increased sodium permeability, potentially leading to cellular damage [38, 39];

◆ arachidonic acid release, eicosanoid and free radical production, causing geometrically progressive lipid peroxidation spreading over the cellular surface, eventually inducing membrane lysis [40-42];

◆ endogenous opioid release and neurotransmitter accumulation, of which glutamate causes excitotoxic (exciting and then poisoning) cell injury [43-45];

◆ oedema, inflammation and loss of adenosine triphosphate-dependent cellular processes [46, 47];

◆ programmed cell death or apoptosis, which by definition is an active process initiated by either internal or external stimuli, characterised by cell shrinking, chromatin aggregation, nuclear pyknosis and eventually phagocytosis without initiating an inflammatory response [48-51].

Primary care

The initial management of ASCI patients is preventive, and aims to resuscitate and to do no further harm. Therefore, an initial professional assessment at the scene is mandatory. All polytraumatised patients with head, thoracic, pelvis and long bone injuries or with focal neurological deficit or pain or tenderness in the spine should be suspected of having occult SCI. Partial cord injury may give rise to peculiar symptoms that may be mistaken for hysteria, or wrongly ignored [3, 52].

In all cases of accidents with potential spinal fractures, patients must be treated spine-in-line until

stability has been confirmed. Physiological instability is as important as biomechanical instability following spinal cord trauma. In all cases of SCI, even when there is musculoskeletal stability, the spine must be immobilised until the secondary changes within the spinal cord have ceased to evolve. Secondary changes within the spinal cord after injury makes it more vulnerable to inappropriate movement across the injury site. In all cases of suspicious SCI, satisfactory blood pressure and oxygenation levels must be maintained. Neurological deterioration occurs in fewer than 5% of traumatic SCI with such care, but in up to 50% of cases where the spinal fracture is missed [3, 35, 52-54] **(IIb/B and III/B)**.

Professional assessment at the scene

When urgent hospital treatment is mandatory, the patient is transferred on a spinal board to the nearest suitable receiving hospital. In the case of a less critical individual, more thorough assessment at the scene, with a brief secondary survey, is performed [3]. The latter includes assessing respiratory rate and volume, equality of air entry, specific indications of spinal cord injury, such as spinal pain, loss of sensation or movement in the limbs, burning and electric shock sensations in the trunk or limbs, and a sensory assessment. If the injury is above the 6th thoracic vertebra, the sympathetic nervous system may be interrupted, resulting in bradycardia and hypotension. This is known as neurogenic shock in contrast to hypovolaemic shock where there is tachycardia [3, 52].

Unconsciousness presents a major problem in assessing for spinal cord injury. Pointers to spinal cord injury include diaphragmatic or abdominal breathing, hypotension with bradycardia, flaccid muscles with absent reflexes and priapism. A high index of suspicion must be maintained in all cases where there is pre-existing spinal disease, such as ankylosing spondylitis. These patients may sustain unstable spinal injuries after trivial falls. In this condition, transportation of the patient on their side is advisable, as supine positioning on any flat surface can displace the broken spine.

Management at the scene

Management includes spinal immobilisation, awareness of inducing bradycardias with airway manoeuvres and giving atropine if required, high flow oxygenation via a non-rebreathing mask, intravenous access, pulse oximetry and ECG monitoring [3, 52]. Assisted ventilation should be considered with respiratory rates of <10 or >30, inadequate lung ventilation expansion or an SaO_2 of <90% on 100% O_2. Intubation at the scene is best performed with a blind naso-endotracheal intubation or with manual inline immobilisation and oral intubation, avoiding neck hyperextension.

Patients with isolated neurogenic shock may require a 200-500ml bolus of IV crystalloid to correct hypotension, but no further fluid should be given if spinal cord trauma is the sole injury. A few degrees of head-down tilt may improve the circulation but in cases of abdominal breathing, this manoeuvre may further compromise respiration and ventilation. If the patient vomits, the whole longboard should be tilted and the airway immediately cleared with suction.

Rescue and transport

An orthopaedic (scoop) stretcher is preferred for lifting a suspected SCI patient who is already on the ground, because a log-roll to turn the patient onto the longboard requires four trained people and is not free from risk [3].

Longboards are extrication devices that make the handling and transfer of patients very much easier. Patients who have spinal cord injury are susceptible to pressure sores, which can develop as little as 45 minutes after the placement on a longboard. Indeed, significant pain can arise in pressure areas even after 30 minutes. They should not be used for transport except in emergency situations.

Vacuum mattresses are not suitable for extrication, but are more comfortable and are effective at spinal immobilisation, although vulnerable to perforation. Wide-bodied vacuum mattresses are the preferred means for transportation for patients with spinal injury, especially over long distances. If it is anticipated that a patient is likely to be on the longboard in excess of 30 minutes then transfer to a vacuum mattress using a scoop [3, 55] **(III/B and IV/C)**.

Collars alone are insufficient in stabilising the cervical spine for transport. In circumstances where a spinal injury is suspected or may have occurred, the only safe form of immobilisation during rescue is the use of a correctly applied semi-rigid collar, a longboard and a head immobilisation device with tape or strapping [3, 55]. It is important that care is taken to ensure that the correct size of collar is selected and properly applied to the skin and not over clothing. There is some evidence that ill-fitting collars cause airway obstruction. In cases of severe head injury (or a Glasgow Coma Score of 8 or less), a collar applied at the scene may be removed as soon as is feasible, for example, once the patient has been immobilised on a longboard. It is inappropriate to routinely apply semi-rigid collars to every conscious patient after low-velocity collisions **(III/B and IV/C)**.

In children, there is no method that has been demonstrated to reliably achieve a neutral position. A collar alone is insufficient and a padded board and straps are usually required. A vacuum mattress may be of benefit in those children suspected to have sustained a significant spinal injury [3, 53].

Accident and emergency care

Approximately 85% of ASCI patients will have injuries that permit their immediate transfer, after resuscitation, to the regional acute spinal cord injury centre. This should be carried out as soon as possible, usually by ambulance, but occasionally by air. The remaining 15% will have specialist problems, such as severe brain injury or suspected aortic rupture that the acute spinal cord injury centres cannot manage. In these instances, immediate transfer to the relevant specialist area should be arranged, whilst simultaneously alerting the regional acute spinal service, so that prompt appropriate SCI care can be established alongside the specialist care [3].

Patients should be moved using a scoop stretcher onto a firm padded trolley after the primary survey has been completed. The ABCs, as outlined by the Advanced Trauma Life Support System, should be implemented [52].

Acute traumatic spinal cord injury care in hospital

Advances in primary care, radiological diagnosis and medical and surgical treatment have made the topic of acute SCI management more important than ever.

It is impossible to distinguish in the acute phase, those patients who might eventually recover meaningful neurological function from those who will not. Therefore, the acute management of ASCI patients requires consideration of two goals: the preservation of the patient's life and to optimise the potential recovery of neurological function.

Life preservation

Acute respiratory and haemodynamic failure is the main cause of early mortality in ASCI. Optimal management is based on an understanding of the causes of these physiologic changes.

Respiratory support

This is a crucial aspect of the prevention of further ischaemic injury to the already damaged spinal cord. Overall, respiratory complications correspond closely to the severity of the SCI and systemic shock [52, 56-58].

Lesions proximal to C3 will have a complete loss of diaphragmatic function and will require an instant ventilatory support at the scene, because of the deficit in respiratory drive. High cervical lesions are prone to develop respiratory problems in the early phase because of the complete loss of the intercostal muscle function. Thoracic injuries often develop an Acute Respiratory Distress Syndrome (ARDS), typically 48 to 96 hours after the onset of the injury, due to severe contusion of lung tissue.

Pulmonary toilet and intensive chest physiotherapy are important measures in preventing the build up of pulmonary secretions and the development of secondary respiratory infections. The ease with which this is performed is significantly helped by early surgical fixation of the unstable spinal elements.

Haemodynamic management

Lesions above T6 can cause a syndrome analogous to a functional sympathectomy; as a result, the cardiac chronotropic and inotropic capacities are decreased, inducing bradycardia [3, 52, 59, 60]. Treatment of bradycardia (less than 40 beats per minute) consists of the intravenous administration of 0.25-0.5mg atropine.

Due to the loss of vasomotor tone, an increase in venous capacity with relative hypovolaemia develops, thereby inducing hypotension. Some authors have referred to this as 'neurogenic shock', not to be confused with the neurological syndrome of 'spinal shock', as described below. Intravenous replacement therapy should maintain systolic blood pressures between 80 and 100mm Hg. One should be careful not to overcompensate and in older patients, Swan-Ganz catheterisation with volume resuscitation up to a pulmonary wedge pressure of 18mm Hg should be used. If hypotension persists, intravenous ß-agonist administration is used in the form of dopamine 5-15µg per kg body weight per minute or dobutamine 3-20µg per kg body weight per minute. The use of α-agonists should be avoided, because of the potential increase of cardiac afterload and impaired cardiac output.

Spinal shock

This is an acute neurological syndrome indicating a complete flaccid paralysis with loss of sensation and absent reflexes at the time of initial evaluation. It is observed in about 50% of ASCI patients.

The aetiologic mechanisms of spinal shock are [61]:

- primary axonal and cellular dysfunction;
- sodium-potassium shifts causing ionic conduction blocks;

- maintenance of spinal inhibitory pathways;
- hyperpolarisation of caudal motor neurones;
- loss of fusimotor drive in caudal spinal segments.

There is no universal agreement on the time at which the phase of the spinal shock ends and this is without any prognostic significance [62]. The bulbocavernosus reflex is regarded as the only reflex that can be found in spinal shock and is usually the first to emerge. Usually within a few days of injury, the delayed plantar response is the second reflex reappearing, followed by the cremaster reflex. Deep tendon reflexes recover randomly within one to two weeks. The reappearance of the delayed plantar reflex has prognostic significance: when its reappearance is delayed for more than 48 hours, it indicates a poor potential for functional recovery. On the contrary, early recovery of direct reflexes in patients with a pre-existing symptomatic spinal stenosis usually is linked to a poorer prognosis for functional recovery [63, 64].

Optimising the potential return of neurological function

The number and the quality of the surviving axons passing the injury site determine the extent of possible neurological recovery after ASCI. The pathophysiological processes responsible for the secondary injury are aggravated by hypoxaemia, hypotension and fever. Immobilisation and stabilisation play an important role in preventing re-injury. Early spine realignment, which causes indirect closed decompression of the spinal canal, may optimise functional recovery.

Immobilisation and care

Until confirmation by imaging studies, we have no information about the stability of the spine and the possible extent of the compression on the spinal cord by displaced spinal elements. For this reason, the patient must be treated as if any significant movement of the spine will cause further damage. This is achieved by transporting the patient in a supine position with every attempt to immobilise the spine.

Any movement of the patient has to be performed spine-in-line and the patient has to be log-rolled, which requires a minimum of four persons.

An indwelling catheter is inserted. A nasogastric tube may prevent aspiration in high lesions and is mandatory in case of the development of a paralytic ileus. Oral intake is completely restricted until bowel sounds reappear, which is usually within 48 hours.

Clinical and neurological examination

A thorough and comprehensive neurological examination is mandatory. The head, thorax, abdomen and extremities are examined. This is helpful in reconstructing the impact of the accident. The patient is turned on their side maintaining the spine in line and the back is examined including the sacral area.

Because sacral sparing indicates an incomplete lesion the voluntary anal sphincter contraction and anal sensation are crucial in determining the completeness of the lesion. The presence or absence of anal sphincter tone, bulbocavernosus and cremaster reflexes are checked. The skin is inspected for early pressure signs or decubitus. Voluntary movements of the extremities are grossly tested and subsequently, careful inspection and power grading of the segmental key muscle groups is performed. The borders of the sensory level are noted and the specific key sensory points of all dermatomes are tested on pinprick and light touch. Plantar, abdominal and deep tendon reflexes, as well as muscle tone in upper and lower limbs, are assessed. This enables an exact ASIA classification and grading of the neurological deficit.

This initial examination is compared with subsequent neurological examination at determined intervals, in order to detect any improvement or deterioration at an early stage.

Pharmacological treatment

Secondary tissue damage after ASCI is time-dependent and, therefore, potentially treatable. This led to a trial of several pharmacologic agents in the last two decades of which glucocorticoids were the most important. Their use is still controversial. Other agents such as the potent lipid peroxidase inhibitor, Lazaroid, and Ganglioside, were examined but no benefit has been proven [52, 65].

Experimental evidence from animal studies pointed to the beneficial effect of steroids on spinal cord neurological outcome, following ASCI, especially when administered in pharmacological doses [66, 67]. These animal-based findings were evaluated in humans through the prospective multicentre, double-blind, placebo-controlled National Acute Spinal Cord Injury Studies (NASCIS I - III) [68-72]. Since 1990, the results from the NASCIS II trial have changed the way patients suffering ASCI are treated. More recently, institutions around the world adopted recommendations from the NASCIS III trial, published in 1997. These studies have concluded that treatment with an intravenous methylprednisolone (MP) loading dose of 30mg per kg is beneficial when started within eight hours of the ASCI. When the loading dose is given within three hours of injury, the patients require a 24-hour intravenous drip of 5.4mg per kg per hour. If the loading dose is given between three and eight hours the identical drip is given for 48 hours. There is no beneficial effect of MP if given later than eight hours after injury or in patients with a penetrating SCI. The published results from NASCIS II and III were reviewed in the context of the original study design, including primary outcomes with post-hoc comparisons [73-76]. Although well designed, and well executed, both NASCIS II and III failed to demonstrate improvement in primary outcome measures as a result of the administration of MP. Post-hoc comparisons, although interesting, did not provide compelling data to establish a new standard of care in treatment of patients with ASCI. A deleterious effect of MP on early mortality and morbidity cannot be excluded.

Whilst the methodology of the NASCIS investigations is of the highest order and the gold standard of how such ASCI studies should be conducted, the interpretation of the results has been debated vigorously from the outset. The initial view of most SCI specialists was that the administration of MP was mandatory following ASCI, unless specifically contraindicated [71]. This view has been gradually replaced in many instances by either scepticism or outright opposition to the use of MP in ASCI. The early euphoria for MP as a breakthrough in the treatment of ASCI was slowly revised by the realisation that any neurological benefit was only short term [76]. Although some physicians continue to report the beneficial effects of MP, the evidence base of such reports is, in general, uncontrolled and of low scientific value. More important than the lack of firm evidence for the benefit of MP, has been the emergence of positive evidence for its harmful effects. The early anecdotal evidence of idiosyncratic life-threatening abdominal, septic, cardiovascular and respiratory complications, has been supplemented by firmer published evidence, such as the development of acute myopathy in some patients who receive MP following ASCI [77].

The current specialist majority view in the UK is that MP should not be given [3, 75] **(III/B)**, although some sources still advocate its use, such as the University of York NHS Centre for Reviews and Dissemination that carried out the 2003 audit of effectiveness and cost-effectiveness of acute hospital-based spinal cord injury services.

In its guidelines, the National Spinal Injuries Centre (NSIC) in Stoke Mandeville does not recommend the use of MP following ASCI, believing that the current evidence points to the potentially adverse effects for the patient, outweighing the potentially beneficial ones. Informed consent should always be obtained prior to administration, bearing in mind that: firstly, the drug is unlicensed for the use in ASCI; secondly, that there are potential serious adverse consequences; and thirdly, that the benefits are at best uncertain.

Radiological imaging

Although proper identification of the patient's spinal fractures is a priority, it should not interfere with ongoing resuscitative measures.

The lateral cervical radiograph obtained in the emergency room is a primary basic assessment. Visualisation of C1 through to the top of T1 is necessary, performed at the earliest convenient time.

Dynamic flexion extension studies are reserved for neurologically intact patients with significant axial pain [78-82].

The development of the powerful fourth generation of computed tomography (CT) scans, with the ability to do a spiral whole body CT scan in virtually less than one minute, has radically changed the efficiency and precision of early diagnostics in polytraumatised patients. The ability to immediately reconstruct a spinal fracture in the sagittal, axial and frontal planes is very helpful in determining the further therapeutic options **(III/B)** [83].

Urgent magnetic resonance imaging (MRI) is indicated for unexplained neurological deficit, discordant skeletal and neurological levels and in neurological deterioration. It allows a detailed assessment of discal and ligamentous injuries, intracanal fragments, canal diameter, epidural or intramedullary haemorrhage, CSF leaks and cord oedema, laceration or transection. In the presence of Jefferson fractures, C2 fractures and fractures of the transverse foramen, it may be helpful, to combine the study with an MR angiogram (MRA) to assess the status of the vertebral arteries **(III/B)** [84-86].

Non-operative treatment and pre-operative immobilisation

Immobilisation of the injured spinal segment and closed decompression of the spinal canal through axial traction or through postural reduction are mandatory, until the decision on further treatment has been taken **(IIb/B)**.

Traction

Skull traction is a therapeutic option in injuries affecting the mobile segments from C0-C1 to T2-3. Cervical dislocations and severe compression fractures are considered for reduction by axial traction. Traction is contraindicated in patients with pre-existing fixed spinal deformity, such as ankylosing spondylitis. Overdistraction may occur in unsuspected disruptive disco-ligamentous injuries and may worsen spinal cord damage [87-89].

The method can be used for closed reduction of dislocations. In acute injuries, skull traction may be applied as an emergency procedure. Traditional Crutchfield tongs are rarely used. Vinke-type tongs do not need pre-drilling and are inserted 90° to the cranium's surface but still cause artefacts in MRI. If the need for MRI during skull traction cannot be excluded, Gardner-Wells-type clamps made from carbon fibre may be chosen. If a full course of conservative treatment is planned, including later mobilisation in a halo-vest, the use of a halo-ring for the initial traction should be considered [90, 91].

Before applying skull traction, a thorough analysis of the pattern of injury has to be performed and the direction of traumatic instability must be identified. The two main components of traction are the direction of the applied force and the amount of weight. The insertion points of the pins will depend on the appropriate direction of traction: co-axial in fractures of the occipital condyles and atlas, reclining in Hangman's fractures and AO classified A and B injuries, with flexion of about 20° for the reduction of facet dislocations. In AO type B injuries and bi-facet dislocations without rotation (which are in fact B type injuries), extra care should be taken because there is a disruptive component, which might be potentially dangerous when traction is performed [89, 91]. Accordingly, the possible insertion points of the pins will be located 3cm vertically above the external auditory meatus and from there a maximum of 2cm forwards or backwards. Before applying weight, a lateral fluoroscopy is performed. A pull on the patient's arms may be needed to visualise the region of interest. A weight of 1.5kg is fitted and this is documented with fluoroscopy. The procedure must be interrupted in the case of over-distraction. Following this, 10% of the patient's body weight is applied and increased in steps of 5kg every ten minutes, with fluoroscopy after each weight change, until the desired effect is achieved. It is mandatory to monitor the patient's neurological function continuously. Half of the patient's body weight should not be exceeded in adults. The maximal traction weight in children is a quarter of the body weight. After the successful reduction of a facet dislocation, the direction of the traction force is changed to lordosing and the traction weight is reduced to 10% of the bodyweight [92].

Postural reduction

Postural reduction is a therapeutic option in injuries affecting the mobile segments from the thoracic, thoracolumbar, lumbar and lumbosacral spine.

Various authors in the 20th century have proposed postural reduction on frames with prolonged bed rest as a means of achieving spinal stability [93-95]. These techniques were designed to reduce and to stabilise the thoracic and lumbar spine, but with the rapid development of spinal surgical techniques in the last 30 years they are much less frequently used. Postural reduction techniques are still extremely worthwhile in the pre-operative phase or in cases where it is decided to treat the fracture conservatively.

The methods of postural reduction techniques were described by Guttmann in the 1950s. Patients were placed on turning beds to prevent decubital complications, and pillows and rolls were used in addition at the appropriate sites to try to reduce the fracture or fracture dislocation. In this way, varying degrees of extension could be achieved, and when indicated, also a neutral or flexed position. Progress was checked by frequent X-ray control and according to this information the position was changed if necessary. Once the patient had started to mobilise after 6-12 weeks, (s)he was fitted with a light plastic jacket for several weeks [1, 2, 4, 96].

Conservative versus surgical treatment

Background

Sir Ludwig Guttmann had stressed the principle that the SCI patient needed an anatomically stable and aligned spine to obtain an optimal rehabilitation potential. He developed conservative treatment methods to achieve this aim without creating unnecessary risk or harm to the patient. With his special postural reduction techniques, he obtained very good results after several weeks of consistent treatment in bed. During this period (1950-1980), the majority of surgical techniques were obsolete or had poor late postoperative realignment results. Consequently, Guttmann was a strong opponent of surgical intervention in spinal cord injured patients. He also declined conservative treatment principles in which the spine was not optimally realigned and he rejected immobilisation in a plaster cast, because of the high risk of pressure sores [96-98].

During the past 30 years, the surgical treatment of spinal trauma has radically changed. Several metallic implants have been developed, which in combination with bone grafting, allows immediate stability, with reliable realignment of the fractured spine [99-117]. The advantage of these procedures is, that long periods of bed immobilisation can be avoided and the active rehabilitation of the patients can start several weeks earlier than with conservative treatment. The earlier the spine is stabilised, so the number of complications of bed rest will be reduced. Early complications include deep venous thrombosis, pulmonary embolism, decubital skin lesions, chest and urinary tract infections. Late complications of poor spinal alignment comprise degenerative change in adjacent segments, progressive deformity and syringomyelia [3, 52, 63].

The one-roof model of spinal care

All patients with traumatic spinal cord injuries ideally should be in a spinal injuries unit within 24 hours of injury. This has been shown to produce the best outcome for patients [118] **(IIb/B)**.

Following this guideline, all patients with spinal cord injury would have their treatment, including surgery and multidisciplinary rehabilitation, in the setting of a specialised spinal unit. Such a unit requires an adequate number of appropriately trained spinal surgeons, 24-hour access to imaging facilities, ITU and HDU. All other appropriate surgical expertise such as, neuro, thoracic and abdominal should be readily available [3].

The above-mentioned 24-hour rule does not apply when:

◆ urgent decompression is required for deteriorating neurology and the delay in transfer would be detrimental to the patient;

- the spinal column is considered to be so unstable that transfer would place the spinal cord at further risk.

About 15% of ASCI patients are unsuitable for acute treatment within the spinal injury units; for example, cases with polytrauma or severe head injury requiring intracranial pressure management.

Non-operative versus operative care of the spine

Opinion as to the role of surgery following spinal cord injury remains divided. A number of studies have shown no significant difference in neurological outcome irrespective of surgical intervention [119-123].

Surgery has some potential advantages over recumbent care, such as rapid mobilisation, thereby hastening entry into the rehabilitation process [124]. The surgical approach, timing and type of instrumentation remain controversial, but in general terms, the aim is to preserve as many motion segments as possible by short segment fixation. Whilst the timing of decompressive surgery is controversial, a widely accepted indication for emergency decompression is progressive neurological deterioration due to spinal cord compression [3].

Non-operative care

Numerous authors have reported excellent results after non-operative management of thoracic, thoracolumbar and lumbar fractures with and without closed reduction [1, 2, 96-98, 120, 125-129]. Although bony deformity often recurs after closed reduction, the eventual residual deformity frequently seems to be well tolerated [120, 124, 125]. If the residual kyphosis angle in the thoracic, thoracolumbar or lumbar spine exceeds 35°, 20° or 10° Cobb respectively, it is proposed that the biomechanical environment favours progression of kyphosis and surgery is indicated [130, 131]. Reports of non-operative treatment versus posterior internal fixation have demonstrated comparable functional outcomes at long-term follow-up; however, in the

latter, the loss of correction is smaller [122-124]. In many studies a positive association was observed between the degree of kyphotic deformity, and back pain. Spinal kyphosis leads to compensatory hyperlordosis, contracture of the posterior ligaments, facet joint arthrosis and accelerated disc degeneration in adjacent segments [3, 95, 131, 132]. These cases then often require later surgical spinal realignment [130].

The short and long-term results of closed reduction in the thoracolumbar fractures are superior to those in lumbar fractures [95]. Reasons for this are:

- the thoracic spine is relatively inflexible compared to the lumbar spine, where mobile segments surround the fracture site;
- the loss of reduction due to protrusion of disc material through the damaged endplate, which has more impact in the bigger lumbar discs;
- the compensatory stress focuses on less motion in units below the lesion.

The conservative treatment takes about 10 to 12 weeks and includes immobilisation, positioning and log-rolling in a spinal bed, the provision of traction or postural reduction and the administration of a halo-vest, brace, orthosis or collar when mobilisation is started [1-4, 96, 128].

Non-operative management plays an important part in the treatment of some vertebral injuries (IIb/B), especially in [128, 130]:

- fractures of the occipital condyles in children;
- C0-C1 ligamentous disruption in children;
- Jefferson fractures with less than 5mm dislocation;
- Dens Axis fractures Anderson type I;
- Hangman fractures Effendi type I;
- unilateral non-dislocated fracture en séparation;
- thoracic and thoracolumbar compression fractures without major encroachment of neural elements, where the post-traumatic deformity is estimated to be lower than 35° and 20° Cobb respectively;

Chapter 5

◆ thoracic and thoracolumbar Chance fractures without dislocation, but here there is a high risk of dislocation with neurological deterioration or development of pseudarthrosis during the conservative treatment.

Principles of surgery in SCI

Surgery should be performed by, or under the appropriate supervision of, a consultant surgeon in whose practice a significant part of the workload is spinal surgery. The expertise of the surgeon should be sufficient that the operation performed should be determined by what is most appropriate for the patient. It should not be compromised by the inability of the surgeon to perform a specific approach. If surgery is to be used, it should be of the highest quality **(IV/C)**. The following principles apply [3, 130]:

◆ compromised, symptomatic neural structures should be decompressed;
◆ rigid fixation of the fewest number of spinal segments should be employed;
◆ the aim is restoration of anatomical alignment. Deformity is particularly difficult to compensate for in the wheelchair-bound patient;
◆ following fixation, early mobilisation should be encouraged;
◆ following complete lesions or partial lesions with marked sensory loss, as long as fixation is adequate, orthoses should be avoided due to the additional problems with skin care that they may cause;
◆ posterior decompression without stabilisation is rarely appropriate for the management of spinal injuries.

Urgent surgery

Urgent surgical intervention should be reserved for those patients with deteriorating neurology and cord compression consistent with that deterioration. There is no evidence that emergency surgery outside of this group improves neurological recovery [3, 124, 130] **(IIb/B)**.

Early surgery

In general, surgery as early as possible is preferred for [3, 98, 124, 130]:

◆ decompression: decompression of the spinal cord for a static neurological deficit is less urgent, but should also be performed early **(III/B)**;
◆ fixation: in most instances, fixation should be performed early, in order to start the rehabilitation process early. Early surgery improves the chance of good correction. Unstable spines in the non-compliant, especially those with psychiatric disorders should be stabilised with high priority **(III/B)**;
◆ severe thoracic injury: this may be associated with lung contusion and ARDS. Fixation prior to the onset of ARDS, typically at 48 to 96 hours post-injury, may help management of the chest contusion **(III/B)**.

Delayed surgery

Delay in surgery may be appropriate in certain instances [3, 130]:

◆ other injuries: if injuries outside the spine have clinical precedence and spinal fixation is felt to carry a risk of worsening the overall clinical picture **(III/B)**;
◆ spinal injury with improving neurological deficit: surgical intervention may be delayed until recovery appears to have reached a plateau. Once that has been reached, there is generally no reason for delaying surgery further **(III/B)**.

The Stoke Mandeville approach to the spine

Restoration of alignment and reconstruction of canal size will not improve neurological function in the short term, but may reduce the risk of syrinx formation in the chronic phase, as well as minimise those musculoskeletal symptoms and changes that emanate from poor posture. Long spinal fixations should always be avoided as they reduce spinal mobility and increase dependence, especially in the later years. A long cervical immobilisation can gravely affect the quality of life of a tetraplegic whose only means of looking around him is by rotation of his head on his neck.

Around 10%-15% of traumatic spinal cord injured patients have fractures at multiple levels [3, 52]. The fractures below the main fracture must be treated on their merits, even in complete spinal cord injury, because these lower level fractures can have important potential neurological and musculoskeletal consequences. Due to the absence of pain as a tool for diagnosis and protection, concomitant fractures below the level of neurological deficit carry an increased risk of pseudoarthrosis. When an unstable fracture unsupported by muscles does not heal satisfactorily, significant spinal deformity can arise, increasing the risk of pressure sores, impairing respiration and reducing independence by producing poor posture [3, 130].

The pattern applied in the NSIC at Stoke Mandeville has been introduced since 2000 by Kluger and is described in Table 2. It is important to stress that the indication for surgery is not solely defined by the type of injury, but also by multiple other variable and important factors such as: neurological deterioration, concomitant injuries, pre-existing medical or psychiatric conditions, compliance and mental state. In this context it is essential to mention that the appended table (Table 2) is only intended for reference in cases where surgery is considered.

Affected systems and associated injuries

It is essential that these be well treated to ensure optimum outcome of the spinal cord injury [3, 10, 52, 96, 129] (IIb/B).

Management of affected body systems

Respiratory system

Respiratory problems are the main cause of morbidity and mortality following spinal cord injury [10, 52, 53, 133, 134]. Mid and low cervical tetraplegic patients have good diaphragmatic breathing but no intercostal muscle control. Pulmonary and chest wall compliance becomes increasingly impaired. High paraplegics have some upper intercostal muscle control, but lack the abdominal muscle control that is indispensable in producing an effective cough [135]. As a result, these groups have a weak cough and require assistance with bringing up secretions. The cough-assist machine should be considered early for all spinal cord injured patients, who have chest secretions that are difficult to clear [3, 136].

For high cervical lesions, tracheal ventilation remains the norm; oronasal ventilation is becoming increasingly popular. A tracheostomy should only be performed after eventual anterior surgery to the cervical spine has been accomplished, to avoid difficulties and complications during the anterior approach [3, 52, 137-140].

Cardiovascular system

Postural hypotension is a common problem in the early stage after a spinal cord injury. It persists less frequently into the chronic phase [3, 141-143].

Autonomic dysreflexia is a serious potential complication in all patients with spinal cord injuries at T6 or above. The syndrome is caused by an abrupt and excessive discharge from the sympathetic nervous system causing headache, profuse sweating, piloerection, cardiac rhythm changes and high blood pressure. It can be precipitated by any stimulus arising below the level of injury, but most commonly from the bladder or the bowels. The condition is not only excruciatingly painful, but also dangerous. Initial treatment includes eradication of the cause, sitting the patient upright and vasodilators such as sublingual nifedipine and glyceryl trinitrate [3, 143-146].

Deep venous thrombosis and pulmonary emboli are important potential early complications. Anticoagulation in the form of low-molecular-weight heparin should be started 48 hours after the ASCI and is required during the first 12 weeks following injury. Thereafter, it can be discontinued. It has to be taken with a drug providing gastric protection [3, 52, 143, 147].

Skin

Pressure sores can largely be avoided by disciplined care, supplemented by suitable equipment. Shearing forces are as important as direct pressure in causing tissue damage. The insensitive skin should be inspected regularly. Red marks and abrasions should be treated by avoiding further direct pressure and the appropriate positioning of

Table 2. The pre-operative conservative management and surgical treatment pattern as it is applied at the NSIC in Stoke Mandeville.

Type of injury	Pre-surgical care/non-operative management	Method of surgery, if needed	Post-surgical care
Injuries C0-T2			
Fractures of the occipital condyles / occipito-cervical disruptions in children	Halo vest in compressive lesions SOMI brace in distractive lesions Minimum 6 wk	Surgical intervention rarely required	
Fractures of the occipital condyles / occipito-cervical disruptions in adults	Skull traction (in compressive displacements only) SOMI brace (Minerva orthosis)	Fusion and instrumentation C0-C1 If Jefferson fracture concomitant: fusion C0-C2 (Magerl screws C1-C2)	No orthosis
C1 Jefferson fractures with dislocation < 5mm	Halo vest Minimum 6 wk	Surgical intervention rarely required	
C1 Jefferson fractures with dislocation > or = 5mm	Skull traction	Clamp fixation with lateral mass screws and connecting rod	No orthosis / soft collar 4 wk
C2 Dens fractures Anderson 1	SOMI brace Minimum 6 wk	Surgical intervention rarely required	
C2 Dens fractures Anderson II	Philadelphia collar / SOMI brace	1 or 2 Böhler screws	1 screw: Philadelphia collar or SOMI brace 4 wk 2 screws: no orthosis
C2 Dens fractures Anderson III	Skull traction	Anterior fixation with mini T-plate / posterior fixation with C1-2 Magerl screws	T-plate: Philadelphia collar 4 wk C1-2 fusion: no orthosis
C2 Hangman fractures Effendi I	Halo vest minimum 6 wk	Surgical intervention rarely required	
C2 Hangman fractures Effendi II & Effendi III	Skull traction	Posterior C2 Judet pedicle screw fixation, then anterior discectomy and fusion with autogenic iliac crest graft and screw plate fixation C2-3 within the same anaesthesia	No orthosis
Burst and wedge fractures C2 to T2 (AO type A & B)	Skull traction	Anterior decompression (discectomy and corpectomy) and fusion with autogenic iliac crest graft and screw plate fixation	AO A: no orthosis AO B: soft collar / Philadelphia collar 4-6 wk
Fracture dislocations C3 to T1 (AO type C)	Closed reduction by skull traction (AO C in T1-2 is rarely reducible by skull traction)	If reduction succeeds: anterior decompression (discectomy and corpectomy) and interbody fusion (s. above). If attempt at closed reduction fails: posterior open reduction, posterior tension band fixation, anterior decompression and interbody fusion (s. above) within the same anaesthesia	Solely anterior fixations: Philadelphia collar 4-6 wk Posterior-anterior fixations: no orthosis

Table 2. *Continued:*

Type of injury	Pre-surgical care/non-operative management	Method of surgery, if needed	Post-surgical care
Special cases cervical spine			
Fractures in ankylosing spondylitis	*In situ* immobilisation with cushions, head support *Skull traction is extremely dangerous!*	Posterior and anterior instrumentation, if possible, in same anaesthesia, always posterior first with V-shaped interlaminar resection, to allow correction of the disease-related deformity and to make anterior approach accessible	SOMI brace 4 wk
Unilateral non-dislocated fractures through the base of cervical pedicles and through lamina (fracture en séparation [fes])	Philadelphia collar Minimum 6 wk	Surgical intervention rarely required	
Fractures through the base of cervical pedicles and through lamina (fracture en séparation [fes])	Skull traction, preferably by Halo / Trippi-Wells, to control rotation	If fes is bilateral: anterior interbody fusion with screw plate fixation of both affected (dislocated) segments In cases of unilateral fes: generally one segment is dislocated and may be fused	No orthosis in 2-segmental fusion Philadelphia collar 6 wk in single-level fusions
Injuries to the trunk spine (T2-S1)			
Injuries T2 to T5 (AO type A, B & C)	Postural reduction	Posterior open reduction, decompression via mini-costotransversectomy, and fixation with Fixateur Interne (pedicle screws 1 above and 1 below injured mobile segment(s)). Interbody fusion of injured mobile segments with autogenic graft via mini-costotransversectomy In children / patients with pedicle diameters less than 4mm: hook fixation (2 above, 2 below), bony fusion is restricted to injured motion segment(s). If non-fused motion segments are fixed by instrumentation, implant removal is mandatory	No orthosis
Injuries T5 to L2 (AO type A, B & C)	Postural reduction	Posterior open reduction and fixation with Fixateur Interne (pedicle screws 1 above and 1 below injured mobile segment(s)), decompression via mini-costotransversectomy (T5-T11) or via interlaminotomy / laminectomy (T12-L2). Secondary (0-6 wk) interbody fusion via intercostal mini-thoracotomy (endoscopically optional), if post-op imaging leads to anticipation of late loss of correction with non-acceptable outcome. If non-fused motion segments are fixed by instrumentation, implant removal is mandatory	No orthosis
Injuries L2 to L5 (AO type A, B & C)	Postural reduction	Posterior open reduction and fixation with Fixateur Interne (pedicle screws 1 above and 1 below injured mobile segment(s)), decompression via interlaminotomy / laminectomy. Secondary (0-6 wk) non-instrumented interbody fusion via retroperitoneal minimal invasive approach (Mini-ALIF), if post-op imaging leads to anticipation of late loss of correction with non-acceptable outcome. If non-fused motion segments are fixed by instrumentation, implant removal is mandatory	No orthosis

Chapter 5

Table 2. *Continued:*

Type of injury	Pre-surgical care/non-operative management	Method of surgery, if needed	Post-surgical care
Special cases trunk spine			
Thoracic and thoracolumbar compression fractures (AO type A) without impairment of neural elements and long-term post-traumatic deformity is estimated < 35° and 20° Cobb* respectively	Postural reduction Bed rest on spinal bed minimum 8 wk. Thereafter, mobilisation in Atlantis brace 4-6 wk	Surgical intervention rarely required Exception: Pincer fracture (A2.2, A2.3)	
Chance fractures	Postural reduction	Posterior open reduction and fixation with Fixateur Interne (pedicle screws 1 above and 1 below) In children / patients with pedicle diameters less than 4mm: compressive hook fixation (1 above, 1 below). No fusion. Implant removal is mandatory	No orthosis Contact brace if hook fixation is used
Thoracic and thoraco-lumbar Chance fractures without dislocation	Postural reduction Bed rest on spinal bed Minimum 8 wk. Thereafter mobilisation in Atlantis brace 4-6 wk	There is a high chance of dislocation during conservative treatment. Therefore recommended: posterior open reduction and fixation with Fixateur Interne (pedicle screws 1 above and 1 below)	
Fractures in ankylosing spondylitis	*In situ* immobilisation with cushions *No postural reduction!*	Posterior open reduction with corrective interlaminar resection and fixation with Fixateur Interne (pedicle screws 2+ above, 2+below), anterior grafting and additional screw-rod instrumentation as staged procedure. No mobilisation between stages.	No orthosis
Sacral fractures	Bed rest, no postural reduction	Posterior open decompression and revision of sacral roots, no forced reduction. Fixation with Fixateur Interne L5 to ileum, with cross-link. Only grafting on Os sacrum. Implant removal mandatory	No orthosis

* The Cobb angle is obtained by the Cobb method concept. It is the angle between perpendiculars to the vertebral body line at inflectional points in a specified planar projection; it is the measure of the magnitude of a scoliotic curve; the angle is formed by the intersection of two perpendicular lines, each of which is parallel to the top and bottom vertebra of the scoliotic curve, respectively.

unaffected areas. In the early stages, two-hourly turns in bed are required, although the period between turns can be gradually increased [3, 52, 148].

Urinary system

In the acute phase patients are treated with an indwelling catheter. As soon as medically possible, regular and sterile intermittent catheterisation should replace the indwelling catheter. According to the video-urodynamic parameters obtained and the patient's compliance, these modalities are switched to self-intermittent catherisation, sheet drainage with or without chemical or surgical sphincter weakening, reflex voiding or a suprapubic catheter. In patients with high lesions with impaired upper limb function in the early stages, a suprapubic catheter should be considered. Life-long regular urologic follow-up is mandatory. In this way, long-term complications affecting the urinary tract can be significantly reduced [3, 149-151].

Bowel

In the early phase after a spinal cord injury, oral intake should be completely restricted until bowel sounds reappear. In high lesions, a nasogastric tube is inserted to prevent aspiration and ileus. A personalised bowel regime is established in which digital evacuation is often required [3].

Joints

Heterotopic ossification (HO) is usually confined to the early stages following SCI and mainly affects hip, elbow and shoulder joints. It presents often with a hot swollen extremity and reduced range of motion in the affected joint. In the early stages, an ultrasound will reveal tissue changes without any evidence of venous thrombosis. In the active phase the alkaline phosphatase blood levels will be increased. Treatment with non-steroidal anti-inflammatory drugs and bisphosphonates can partially contain the process, although this is rather empiric. The efficiency of low-dose radiation in the early stages of HO is clinically proven. Active physiotherapy is mandatory to preserve the joint mobility. Surgical excision of the HO occasionally has to be performed, but is contraindicated when the process is still active. Early postoperative radiotherapy reduces the recurrence significantly [3, 152-155].

Spasms and spasticity

These are a normal accompaniment of spinal cord injury and begin to appear after the spinal shock phase. When a sudden increase in spasms or spasticity is observed, all irritative foci below the level of injury have to be excluded, such as skin problems, a bladder stone, constipation or a fracture. Physiotherapeutic measures including standing, joint ranging and hydrotherapy may have a relieving effect [156]. Oral medications such as Baclofen, Dantrium and Tizanidine all have certain potential side effects and are only used when the spasms or spasticity interfere with the activities of daily life. In exceptional cases of spasm within defined muscle groups, Botulinum toxin may be beneficial. In a small number of patients with severe, intractable, disabling and generalised spasticity, intrathecal administration of Baclofen by means of a subcutaneous implanted pump is required [157, 158].

Contractures can cause major problems. Good physiotherapy, satisfactory positioning and expert splinting can usually prevent them [3, 96].

Management of associated injuries

Brain injuries

Successful rehabilitation after spinal cord injury is dependent on the total involvement of the paralysed person [3, 96, 129]. Even minor impairment of executive function, personality, memory, concentration and intellect can interact with other aspects of the spinal cord injury to make successful independent living and employment impossible.

Limb injuries

Arm function is essential for paraplegic and low tetraplegic patients to retain optimum independence in transfers and activities of daily living. Upper limb joints, especially the shoulder girdle, are put under greater physical stress during day-to-day activities. As a result they degenerate prematurely. Any upper limb damage sustained at injury will compound and expedite these changes. Where there are brachial plexus or other upper limb peripheral nerve injuries, the affected arm is less useful. Trick movements limit the functional impact but can take years to develop [3].

Joint damage, and to a lesser extent, long bone fractures, can severely impair transfers, wheelchair skills and the ability to use a standing frame, callipers, Zimmer frame or crutches. These problems will also need to be addressed in the early stages.

Chest and abdominal injuries

These injuries can initially be life-threatening, but are seldom functionally relevant thereafter.

Conclusions

The recent insights into the pathophysiological aspects of SCI show that the clinical neurological outcome depends directly upon the extent of the primary and secondary damage to the spinal cord.

Chapter 5

The acute management comprises proper resuscitation techniques consisting of the combination of acute life-saving measures and protection of the spinal cord. All patients with ASCI should ideally be in a spinal injuries unit within 24 hours of injury. This guarantees a specialised and comprehensive approach from the early stages, comprising spinal surgery, multidisciplinary rehabilitation and all relevant associated medical, surgical and psychological specialties. The combined approach of these professionals will minimise the morbidity and mortality and help the SCI patients to reach their full potential for recovery.

Recommendations	Evidence level
◆ In all cases of accidents with potential spinal fractures, patients must be treated spine-in-line until stability has been confirmed.	IIb/B
◆ Scoops are used for roadside victims; longboards are suitable for extrication; and vacuum mattresses for transportation of patients with a spinal injury.	III/B
◆ Collars alone are insufficient in stabilising the cervical spine for transport. A head immobilisation device and tape or strapping should be used to secure the head.	III/B
◆ All patients with traumatic spinal cord injuries ideally should be in a spinal injuries unit within 24 hours of injury.	IIb/B
◆ Immobilisation of the injured spinal segment and closed decompression of the spinal canal through axial traction or through postural reduction are mandatory until the decision upon further treatment has been taken.	IIb/B
◆ The current specialist majority view in the UK is that MP should not be given, although some sources still advocate its use.	III/B
◆ Spiral whole body CT is superior to conventional radiological examinations in early diagnostics in polytraumatised ASCI patients.	III/B
◆ Urgent magnetic resonance imaging (MRI) is indicated in ASCI with unexplained neurological deficit, discordant skeletal and neurological levels and in neurological deterioration.	III/B
◆ Non-operative management plays an important part in the treatment of some vertebral injuries.	IIb/B
◆ If surgery is to be used, it should be of the highest quality and includes: decompression, rigid fixation, anatomical alignment, and least number of segments.	IV/C
◆ Urgent surgical intervention should be reserved for those patients with deteriorating neurology and cord compression consistent with that deterioration.	IIb/B
◆ Early surgery is preferred in situations where conservative treatment is not practicable, e.g. in patients with confusion, epilepsy or at risk of drugs or alcohol withdrawal.	III/B
◆ Fixation prior to the onset of ARDS, typically at 48 to 96 hours post-injury, may help management of the chest contusion.	III/B
◆ Delay in surgery may be appropriate in severe polytrauma and patients with improving neurology.	III/B
◆ A specialised, holistic and comprehensive approach from the early stages in the setting of a specialised spinal unit, will minimise the morbidity and mortality and enable the highest possible levels of recovery.	IIb/B

References

1. Guttmann L. Statistical survey on one thousand paraplegics. *Proc R Soc Med* 1954; 47: 1099-1103.

2. Guttmann L. The management of paraplegia. *Med Annu* 1961; 79: 19-31.

3. Gardner B, Kluger P. Mini-Symposium: Spinal Trauma. (iv) The overall care of the spinal cord injured patient. *Curr Orthop* 2004; 18: 33-48.

4. Frankel HL, Hancock DO, Hyslop G, *et al*. The value of postural reduction in the initial management of closed injuries of the spine with paraplegia and tetraplegia. *Paraplegia* 1969; 7: 179-92.

5. Ditunno JF, Young W, Donovan WH, *et al*. The international standards booklet for neurological and functional classificaiton of spinal cord injury. *Paraplegia* 1994; 32: 70-80.

6. Bode RK, Heinemann AW, Chen D. Measuring the impairment consequences of spinal cord injury. *Am J Phys Med Rehabil* 1999; 78: 582-94.

7. Botterell EH, Jousse ET, Kraus AS, *et al*. A model for the future care of acute spinal cord injuries. *Can J Neurol Sci* 1975; 2: 361-80.

8. Kraus JF, Silberman TA, McArthur DL. In: *Principles of spinal cord injury: epidemiology of spinal cord injury*. Benzel EC, Cahill DW, McCormack P, Eds. New York: McGraw-Hill, 1996: 41-58.

9. Burney RE, Maio RF, Maynard F, *et al*. Incidence, characterisics and outcome of spinal cord injuries at trauma centers in North America. *Arch Surg* 1993; 128: 596-9.

10. Sekhon LHS, Fehlings MG. Epidemiology, demographics, and pathophysiology of acute spinal cord injury. *Spine* 2001; 26 (Suppl): S2-S12.

11. Anderson DW, Kalsbeek WD. The National Head and Spinal Cord Injury Survey: assessment of some uncertainties affecting the findings. *J Neurosurg* 1980; (Nov suppl): S32-S34.

12. DeVivo MJ, Fine PR, Maetz HM, *et al*. Prevalence of spinal cord injury: a re-estimation employing life table techniques. *Arch Neurol* 1980; 37: 707-8.

13. Ergas Z. Spinal cord injury in the United States: a statistical update. *Cent Nerv Syst Trauma* 1985; 2: 19-32.

14. Harvey C, Wilson SE, Greene CG, *et al*. New estimates of the direct costs of traumatic spinal cord injuries: results of a nationwide survey. *Paraplegia* 1992; 30: 834-50.

15. Kraus JF, Franti CE, Riggins RS, *et al*. Incidence of traumatic spinal cord lesions. *J Chronic Dis* 1975; 28: 471-92.

16. Kraus JF. Injury to the head and the spinal cord: the epidemiological relevance of the literature published from 1960 to 1978. *J Neurosurg* 1980; (Suppl): S3-S10.

17. DeVivo MJ, Kartus PL, Stover SL, *et al*. Cause of death for patients with spinal cord injuries. *Arch Intern Med* 1989; 149: 1761-6.

18. Tator CH. Epidemiology and general characteristics of the spinal cord-injured patient. In: *Contemporary Management of Spinal Cord Injury: From Impact to Rehabilitation*. Tator CH, Benzel EC, Eds. 3rd ed. Park Ridge, IL: American Association of Neurological Surgeons, 2000: 15-9.

19. Sutherland MW. The prevention of violent spinal cord injuries. *SCI Nurs* 1993; 10: 91-5.

20. Claxton A, Wong DT, Chung F, *et al*. Factors predictive of hospital mortality and mechanical ventilation in patients with cervical spinal cord injury. *Can J Anaesth* 1998; 45: 144-9.

21. DeVivo MJ, Stover SL, Black KJ. Prognostic factors for 12-year survival after spinal cord injury. *Arch Phys Med Rehabil* 1992; 73: 156-62.

22. Tator CH, Duncan EG, Edmonds VE, *et al*. Changes in epidemiology of acute spinal cord injury from 1947 to 1981. *Surg Neurol* 1993; 40: 207-15.

23. Hachen HJ. Idealized care of the acutely injured spinal cord in Switzerland. *J Trauma* 1977; 17: 931-6.

24. Harris P, Karmi MZ, McClemont E, *et al*. The prognosis of patients sustaining severe cervical spine injury (C2-C7 inclusive). *Paraplegia* 1980; 18: 324-30.

25. Meyer PR Jr, Sullivan DE. Injuries to the spine. *Emerg Med Clin North Am* 1984; 2: 313-29.

26. Zäch GA, Koch HG, Wolfensberger M, *et al*. In: *Querschnittslaehmung-ganzheitliche Rehabilitation: Demographie und Statistik der Querschnittlaehmung*. Zäch G, Ed. Küsnacht, Switzerland: Verlag Dr Felix Würst AG, 1995: 16-9.

27. Stover SL, Fine PR. The epidemiology and economics of spinal cord injury. *Paraplegia* 1987; 25: 225-8.

28. Exner G, Meinecke FW. Trends in the treatment of patients with spinal cord lesions seen within a period of 20 years in German centers. *Spinal Cord* 1997; 35: 415-9.

29. Harris P. Acute spinal cord injury patients: who cares? *Paraplegia* 1985; 23: 1-7.

30. Meguro K, Tator CH. Effect of multiple trauma on mortality and neurological recovery after spinal cord or cauda equina injury. *Neurol Med Chir* (Tokyo) 1988; 28: 34-41.

31. Meinecke FW. Pelvis and limb injuries in patients with recent spinal cord injuries. *Proc Veterans Admin Spinal Cord Inj Conf* 1973: 205-13.

32. Poonnoose P, Ravichandran G, McClelland M. Missed and mismanaged injuries of the spinal cord. *J Trauma* 2002; 53: 314-20.

33. Tator CH. Update on the pathophysiology and pathology of acute spinal cord injury. *Brain Pathol* 1995; 5: 407-13.

34. Fehlings MG, Sekhon LHS. In: *Contemporary Management of Spinal Cord injury: From Impact to Rehabilitation: Cellular, Ionic and Biomolecular Mechanisms of the Injury Process*. Tator CH, Benzel EC, Eds. New York: American Association of Neurological Surgeons, 2000: 33-50.

35. Tator CH, Fehlings MG. Review of the secondary injury theory of acute spinal cord trauma with emphasis on vascular mechanisms. *J Neurosurg* 1991; 75: 15-26.

36. Tator CH. Review of experimental spinal cord injury with emphasis on the local and systemic circulatory effects. *Neurosurgery* 1991; 37: 291-302.

37. Tator CH, Koyanagi I. Vascular mechanisms in the pathophysiology of human spinal cord injury. *J Neurosurg* 1997; 86: 483-92.

38. Agrawal SK, Fehlings MG. Mechanisms of secondary injury to spinal cord axons *in vitro*: role of Na+, Na+-K+-ATPase, the Na+-H+ exchanger and the Na+-Ca2+ exchanger. *J Neurosci* 1996; 16: 545-52.

39. Young W, Koreh I. Potassium and calcium changes in injured spinal cords. *Brain Res* 1986; 365: 42-53.

40. Demopoulos HB, Flamm ES, Pietronigro DD, *et al*. The free radical pathology and the microcirculation in the major central nervous system disorders. *Acta Physiol Scand Suppl* 1980; 492: 91-119.

41. Hall ED, Yonkers PA, Horan KL, *et al*. Correlation between attenuation of posttraumatic spinal cord ischemia and preservation of tissue vitamin E by the 21-aminosteroid U74006F: evidence for an *in vivo* antioxidant mechanism. *J Neurotrauma* 1989; 6: 169-76.

42. Hung TK, Albin MS, Brown TD, *et al*. Biomechanical responses to open experimental spinal cord injury. *Surg Neurol* 1975; 4: 271-6.

43. Faden AI, Jacobs TP, Holaday JW. Comparison of early and late naloxone treatment in experimental spinal injury. *Neurology* 1982; 32: 677-81.

44. Faden AI, Jacobs TP, Smith MT. Evaluation of calcium channel antagonist nimodipine in experimental spinal cord ischemia. *J Neurosurg* 1984; 60: 796-9.

45. Osterholm JL, Mathews GJ. Altered norepinephrine metabolism, following experimental spinal cord injury: 2. Protection against traumatic spinal cord hemorrhagic necrosis by norepinephrine synthesis blockade with alpha methyl tyrosine. *J Neurosurg* 1972; 36: 395-401.

46. Wagner FC Jr, Stewart WB. Effect of trauma dose on spinal cord edema. *J Neurosurg* 1981; 54: 802-6.

47. Anderson DK, Means ED, Waters TR, *et al*. Spinal cord energy metabolism following compression trauma to the feline spinal cord. *J Neurosurg* 1980; 53: 375-80.

48. Casha S, Yu WR, Fehlings MG. Oligodendroglial apoptosis occurs along degenerating axons and is associated with FAS and P75 expression following spinal cord injury. *Neuroscience* 2001; 103: 203-18.

49. De la Torre JC. Spinal cord injury: review of basic and applied research. *Spine* 1981; 6: 315-35.

50. Lou J, Lenke LG, Ludwig FJ, *et al*. Apoptosis as a mechanism of neuronal cell death following acute experimental spinal cord injury. *Spinal Cord* 1998; 36: 683-90.

51. Lu J, Ashwell KWS, Waite P. Advances in secondary spinal cord injury: role of apoptosis. *Spine* 2000; 25: 1859-66.

52. Nockels RP. Non-operative management of acute spinal cord injury. *Spine* 2001; 26 (Suppl): S31-S37.

53. Proctor MR. Spinal cord injury. *Critical Care Medicine* 2002; 30 (Suppl): S489-S499.

54. Marshall LF, Knowlton S, Garfin SR, *et al*. Deterioration following spinal cord injury. *J Neurosurg* 1987; 66: 400-4.

55. Lorenzo RE. A review of spinal immobilisation techniques. *J Emerg Med* 1996; 14: 603-13.

56. Jackson AB, Groomes TE. Incidence of respiratory complications following spinal cord injury. *Arch Phys Med Rehabil* 1994; 75: 270-5.

57. Lam A. Spinal cord injury: management. *Curr Opin Anesth* 1992; 5: 632-9.

58. Lam AM. Acute spinal cord injury: monitoring and anaesthetic implications. *Can J Anaesth* 1991; 38: 60-73.

59. Schwenker D. Cardiovascular considerations in the critical care phase. *Crit Care Nurs Clin North Am* 1990; 2: 363-7.

60. Walleck CA. Neurologic considerations in the critical care phase. *Crit Care Nurs Clin North Am* 1990; 2: 357-61.

61. Leis AA, Kronenberg MF, Stetkarova I, *et al*. Spinal motoneuron excitability after acute spinal cord injury in humans. *Neurology* 1996; 47: 231-7.

62. Stauffer ES. Neurologic recovery following injuries to the cervical spinal cord and nerve roots. *Spine* 1984; 9: 532-4.

63. Gerner HJ. *Die Querschnittlähmung*. Berlin: Blackwell Wissenschaft, 1992.

64. Ko HY, Ditunno JF Jr, Graziani V, *et al*. The pattern of reflex recovery during spinal shock. *Spinal Cord* 1999; 37: 402-9.

65. Bracken, Michael B. PhD summary statement: the Sygen(R) (GM-1 Ganglioside) clinical trial in acute spinal cord injury. *Spine* 2001; 26 (Suppl): S99-S100.

66. Behrmann DL, Bresnahan JC, Beattie MS. Modeling of acute spinal cord injury in the rat: neuroprotection and enhanced recovery with methylprednisolone, U-74006F and YM-14673. *Exp Neurol* 1994; 126: 61-75.

67. Bracken MB, Collins WF, Freeman DF, *et al*. Efficacy of methylprednisolone in acute spinal cord injury. *JAMA* 1984; 251: 45-52.

68. Bracken MB, Shepard MJ, Hellenbrand KG, *et al*. Methylprednisolone and neurological function 1 year after spinal cord injury: results of the National Acute Spinal Cord Injury Study. *J Neurosurg* 1985; 63: 704-13.

69. Bracken MB, Shephard MJ, Collins WF, *et al*. A randomized, controlled trial of methylprednisolone or naloxone in the treatment of acute spinal-cord injury: results of the Second National Acute Spinal Cord Injury Study. *N Engl J Med* 1990; 322: 1405-11.

70. Bracken MB, Shephard MJ, Holford TR, *et al*. Methylprednisolone or naloxone treatment after acute spinal cord injury: 1-year follow-up data. Results of the Second National Acute Spinal Cord Injury Study. *J Neurosurg* 1992; 76: 23-31.

71. Bracken MB, Shephard MJ, Holford TR, *et al*. Administration of methylprednisolone for 24 or 48 hours or tirilazad mesylate for 48 hours in the treatment of acute spinal cord injury: results of the Third National Acute Spinal Cord Injury Randomized Controlled Trial. National Acute Spinal Cord Injury Study. *JAMA* 1997; 277: 1597-604.

72. Bracken MB, Shephard MJ, Holford TR, *et al*. Methylprednisolone or tirilazad mesylate administration after acute spinal cord injury: 1-year follow up. Results of the Third National Acute Spinal Cord Injury randomized controlled trial. *J Neurosurg* 1998; 89: 699-706.

73. Nesathurai S. Steroids, spinal cord injury: revisiting the NASCIS 2 and NASCIS 3 trials. *J Trauma* 1998; 45: 1088-93.

74. Bracken MB, Aldrich EF, Herr DL, *et al*. Clinical measurement, statistical analysis, and risk-benefit: controversies from trials of spinal injury. *J Trauma* 2000; 48: 558-61.

75. Short D, El Masry WS, Jones PW. High dose methylprednisolone in the management of acute spinal cord injury - a systematic review from a clinical perspective. *Spinal Cord* 2000; 38: 273-86.

76. Hurlbert RJ. Methylprednisolone for acute spinal cord injury: an inappropriate standard of care. *J Neurosurg* (Spine 1) 2000; 93: 1-7.

77. Jinks SL, Dominguez CL, Antogini JF. High-dose methylprednisolone may cause myopathy in acute spinal cord injury patients. *Spinal Cord* 2005; 43: 199-203.

78. Cohn SM, Lyle WG, Linden CH, *et al.* Exclusion of cervical spine injury: a prospective study. *J Trauma* 1991; 31: 570-4.

79. Gehweiler JA Jr, Clark WM, Schaaf RE, *et al.* Cervical spine trauma: the common combined conditions. *Radiology* 1979; 130: 77-86.

80. MacDonald RL, Schwartz ML, Mirich D, *et al.* Diagnosis of cervical spine injury in motor vehicle crash victims: how many X-rays are enough? *J Trauma* 1990; 30: 392-7.

81. Ross SE, Schwab CW, David ET, *et al.* Clearing the cervical spine: initial radiologic evaluation. *J Trauma* 1987; 27: 1055-60.

82. Scher AT. Cervical spinal cord injury without evidence of fracture or dislocation: an assessment of the radiological features. *S Afr Med J* 1976; 50: 962-5.

83. Brown CV, Antevil JL, Sise MJ, *et al.* Spiral computed tomography for the diagnosis of cervical, thoracic, and lumbar spine fractures: its time has come. *J Trauma* 2005; 58: 890-5 and discussion 895-6.

84. Schenker C. In: *Querschnittslaehmung-ganzheitliche Rehabilitation: Akute Rueckenmarkssymptomatik: CT oder MRI?* Zäch G, Ed. Küsnacht, Switzerland: Verlag Dr Felix Würst AG, 1995: 25-9.

85. Fehlings MG, Rao SC, Tator CH, *et al.* The optimal radiologic method for assessing spinal canal compromise, cord compression in patients with cervical spinal cord injury. *Spine* 1999; 24: 605-13.

86. Grunhagen J, Egbers HJ, Heller M, *et al.* Comparison of spine injuries by means of CT and MRI according to the classification of Magerl. *Rofo* 2005; 177: 828-34.

87. Hirsch LF Intracranial aneurysm and hemorrhage following skull caliper traction. Review of skull traction complications. *Spine* 1979; 43: 206-8.

88. Reiss SJ, Raque GH Jr, Shields CB. Cervical spine fractures with major associated trauma. *Neurosurgery* 1986; 18: 327-30.

89. Gruenberg MF, Rechtine GR, Chrin AM, *et al.* Overdistraction of cervical spine injuries with the use of skull traction: a report of two cases. *J Trauma* 1997; 42: 1152-6.

90. Manthey DE. Halo traction device. *Emerg Med Clin North Am* 1994; 12: 771-8.

91. Choo JH, Liu WY, Kumar VP. Complications from the Gardner-Wells tongs. *Injury* 1996; 27: 512-3.

92. Cotler JM, Herbison GJ, Nasuti JF, *et al.* Closed reduction of traumatic cervical spine dislocation using traction weights up to 140 pounds. *Spine* 1993; 18: 386-90.

93. Louis R, Maresca C, Bel P. Réduction orthopédique contrôlée des fractures du rachis. *Rev Chir Orth* 1977; 63: 449-51.

94. Louis R. Les théories de l' instabilité. *Rev Chir Orth* 1979; 63: 423-5.

95. Tropiano P, Huang RC, Louis CA, *et al.* Functional and radiographic outcome of thoracolumbar and lumbar burst fractures managed by closed orthopaedic reduction and casting. *Spine* 2003; 28: 2459-65.

96. Guttmann Sir L. *Spinal cord injuries: comprehensive management and research,* 2nd ed. London: Blackwell Scientific Publishers, 1976.

97. Meinecke FW. Geschichte der Behandlung Querschnittsgelaehmter in der Bundesrepublik Deutschland. *Unfallchirurg* 1988; 14: 64-73.

98. Bötel U. In: *Querschnitt im Laengsschnitt; Erstversorgung-Lebenslange Betreuung: Operative Stabilisierung der verletzten Wirbelsauele bei Ruekenmarkschaedigung.* Zäch GA, Gmünder HP, Koch HG, Eds. Nottwill, Switzerland: Schweizer Paraplegiker Zentrum, 1999: 17-25.

99. Harrington PR. Instrumentation in spine instability other than scoliosis. *S Afr J Surg* 1967; 5: 7-12.

100. Robinson RA, Smith GW. Anterolateral cervical disc removal and interbody fusion for cervical disc syndrome. *Bull Johns Hopkins Hosp* 1955; 96: 223-4.

101. Cloward RB. Treatment of acute fractures and fracture-dislocation of the cervical spine by vertebral body fusion. *J Neurosurg* 1969; 16: 201-9.

102. Magerl F, Worsdorfer O. Long-term results of spondylodeses in the lumbar region. 10-year results of lumbar interbody spondylodeses. *Orthopäde* 1979; 8: 192-203.

103. Bötel U. Die Behandlung der Verrenkungsbrueche der Brust- und Lendenwirbelsaeule mit der Weiss-Feder und ihre Modifikationen. *Hefte zur Unfallheilkunde* 1980; 149: 182-89.

104. Böhler J. Schraubenosteosynthese von Frakturen der Dens Axis. *Unfallheilkunde* 1981; 84: 221-3.

105. Magerl F. Stabilisierung der unteren Brust- und Lendenwirbelsaeule mit dem Fixateur externe. *Acta Chir Austria Suppl* 1982; 43: 78-85.

106. Luque ER, Cassis N, Ramirez-Wiella G. Segmental spinal instrumentation in the treatment of fractures of the thoracolumbar spine. *Spine* 1982; 7: 312-9.

107. Kostuik JP. Anterior spinal cord decompression for lesions of the thoracic and lumbar spine. Techniques, new methods of internal fixation, results. *Spine* 1983; 8: 512-31.

108. Dick W. *Aktuelle Probleme in Chirurgie und Orthopaedie: Innere Fixation von Brust - und Lendenwirbelfrakturen.* Huber, Bern: Band 28, 1984.

109. Cotrel Y, Dubousset J, Guillaumat M. New universal instrumentation in spinal surgery. *Clin Orth* 1984; 227: 10-23.

110. Kaneda K, Abumi K, Fujiya M. Burst fractures with neurologic deficits of the thoracolumbar spine. Results of anterior decompression and stabilisation with anterior instrumentation. *Spine* 1984; 9: 788-95.

111. Daniaux H. Transpedikulaere Reposition und Spongiosaplastik bei Wirbelkörperbrüchen der unteren Brust- und Lendenwirbelsaeule. *Unfallchirurg* 1986; 197-213.

112. Kluger P, Gerner HJ. Das mechanische Prinzip des Fixateur interne zur dorsalen Stabilisierung der Brust- und Lendenwirbelsaeule. *Unfallchirurg* 1986; 12: 68-79.

113. Morsher E, Sutter F, Jenny H, *et al.* Die vordere Verplattung der Halswirbelsaeule mit dem Hohlschrauben-Plattensystem aus Titanium. *Chirurg* 1986; 57: 702-7.

114. Müller M, Allgöwer M, Schneider R, Willenegger H. *Manual of Internal Fixation.* Berlin, Heidelberg, New-York, Tokyo: Springer, 1991.

Chapter 5

115. Jeanneret B, Magerl F. Primary posterior fusion C1/2 in odontoid fractures: indications, technique, and results of transarticular screw fixation. *J Spinal Disord* 1992; 5: 464-75.

116. Verheggen R, Jansen J. Hangman's fracture: arguments in favor of surgical therapy for type II and III according to Edwards and Levine. *Surg Neurol* 1998; 49: 253-61 and discussion 261-2.

117. Richter M, Mattes T, Cakir B. Computer-assisted posterior instrumentation of the cervical and cervico-thoracic spine. *Eur Spine J* 2004; 13: 50-9.

118. Donovan WH, Carter RE, Bedbrook GM, *et al*. Incidence of medical complications in spinal cord injury: patients in specialised, compared with non-specialised centres. *Paraplegia* 1984; 22: 282-92.

119. Jacobs R MD, Asher M, Snider R. Thoracolumbar spinal injuries. A comparative study of recumbent and operative treatment 100 patients. *Spine* 1980; 5: 463-77.

120. Roy-Camille R, Saillant G, Massin P. Traitement des fractures du rachis dorso-lombaire par la méthode de Boëhler. *Rev Chirurg Orth* 1989; 75: 479-89.

121. Domenicucci M, Preite R, Ramieri A, *et al*. Thoracolumbar fractures without neurological involvement: surgical or conservative treatment? *J Neurosurg Sci* 1996; 40: 1-10.

122. Seybold EA, Sweeny CA, Fredrickson BE, *et al*. Functional outcome of low lumbar burst fractures. A multicenter review of operative and nonoperative treatment from L3-L5. *Spine* 1999; 15: 2154-61.

123. Denis F, Armstrong GW, Searls K, *et al*. Acute thoraco-lumbar burst fractures in the absence of neurologic deficit. A comparison between operative and nonoperative treatment. *Clin Orthop* 1984; 189: 142-9.

124. Fehlings MG, Sekhon LHS, Tator C. The role and timing of decompression in acute spinal cord injury: what do we know? What should we do? *Spine* 2001; 26 (Suppl): S101-S110.

125. Böhler L. *Die Technik der Knochenbruchbehandlung.* Vienna, Austria: Maudrich (13. Auflage), 1951.

126. Bedbrook GM. A balanced viewpoint in the early management of patients with spinal injuries who have neurological damage. *Paraplegia* 1985; 23: 8-15.

127. Weinstein JN, Collalto P, Lehmann TR. Thoracolumbar 'burst' fractures treated conservatively: a long-term follow-up. *Spine* 1988; 13: 33-8.

128. Katoh S, El Masry WS, Jaffray D, *et al*. Neurologic outcome in conservatively treated patients with incomplete closed traumatic cervical spinal cord injuries. *Spine* 1996; 21: 2345-51.

129. El Masry WS, Short DJ. Current concepts: spinal injuries and rehabilitation. *Curr Opin Neurol* 1997; 10: 484-92.

130. Kluger P. Good practice in the treatment of acute traumatic spinal cord injury - timing and methods for surgical treatment of the vertebral injury. Internetforum for spine. http://www.ulrich-ulm.de/eng/forum/index.html, 2003.

131. Farcy JP, Veidenbaum M, Glassman S. Sagittal index in management of thoracolumbar burst fractures. *Spine* 1990; 15: 958-65.

132. Oda I, Cunningham BW, Buckley RA, *et al*. Does spinal kyphotic deformity influence the biomechanical characteristics of the adjacent motion segment? An *in vivo* model study. *Spine* 1999; 24: 2139-46.

133. Whiteneck G, Adler C, Carter RE, *et al. The management of high quadriplegia.* New York: Demos Publications, 1989.

134. Fromm B, Hundt G, Gerner HJ, *et al*. Management of respiratory problems unique to high tetraplegia. *Spinal Cord* 1999; 37: 239-44.

135. Bach JR. Alternative methods of ventilatory support for the patient with ventilatory failure due to spinal cord injury. *J Am Paraplegia Soc* 1991; 14: 158-74.

136. Marchant WA, Fox R. Postoperative use of a cough-assist device in avoiding prolonged intubation. *Br J Anaesth* 2002; 89: 644-7.

137. Viroslav J, Rosenblatt R, Tomazevic SM. Respiratory management, survival, and quality of life for high-level traumatic tetraplegics. *Respir Care Clin N Am* 1996; 2: 313-22.

138. Harrop JS, Sharan AD, Scheid EH, *et al*. Tracheostomy placement in patients with complete cervical spinal cord injuries: American Spinal Injury Association Grade A. *J Neurosurg* 2004; 100(Suppl Spine): S20-S23.

139. Nothrup BE. Occurrence of infection in anterior cervical fusion for spinal cord injury after tracheostomy. *Spine* 1995; 20: 2449-53.

140. Tran NV, Vernick J, Cotler JM, *et al*. Lateral tracheostomy in patients with cervical spinal cord injury. *Br J Surg* 1995; 82: 412-3.

141. Illman A, Stiller K, Williams M. The prevalence of orthostatic hypotension during physiotherapy treatment in patients with an acute spinal cord injury. *Spinal Cord* 2000; 38: 741-7.

142. Cariga P, Ahmed S, Mathias CJ, *et al*. The prevalence and association of neck (coat-hanger) pain and orthostatic (postural) hypotension in human spinal cord injury. *Spinal Cord* 2002; 40: 77-82.

143. Bravo G, Guziar-Sahagun G, Ibarra A, *et al*. Cardiovascular alterations after spinal cord injury: an overview. *Curr Med Chem Cardiovasc Hematol Agents* 2004; 2: 133-48.

144. Teasell RW, Arnold JM, Krassioukov A, *et al*. Cardiovascular consequences of loss of supraspinal control of the sympathetic nervous system after spinal cord injury. *Arch Phys Med Rehabil* 2000; 81: 506-16.

145. Jacob C, Thwaini A, Rao A, *et al*. Autonomic dysreflexia: the forgotten medical emergency. *Hosp Med* 2005; 66: 294-6.

146. Sullivan-Tevault M. Autonomic dysreflexia in spinal cord injury. *Emerg Med Serv* 2005; 34: 79-80.

147. Green D, Hartwig D, Chen D, *et al*. Spinal Cord Injury Risk Assessment for Thromboembolism (SPIRATE Study). *Am J Phys Med Rehabil* 2003; 82: 950-6.

148. Ash D. An exploration of the occurrence of pressure ulcers in a British spinal injuries unit. *J Clin Nurs* 2002; 11: 470-8.

149. Stöhrer M, Castro-Diaz E, Chartier-Kastler E, *et al*. Guidelines on neurogenic lower unrinary tract dysfunction. European Association of Urology. http://www.uroweb.org/files/uploaded_files/guidelines/neurogenic.pdf, 2003.

150. Stöhrer M. *Manual neuro-urology and spinal cord lesion guidelines for urological care of spinal cord injury patients.* Burgdoerfer H, Heidler H, Madersbacher H, Palmtag H,

Chapter 5

Sauerwein D, Stoehrer M, Eds. 3rd revised edition. Murnau: Arbeitskkreis Urologische Rehabilitation, 2002.

151. Reitz A, Stöhrer M, Kramer G, *et al.* European experience of 200 cases treated with botulinum-A toxin injections into the detrusor muscle for urinary incontinence due to neurogenic detrusor overactivity. *Eur Urol* 2004; 45: 510-5.

152. Singh RS, Craig MC, Katholi CR, *et al.* The predictive value of creatine phosphokinase and alkaline phosphatase in identification of heterotopic ossification in patients after spinal cord injury. *Arch Phys Med Rehabil* 2003; 84: 1584-8.

153. Banovac K, Sherman AL, Estores IM, *et al.* Prevention and treatment of heterotopic ossification after spinal cord injury. *J Spinal Cord Med* 2004; 27: 376-82.

154. Meiners T, Abel R, Bohm V, Gerner HJ. Resection of heterotopic ossification of the hip in spinal cord injured patients. *Spinal Cord* 1997; 35: 443-5.

155. Maier D. Heterotopic ossification after acute spinal cord injury: early diagnosis and therapy. *Orthopäde* 2005; 34: 120-7.

156. Kesiktas N, Paker N, Erdogan N, *et al.* The use of hydrotherapy for the management of spasticity. *Neurorehabil Neural Repair* 2004; 18: 268-73.

157. Dario A, Tomei G. A benefit-risk assessment of baclofen in severe spinal spasticity. *Drug Saf* 2004; 27: 799-818.

158. Boviatsis EJ, Kouyialis AT, Korfias S, *et al.* Functional outcome of intrathecal baclofen administration for severe spasticity. *Clin Neurol Neurosurg* 2005; 107: 289-95.

Chapter 5

Chapter 6

Total disc replacement in the lumbar spine

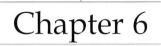

Brian Freeman DM FRCS (Tr & Orth)

Consultant Spinal Surgeon

James Davenport MRCS (Eng)

Clinical Research Fellow

UNIVERSITY HOSPITAL, QUEEN'S MEDICAL CENTRE, NOTTINGHAM, UK

Introduction

The management of discogenic low back pain remains controversial: its accurate diagnosis is difficult and relies on magnetic resonance imaging (MRI) and provocative lumbar discography. Möller *et al* compared posterolateral spinal fusion to an exercise programme for patients with isthmic spondylolisthesis in a randomised controlled trial [1]. The authors showed the functional outcome assessed by the disability rating index and pain reduction was better in the surgically treated group when compared to the exercise group. Fritzell *et al* reported on a randomised controlled multicentre study with two-year follow-up for patients with degenerative disc disease [2]. The authors concluded that lumbar fusion in a well informed and selected group of patients with severe chronic low back pain can diminish pain and decrease disability more efficiently than commonly used non-surgical treatment. These two papers **(Ib/A)** currently place spinal fusion as the gold standard for the treatment of spondylolisthesis and degenerative disc disease. It is this gold standard that total disc replacement should be measured against.

Motion preservation is an intuitively attractive alternative to spinal fusion, theoretically preventing adjacent segment degeneration. However, the long-term stability, endurance and strength of the prostheses are unknown for the majority of implants. Significant facet joint osteoarthritis is a contraindication to the procedure; however, it is difficult to identify this in its early stages. The use of total disc replacement may be limited to the treatment of early degenerative disc disease with preservation of disc height, thereby limiting its use to a minority of patients. Furthermore, the fate of facet joints after a prosthetic disc replacement is unknown and facet joint hypertrophy, which accelerates spinal stenosis, may be a potent long-term complication of motion preservation. Revision procedures will be difficult with a heightened risk of vascular injury, particularly at the L4/5 level. There are numerous types of disc prosthesis either available or in development and well-designed, prospective randomised controlled trials are needed before approval and widespread application. The long-term benefits and complications of total disc replacement may not be known for many years.

Methodology

In order to establish what body of evidence exists to support the use of disc replacement, we conducted a broad search of the literature. As we anticipated the number of prospective, randomised controlled trials (RCTs) to be small, we included relevant retrospective and prospective cohort studies (non-randomised) to increase the yield of information for 'best evidence synthesis'.

Search strategy

The literature was searched using some of the most commonly used medical databases:

- the Cochrane database (to July 2005);
- Medline (1996 to July 2005);
- Embase (1996 to July 2005);
- Cinahl (1982 to July 2005);
- Pubmed (to July 2005).

The same search strings were used for each database, albeit with small modifications for the Cochrane database and Pubmed to take into account differences between search engines. The search strings included the terms (as MeSH headings): 'lumbar disc replacement', 'intervertebral disc', 'disc degeneration', 'joint prosthesis', 'arthroplasty' and 'randomised controlled trials'. These were used individually and as part of complex search terms to give the most relevant results. Thesaurus mapping was used, given the variations of spelling of key terms.

Pubmed produced 125 hits whilst Embase, Cinahl and Medline, using the same search strategy produced 84, 17 and 19 hits respectively. The Cochrane database revealed ten randomised controlled trials; however, this included the guidelines issued by the National Institute for Clinical Excellence (NICE) and several interim results from the larger multicentre trials.

Breaking these down by type and eliminating duplicate studies, the following list was produced:

- randomised controlled trials - two [15-19, 21-25];
- systematic reviews - one [13];
- non-randomised comparative studies - none;
- prospective cohort studies - six [8-12, 29];
- retrospective cohort studies - eight [3-7, 27, 28, 30].

Retrospective cohort studies (III/B)

Cinotti *et al* reported on a retrospective review of 46 patients undergoing artificial disc replacement with a Charité SB III disc prosthesis (DePuy Spine, Raynham, MA) with a mean follow-up of 3.2 years (range 2-5 years) (Figure 1) [3]. Twenty-two patients had degenerative disc disease; 24 patients were post-lumbar discectomy. Thirty-six patients were operated at a single level, ten patients were operated at two levels.

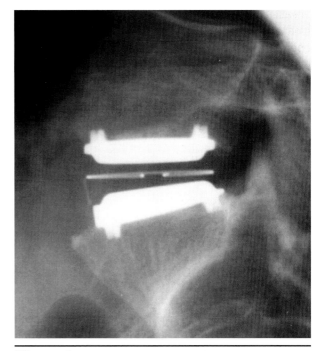

Figure 1. Lateral radiograph of a Charité lumbar disc replacement L5/S1.

Sixty-three percent of patients reported satisfactory results overall. The success rate rose to 69% for patients undergoing single-level disc replacement, but dropped to 40% for those having surgery at two levels. For those patients who had had previous back surgery, 50% reported satisfactory results. For those patients who had not undergone previous back surgery, satisfactory results were obtained in 77%. Four of six patients who were involved in workers' compensation had unsatisfactory outcomes. Seven patients who had unsatisfactory results went on to have a posterolateral instrumented fusion without removal of the artificial disc. Three of these seven patients reported satisfactory results. A further two patients underwent removal of the prosthesis and circumferential fusion. There was no evidence of implant failure, loosening or polyethylene wear. Four patients developed spontaneous fusion at the operated level. The vertebral motion averaged 9° (range 0-15°) at the operated level and 16° (range 10-21°) at adjacent levels.

Van Ooij et al reported on 27 patients presenting to their institution over an eight-year period with unsatisfactory results or complications following SB Charité disc replacement [4]. These patients had been operated on at a different institution. There was no information given regarding the total number of patients undergoing total disc replacement over that period, the report being confined to the 27 patients presenting with complications. There were 15 women and 12 men; the mean age was 40 (range 30-67 years). Four patients had their implant removed and a total of 11 patients required a second spinal reconstructive salvage procedure. Implant-related complications included anterior subluxation of the prosthesis in two cases, subsidence of the prosthesis in 16 cases and polyethylene wear in one patient. There were two approach-related complications: abdominal wall haematoma and retrograde ejaculation. Further problems arose from disc degeneration at other lumbar discs and facet joint arthrosis at the same or other levels. The authors expressed concern regarding the survivorship of the SB Charité disc prosthesis, expecting that many more patients would be seen with late problems.

Huang et al studied the prevalence of contraindications to total disc replacement in a cohort of lumbar surgical patients [5]. The authors reviewed 100 consecutive patients who had lumbar surgery carried out by one surgeon in 2002. The procedures performed and the contraindications to total disc replacement were recorded. Contraindications to total disc replacement included: central or lateral recess stenosis, facet joint arthrosis, spondylolysis or spondylolisthesis, herniated nucleus pulposus with radiculopathy, scoliosis, osteoporosis, post-surgical pseudarthrosis and deficiency of the posterior elements. Patients were divided into fusion or non-fusion groups and the percentage of patients without

contraindications to total disc replacement was calculated. From 100 patients, 56 underwent spinal fusion and 44 underwent non-fusion surgery. In the fusion group, 56 of 56 patients had contraindications to total disc replacement. In the non-fusion group, 11% (5/44) were considered candidates for total disc replacement. Overall, 5% of patients in this selected series were candidates for total disc replacement. The average number of contraindications to total disc replacement was 2.48 (range 0-5). Predictions that total disc replacement will replace fusion would appear premature.

Tropiano et al reported on 64 patients undergoing lumbar total disc replacement with the Pro-Disc (Synthes Inc., Paoli, PA) (Figure 2) in a retrospective study [6]. Sixty-four patients had a single or multi-level implantation of a total disc replacement between 1990 and 1993 performed by one surgeon. The mean duration of follow-up was 8.7 years. The authors reported significant improvements in back pain, radiculopathy, disability and modified Stauffer-Coventry scores. Fifty-five patients were available for follow-up (86%), 33 had an excellent result, eight had a good result and 14 had a poor result. The authors found gender and multi-level surgery did not appear to affect the outcomes. Radiographs showed no evidence of loosening, migration or mechanical failure. There were five approach-related complications, including one deep venous thrombosis, one iliac vein laceration, one transient retrograde ejaculation and two incisional hernias. The study has limitations in that it was retrospective and did not use validated outcome measures. Nevertheless, the authors concluded that the data indicated that the prosthesis was safe with a low rate of complications.

Huang et al attempted to correlate a range of motion and clinical outcome after lumbar total disc replacement [7]. This was a retrospective review of 38 patients undergoing one or two-level total disc replacement with the Pro-Disc I implant (part of the same cohort previously described by Tropiano et al [6]). The flexion / extension range of motion was measured on lateral radiographs; the mean range of motion was 4.0° + or - 3.9° (range 0-18°). The clinical outcome was measured at a mean of 8.6 years (range 6.9-10.7 years) by the modified Stauffer-Coventry scores, Oswestry Disability Questionnaire, subjective rating of

Chapter 6

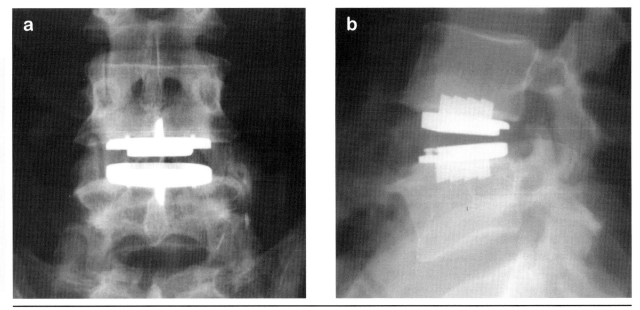

Figure 2. a) **Anteroposterior radiograph of a ProDisc lumbar disc replacement L4/5. b) Lateral radiograph of a ProDisc lumbar disc replacement L4/5.**

back pain, leg pain and disability. Spearman correlation revealed a weak to moderate, but statistically significant, association between the range of motion and outcome for back pain, Oswestry Disability Questionnaire and modified Stauffer-Coventry scores. Patients with motion of more than 5° had superior outcomes in the Oswestry Disability Questionnaire (mean difference 12.6 points) and Stauffer-Coventry scores (mean difference 2.2 points). Although differences were statistically significant, they were clinically modest.

Prospective cohort studies (IIa & b/B)

Mayer *et al* reported the preliminary results of the first 34 consecutive patients treated with the Pro-Disc total disc replacement [8]. The indications included degenerative disc disease (61.8%), degenerative disc disease plus disc herniation (11.8%), post-discectomy (14.7%), adjacent level degeneration (8.8%) and degeneration following nuclear replacement (2.9%). Of the 34 patients, 26 (76.5%) had attended at least one follow-up visit for evaluation. The average follow-up was very short at 5.8 months. The mean Visual Analogue Score (VAS) for low back pain dropped from 6.3 points

to 2.4 points and the mean Oswestry Disability Index (ODI) dropped from 19.1 points to 11.5 points. Three patients suffered complications, including an anterior dislocation of the polyethylene inlay, one L5 nerve root irritation and one retrograde ejaculation.

Bertagnoli and Kumar reported on 108 patients undergoing total disc replacement with the Pro-Disc II implant [9]. Ninety-four patients underwent total disc replacement at one level, 12 patients at two levels and two patients at three levels. The range of follow-up varied from three months to two years with 54 patients having more than one-year follow-up. The ODI, VAS and Short-Form 36 questionnaire was used for clinical evaluation; however, in the results section these figures were not available. The authors categorise their results into excellent, good, fair and poor, stating that 90.8% of patients achieved an excellent result, 7.4% a good result, 1.8% a fair result and no patients with a poor result. However, the method of categorisation is not discussed. The authors stated that ten of the 108 patients had progression of disc degeneration at an adjacent level following surgery. There were no implant failures and the average range of motion at L5-S1 was 9° (range 2-13°) and at L4-5 was 10° (range 8-15°).

Tropiano *et al* reported on the preliminary results with Pro-Disc II lumbar disc replacement in 53 patients [10]. Forty patients underwent total disc replacement at one level, 11 patients at two levels and two patients at three levels. The mean follow-up was 1.4 years (range 1-2 years). The indications included degenerative disc disease in 33 patients and failed spine surgery in 20 patients. The mean VAS for back pain improved from 7.4 to 1.3 at final follow-up, the mean VAS for leg pain improved from 6.7 to 1.9 and the mean ODI improved from 56 points to 14 points. There was no implant failure or loosening. There was no significant difference in the clinical outcome between the single or multi-level groups. Satisfactory clinical results were obtained in 90% of patients who had had previous lumbar surgery. Complications occurred in five patients (9%) and included a vertebral body fracture in one, transient radicular pain in two, and an implant malposition in two. One patient complained of transient retrograde ejaculation. Three of 53 patients required re-operation. At L5-S1, the flexion / extension range of motion averaged 8° (range 2-12°) at the operated level. In patients who had an implantation at L4-5 the range of motion averaged 10° (8-18°). The mean lumbar lordosis was 56.7° before surgery (range 30-72°) and 61.9° at final follow-up

(range 46-72°). The authors concluded that the results obtained with Pro-Disc II were satisfactory in over 90% of patients.

Fraser *et al* prospectively evaluated the AcroFlex total disc replacement (DePuy Acromed, Raynham, MA)(Figure 3) [11]. This implant differs from the low friction devices such as the Charité and the Pro-Disc in that it uses an elastomer to replicate the elasticity of the normal human intervertebral disc. The AcroFlex prosthesis consists of two titanium endplates bound together by a hexane-based polyolefin rubber core. A pilot study was carried out on 28 patients suffering from one or two-level symptomatic disc degeneration proven on discography. Twenty-four procedures were carried out at a single level (19 at L5-S1 and five at L4-5), four were carried out as double procedures at L4-5 and L5-S1. For the whole group, the ODI improved from 49.3 to 34.4 at 24-month follow-up. The Low Back Outcome Score (LBOS) improved from 17.7 to 33 at 24-month follow-up and there was improvement in five of the eight subscales of the Short Form-36 general health questionnaire. Complications included: nerve root irritation in two, auto-fusion in one, partial anterior expulsion in one, minor anterior polyolefin tears in seven, large anterior polyolefin tears

Chapter 6

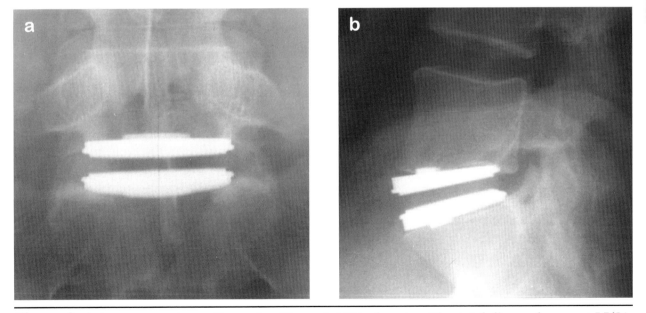

Figure 3. a) Anteroposterior radiograph with caudal tilt of an AcroFlex total disc replacement L5/S1. b) Lateral radiograph of an AcroFlex total disc replacement L5/S1.

in three, pulmonary embolus in one and retrograde ejaculation in one. Of particular concern was the demonstration on fine-cut computed tomography of rubber tears in 36% of patients. The majority were antero-inferior peripheral tears. Seven patients required revision between two and four years after disc replacement. In three cases, an anterior revision was performed with removal of the implant, insertion of an interbody fusion device and posterior supplementation with pedicle screws. In two of these three procedures, a tear to the left common iliac vein occurred which was difficult to repair. In the remaining four, the implant was left *in situ* and an instrumented posterolateral fusion was carried out. The discovery of the anterior disruption of the rubber with associated osteolysis led to cessation of the trial and the withdrawal of the AcroFlex total disc replacement from the market. This study illustrates the need for long-term follow-up of all implants in this class.

Le Huec *et al* reported the two-year clinical results of the Maverick (Medtronic Sofamor Danek, Memphis, TN) lumbar total disc replacement [12]. Sixty-four Maverick devices were implanted between January 2002 and November 2003. The authors noted a degree of improvement equivalent to that obtained with anterior fusion cages, using a minimally invasive technique. The ODI improved for 75% of patients.

Systematic review of the literature (IIa & b/B and III/B)

Marinus de Kleuver *et al* conducted a systematic review of the literature pertaining to total disc replacement for chronic low back pain [13]. The authors employed a 'best evidence synthesis' technique, stratifying each study according to the level of evidence. De Kleuver (2003) searched the Cochrane database (2001-2004), MEDLINE (1966-2002) and CINAHL (1982-2001). Studies were ranked from strong to weak according to Shekelle in the following order: randomised controlled trials, other controlled trials and non-experimental studies (cohort studies, cross-sectional studies) [14]. The search resulted in 430 references of which nine articles were found to be relevant and fully evaluated. There were no controlled trials comparing intervertebral disc replacement with

arthrodesis. The nine articles consisted of six retrospective cohort studies, one cross-sectional study and two prospective cohort studies. Eight studies involved the Charité total disc replacement and one study involved the AcroFlex total disc replacement. A total of 411 patients were represented in these nine articles. The follow-up was generally short with a mean of 28 months. There was a high rate of secondary arthrodesis observed across all studies. The short-term results (one to 68 months) appeared to be comparable to the results of arthrodesis; however, the authors stated that only a very limited number of articles concerning total disc replacement were available. All were non-controlled case series with many methodological flaws. Few of the papers commented on radiological results such as loosening, subsidence, polyethylene wear, maintenance of motion and adjacent level disc degeneration. Finally, the authors concluded that despite almost 15 years of clinical application, there are insufficient data to assess the performance of total disc replacement adequately and that total disc replacement should still be considered an experimental procedure.

Randomised controlled trials (Ia & b/A)

There are now two randomised controlled trials (RCTs) comparing total disc replacement with spinal fusion. The first of these involves the Charité artificial disc [15] and the second involves the ProDisc II total disc replacement [16].

The Food and Drug Administration investigational device exemption multicentre trial of the Charité artificial disc involved 14 centres across the USA [15]. A single participating centre published its early results in two journals [17, 18]. The inclusion criteria for the multicentre study, reported by Geisler *et al,* listed single-level symptomatic degenerative disc disease either at L4-5 or L5-S1 [15]. Patients were aged between 18 and 60 years of age. The ODI on entry was greater or equal to 30. The VAS for low back pain was greater or equal to 40 points (on a 100-point scale). All patients had failed conservative measures and had chronic low back pain for at least six months duration. The randomisation involved a 2:1 schedule in favour of the Charité disc. Two hundred and five patients were randomised to receive the Charité disc and 99 patients were randomised to receive the BAK cage as part of an anterior lumbar interbody fusion using iliac crest autograft. There were no significant intergroup differences at baseline. Neurological status was equivalent between the two groups at 6, 12 and 24 months postoperatively. Major neurological events occurred in ten (4.9%) of the Charité and four (4%) of the BAK fusion group. For the Charité group, the ODI improved from 50.6 pre-operatively to 25.8 at 24 months, an improvement of 24.8 points. For the BAK fusion group, the ODI improved from 52.1 to 30.1, an improvement of 22 points. The intergroup change in ODI was not significantly different at 12 or 24 months. The VAS improved from 72 points in the Charité group to 30.6 points at 24 months, an improvement of 41.4 points. For the BAK fusion group, the VAS improved from 71.8 points to 36.3 points, an improvement of 35.5 points. The flexion / extension range of motion in the Charité disc replacement group was a mean of 7.4 +/- 5.28° (mean +/- standard deviation) whereas in the BAK fusion group it was 1.1 +/- 0.87° (mean +/- standard deviation). The authors concluded the Charité intervertebral disc is safe and effective for the treatment of mechanical back pain caused by one-level degenerative disc disease either at L4/5 or L5/S1. The clinical outcomes at two years are equivalent to those resulting from a one-level anterior interbody fusion using the BAK cage.

Blumenthal *et al* reported further on the same cohort of 304 patients [19]. In this paper the criteria for success included all of the following: greater than 25% improvement in ODI at 24 months, no device failure, no major complications and no neurological deterioration. There was no difference observed between the two groups with respect to operative time, blood loss or level of implantation. The duration of hospital stay was significantly lower in the investigational group (mean of 3.7 days compared to a mean of 4.2 days for the fusion group, p=0.0039). At all follow-up time points, patients in both groups demonstrated significant improvements in ODI and VAS. One hundred and eighty-five patients from 205 patients in the investigational group were followed-up at 24-months, compared to 82 of 99 patients in the fusion group. At 24 months, the investigational group demonstrated a higher rate of satisfaction (73.7%),

compared to the control group (53.1% satisfaction, p=0.0011). All four criteria for clinical success were met in 57.1% of patients in the investigational group and 46.5% in the control group (p<0.0001). For those patients completing 24 months of follow-up the overall clinical success was reported at 63.6% in the investigational group compared to 56.8% in the control group (p=0.0004). Narcotic usage decreased in both groups at 24 months and there was a 9.2% improvement in employment in the investigational group compared to a 7.4% improvement in the control group. The authors conclude that the Charité artificial disc yielded clinical results equivalent to those obtained with anterior lumbar interbody fusion. Significant clinical improvements were observed in the early postoperative period and maintained through the 24-month follow-up period and there were no cases of catastrophic device failure. The Charité artificial disc would appear to be safe and effective for the treatment of single-level lumbar degenerative disc disease, either at L4/5 or L5/S1 as an alternative to fusion in properly indicated patients.

Mirza criticised the study for comparing total disc replacement to an operation that has largely been abandoned, because surgeons saw first-hand that it failed frequently [20]. Few surgeons now perform anterior lumbar interbody fusion with stand-alone cages. Also of concern was the meagre success rate observed in both the artificial disc and the lumbar fusion groups. Only 57% of patients with disc replacement and 46% of those with interbody fusion met all four criteria for success.

McAfee *et al* evaluated the radiographic outcomes in both the investigational group and the control group [21]. The technical accuracy of the Charité artificial disc replacement was divided into three groups: I, ideal (83%); II, sub-optimal (11%); and III, poor (6%). Those with sub-optimal and poor implant positioning resulted in sub-optimal or poor clinical outcome. The authors reported that total disc replacement with the Charité artificial disc resulted in restoration and maintenance of flexion / extension range of motion 24 months following surgery. The investigational group had significantly better restoration of disc height when compared to the fusion group. The total disc replacement group had significantly less subsidence than the anterior lumbar interbody fusion group. The ideal surgical placement of the Charité artificial disc prosthesis correlated with improved clinical outcomes and improved flexion / extension range of motion compared to poor or sub-optimal surgical placement of the prosthesis.

The second RCT is an investigational device exemption study carried out in the USA prospectively, comparing implantation of the Pro-Disc II with a 360° fusion with both single and double-level study arms. The study involved 18 sites within the USA and has recently completed [22]. Two sites have reported their preliminary results [16, 22-25]. There are a number of interim results published, the most recent of which is by Zigler *et al* with 54 patients having one-year follow-up [16]. Significant reductions in ODI and VAS have been reported for both groups. The definitive results from all 18 centres are eagerly awaited.

The National Institute for Clinical Excellence Review

In November 2004, the National Institute for Clinical Excellence published interventional procedure guidance on prosthetic intervertebral disc replacement [26]. The Institute stated that current evidence of the safety and efficacy of prosthetic intervertebral disc replacement appears adequate to support the use of this procedure. However, there is little evidence on outcomes beyond two to three years and collection of long-term data are, therefore, particularly important.

The review discusses two studies reporting good or excellent clinical results in 63% (29/46) [3] and 79% (83/105) [27]. The percentage of patients able to return to work was reported to be 67% (31/46) and 87% (91/105), respectively. A third study, however, with 93 patients found no increase in patients returning to work [28]. The same multicentre study reported on leg pain and found a statistically significant improvement in patients at 12 months compared with baseline. The recent RCT reported by Geisler *et al* was discussed [15]. The specialist advisors expressed concern about the lack of good-quality, long-term evidence. They stressed the importance of training.

Complication rates in the studies range from 16% (8/50) [29] to 45% (9/20) [30]. The wide variation may in part be explained by differing definitions of complications. These included implant-related problems such as migration and dislocation. Re-operation rates varied between 3% (3/93) [28] and 24% (12/50) [29]. The RCT of 304 patients reported major neurological events by 24 months in 5% (10/205) of patients receiving an artificial disc compared with 4% (99) of patients undergoing spinal fusion [15]. The specialist advisors listed the potential complications as pain, spinal infection, vascular damage and damage to the pre-sacral plexus that may cause retrograde ejaculation.

Conclusions

Total disc replacement in the lumbar spine has been in use in Europe since 1988 [31]. In 2004, the first RCT comparing the Charité lumbar disc replacement to anterior interbody fusion for single-level degenerative disc disease, demonstrated equivalent clinical outcomes at two years. However, the overall results remain disappointing, with only 57% of patients with disc replacement and 46% of those with interbody fusion meeting all four criteria for success [20]. Results of the second RCT for one and two-level degenerative disc disease are eagerly awaited. The long-term benefits of total disc replacement in preventing adjacent level disc degeneration remain unproven. Current contraindications to total disc replacement suggest it is unlikely that this procedure will replace spinal fusion.

Recommendations	Evidence level

- The Charité lumbar disc replacement appears safe and effective for the treatment of mechanical low back pain caused by one-level degenerative disc disease at L4/5 or L5/S1. Ib/A
- Clinical results at two years are equivalent to those resulting from single-level anterior lumbar interbody fusion. Ib/A
- The incidence of major neurological complications is low and equivalent to those observed following a single-level anterior lumbar interbody fusion. Ib/A
- Total disc replacement with the Charité artificial disc results in restoration and maintenance of flexion/extension range of motion 24 months following surgery. Ib/A
- Ideal placement of the Charité artificial disc prosthesis correlates with improved clinical outcome and flexion / extension range of motion. Ib/A
- The role for two-level total disc replacement has not yet been proven. Ib/A
- The long-term benefits of total disc replacement in preventing adjacent level disc degeneration are not yet proven. Ib/A

Chapter 6

References

1. Möller H, Hedlund R. Surgery versus conservative management in adult isthmic spondylolisthesis. *Spine* 2000; 25: 1711-5.

2. Fritzell P, Hägg O, Wessberg P, *et al*. Volvo award winner in clinical studies: lumbar fusion versus non-surgical treatment for chronic low back pain. A multi-centre randomised controlled trial from the Swedish Lumbar Spine Study Group. *Spine* 2001; 26: 2521-34.

3. Cinotti G, David T, Postacchini F. Results of disc prosthesis after a minimum follow-up period of two years. *Spine* 1996; 21: 995-1000.

4. Van Ooij A, Oner FC, Verbout AJ. Complications of artificial disc replacement; a report of 27 patients with the SB Charité disc. *Journal of Spinal Disorders and Techniques* 2003; 16: 369-83.

5. Huang RC, Lim MR, Girardi FP, *et al*. The prevalence of contraindications to total disc replacement in a cohort of lumbar surgical patients. *Spine* 2004; 29: 2538-41.

6. Tropiano P, Huang RC, Girardi FP, *et al*. Lumbar total disc replacement. Seven to eleven-year follow-up. *J Bone Joint Surg Am* 2005; 87A: 490-6.

7. Huang RC, Girardi FP, Cammisa FP, *et al*. Correlation between range of motion and outcome after lumbar total disc replacement: 8.6-year follow-up. *Spine* 2005; 30: 1407-11.

8. Mayer HM, Wiechert K, Korge A, *et al*. Minimally invasive total disc replacement: surgical technique and preliminary clinical results. *Eur Spine J* 2002; 11: S124-S130.

9. Bertagnoli R, Kumar S. Indications for full prosthetic disc arthroplasty: a correlation of clinical outcome against a variety of indications. *Eur Spine J* 2002; 11: S130-S136.

10. Tropiano P, Huang RC, Girardi FP *et al*. Lumbar disc replacement: preliminary results with ProDisc II after a minimum follow-up period of one year. *Journal of Spinal Disorders & Techniques* 2003; 4: 362-8.

11. Fraser RD, Ross ER, Lowery GL, Freeman BJ, *et al*. Lumbar disc replacement. AcroFlex design and results. *The Spine J* 2004; 4: 245S-251S.

12. Le Huec JC, Mathews H, Basso Y, *et al*. Clinical results of Maverick lumbar total disc replacement: two-year prospective follow-up. *Orthop Clin North Am* 2005 36: 315-22

13. De Kleuver M, Oner FC, Jacobs WCH. Total disc replacement for chronic low back pain: background and a systematic review of the literature. *Eur Spine J* 2003; 12: 108-16.

14. Shekelle PG, Woolf SH, Eccles M, *et al*. Clinical guidelines; Developing Guidelines. *Br Med J* 1999; 318: 593-6

15. Geisler FH, Blumenthal SL, Guyer RD, *et al*. Neurological complications of lumbar artificial disc replacement and comparison of clinical results with those related to lumbar arthrodesis in the literature: results of a multicentre, prospective, randomized investigational device exemption study of Charité intervertebral disc. *J Neurosurg (Spine 2)* 2004; 1: 143-54.

16. Zigler JE. Lumbar spine arthroplasty using the Pro-Disc II. *The Spine Journal* 2004: 4: 260S-267S.

17. McAfee PC, Fedder IL, Saiedy S, *et al*. Experimental design of total disc replacement: experience with a prospective randomized study of the SB Charité. *Spine* 2003; 28: S153-S162.

18. McAfee PC, Fedder IL, Saiedy S, *et al*. SB Charité disc replacement. Report of 60 prospective randomized cases in a US Centre. *Journal of Spinal Disorders & Techniques* 2003; 4: 424-33.

19. Blumenthal S, McAfee PC, Guyer RD, *et al*. A prospective, randomised multi-centre Food and Drug Administration investigational device exemption study of lumbar total disc replacement with the Charité artificial disc versus lumbar

fusion. Part I: evaluation of clinical outcomes. *Spine* 2005; 30: 1565-75.

20. Mirza SK. Point of view: commentary on the research reports that led to Food and Drug Administration approval of an artificial disc. *Spine* 2005; 30: 1561-4.

21. McAfee PC, Cunningham B, Holsapple G, *et al*. A prospective, randomised, multi-centre Food and Drug Administration investigational device exemption study of total lumbar disc replacement with the Charité artificial disc versus lumbar fusion. Part II: evaluation of radiographic outcomes and correlation of surgical technique with clinical outcomes. *Spine* 2005; 30: 1576-83.

22. Delamarter RB, Bae HW, Pradhan BB. Clinical results of ProDisc II lumbar total disc replacement: report from the United States Clinical trial. *Orthop Clin North Am* 2005; 36: 301-13.

23. Zigler JE, Burd TA, Vialle EN, *et al*. Lumbar spine arthroplasty. Early results using the ProDisc II: a prospective randomized trial of arthroplasty versus fusion. *Journal of Spinal Disorders & Techniques* 2003; 4: 352-61.

24. Zigler JE. Clinical results with ProDisc: European experience and US Investigation Device Exemption Study. *Spine* 2003; 28: S163-S166.

25. Delamarter RB, David MF, Linda EAK. ProDisc artificial total lumbar disc replacement: introduction and early results from the United States clinical trial. *Spine* 2003; 28: S167-S175.

26. Interventional Procedure Guidance 100. Prosthetic intervertebral disc replacement. National Institute for Clinical Excellence, November 2004. ISBN: 1-84257-817-0 (www.nice.org.uk).

27. LeMaire JP, Skalli W, Lavaste F, *et al*. Intervertebral disc prosthesis: results and prospects for the year 2000. *Clin Orthop Relat Res* 1997; 337: 64-76.

28. Griffith SL, Shelokov AP, Buttner-Janz K, *et al*. A multi-centre retrospective study of the clinical results of the link SB Charité intervertebral prosthesis. *Spine* 1994; 19: 1842-9.

29. Zeegers WS, Bohnen LMLG, Laaper M, *et al*. Artificial disc replacement with the modular type SB Charité III: two-year results in 50 prospectively studied patients. *Eur Spine J* 1999; 8: 210-7.

30. Buttner-Janz K, Hahn S, Schikora K, *et al*. Principles for successful application of the Link SB Charité artificial disc. *Orthopade* 2002; 31: 441-53.

31. Buttner-Janz K, Schellnack K, Zippel H, *et al*. Experience and results with the SB Charité lumbar intervertebral endoprosthesis. *Z Klin Med* 1988; 43: 1785-9.

Chapter 6

Chapter 7

The glenoid component of total shoulder replacements

Robert Bethune MRCS, Research Fellow [1]
Ulrich Hansen PhD, Lecturer [2]
Roger Emery MS FRCS, Reader, Orthopaedic Surgery [3]
Andrew Amis PhD DSc, Professor [2, 3]

1 St. Mary's Hospital, London, UK
2 Department of Mechanical Engineering, Imperial College London, UK
3 Department of Orthopaedic Surgery, Imperial College London, UK

Introduction

Shoulder arthroplasty has evolved significantly over the last 30 years, but there are many questions that have not been completely answered. In this chapter we will briefly look at the development of the types of replacement, before looking at the evidence for the various controversial issues, what kind of replacement to use, what fixation to use, what to do in rotator cuff-deficient shoulders and finally, when to replace the glenoid.

In the 1950s, Neer [1] started the modern era of shoulder replacements by performing hemi-arthroplasties initially for fracture-dislocations of the humeral head, and then later for osteoarthritis. In a series of hemi-arthroplasties for primary osteoarthritis published in 1974 [2], he did not take the view that the glenoid was a source of pain, citing the impressive radiological appearance, with no flattening, sclerosis or enlargement of the glenoid, after six years.

Attempts were made to reflect developments in total hip replacement in the shoulder over the next 20 years, using fixed fulcrum devices, which were largely unsuccessful. Lettin *et al* [3] reported a series of 50 cases in 1982; 44% showed signs of loosening and ten cases required revision. These findings were in keeping with studies from the USA and led to the discontinuation of these implants. The first report of successful total shoulder replacements (TSR) was again by Neer [4] in 1982, describing a large series using polyethylene glenoid components. In these cases he had introduced the glenoid component for difficult technical problems encountered in cases of erosion.

The indications for glenoid replacement are controversial, and the procedure is not without risks. It increases the operation time and is technically difficult, as well as being a source of complications: glenoid fracture, misalignment, vault perforation, overstuffing, and the need for complex bone grafting. The questions to be addressed are: what kind of replacement?; what to do in particular situations?; and, most importantly, when to do a total shoulder replacement?

Methodology

Most of the literature was found by searching the Pubmed online database of the National Library of Medicine at the NIH in the USA, but the senior authors were also in possession of extensive collections and knowledge of the literature. Imperial College maintains online access to the majority of important medical journals, so it was easy to obtain pdf copies of papers.

Others could be obtained via the UK inter-library loan service, linked into the national lending library at Boston Spa.

The glenoid component

By its very nature glenoid resurfacing during total shoulder replacement brings inherent difficulties. It is a small surface, it does not have a large bone stock, and in most cases, there will be disease that will be altering the structure of the glenoid (Figure 1).

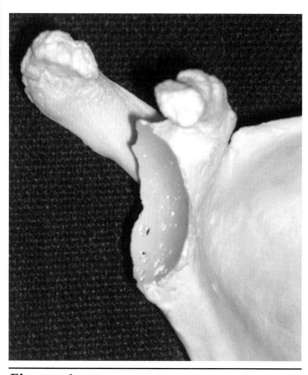

Figure 1. Rheumatoid scapula with medial erosion to the base of the coracoid and loss of the glenoid vault.

Unconstrained replacements have been shown to be superior to constrained devices [5], but there are many different choices among these devices. There are also different materials to consider: all-polyethylene or metal-backed polyethylene; and different fixation methods: keel, pegs, or screw. Additionally, fixation methods can include cement of various types and uncemented components with various coatings and methods of initial fixation.

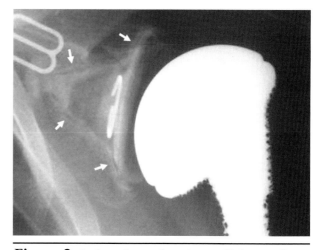

Figure 2. Arthroplasty showing radiolucent lines all around the keel. *Reproduced with permission from P. Rozing, Leiden University Medical Center.*

Radiolucent lines (Figure 2) are used in many studies as a marker for progressive failure and loosening of the glenoid component; however, no consensus exists as to whether there is a clear correlation. In fact there is no defined agreement on how wide the radiolucencies need to be before they are considered significant.

Torchia *et al* [6] followed-up 113 Neer prostheses and, using a figure of greater than 1.5mm, found a statistical correlation between radiolucent lines and pain. Other clinical reports have disagreed, finding no correlation [7]. Using radiostereophotogrammetric (RSA) techniques, Rahme *et al* [8] also found no correlation between migration and the presence of radiolucencies. This is an important issue, as the incidence of radiolucencies varies between 30%-90% [4, 8-11]. Loosening is not an event but rather a continuous process. The immediate postoperative radiolucencies are probably not significant; however, the progression in size of radiolucencies is thought to be significant **(IV/C)**.

Neer's initial design, which continues to be most widely used, consists of an all-polyethylene keeled component. Since then, metal backing, and screws and pegging for the polyethylene component, have been tried. Controversy exists as to whether metal-backed glenoids are better. Metal backing offers possible advantages. Bone is able to grow into porous-surfaced metal forming a tight bond, particularly if the proximal part of the metal is coated with hydroxyapatite.

Finite element analyses (FEA) have shown metal backing to improve stress transfer [12]; however, metal backing has shown higher peak stresses [13]. In a randomised, prospective, double-blind study, Boileau et al [14] showed that cementless, metal-backed glenoids had a statistically higher rate of loosening and revision than all-polyethylene components, despite a lower rate of observed radiolucent lines in the metal-backed group. This lower rate might be a result of the difficulty in comparing radiographs of polyethylene and metal, as the appearances are different.

As with most surgery, an important component of the success of the operation is the skill of the surgeon. Lazarus et al [15] found that more experienced surgeons achieved better seating and cementing of the glenoid component. This is additionally important as the angle of the replacement has been shown to make a significant difference to cement mantle stresses and to other mechanical measures of loosening [16, 17]. Hopkins et al [16] used finite element analysis to show that the alignment of the glenoid component had a large effect on the survival of the cement mantle. Retroversion was worse than anteversion and supero-inferior misalignment was worse than anteroposterior.

Should the replacement be pegged or keeled?

Two main anchorage systems have been designed to reduce loosening rates: keeled and pegged, and research has been carried out to see which is superior. The results of in vitro mechanical experiments [18] indicated that keeled implants were more prone to fixation failure than pegged components. Lacroix et al [19], using finite element analysis, showed that a pegged glenoid was superior in normal bone but a keeled glenoid was better in rheumatoid bone.

Two clinical studies [15, 20] have verified these findings using the evidence of radiolucent lines in follow-up of TSRs. Lazarus et al [15] retrospectively reviewed 328 initial postoperative radiographs and found that pegged components had better cement seating and fewer radiolucent lines. In a more recent study, Gartsman et al [20] performed a randomised study on radiographs taken six weeks after surgery, and again found less radiographic lucency with the pegged fixation. This result is difficult to interpret, as

mentioned before the significance of radiolucency is not certain and in addition, the interpretation of radiolucencies around pegged and keeled components is inherently different.

An additional point was demonstrated by FEA by Murphy et al [21] who showed that a keel offset in an anterior manner had lower cement stresses.

Should the replacement be cemented in place?

This is a similar question to whether the glenoid should be metal-backed or all-polyethylene. Boileau et al [14] conducted a prospective, double-blind randomised study of 40 shoulders and statistically showed that the cementless, metal-backed components were inferior (at three years) to the cemented all-polyethylene components.

However, Wallace et al [22] retrospectively reviewed 58 shoulders and found no difference after four to seven years of follow-up, but this was not a randomised study.

There is no firm consensus on the exact thickness of the cement to be used. However, using a thick cement mantle may lead to overstuffing of the joint or alternatively, removal of too much of the subchondral bone has been found to be detrimental to the fixation strength of the implant (Frich [23]). Terrier et al [24], based on FEA of the stresses in the cement mantle and bone-implant interface, recommended a thickness of 1-1.5mm. Nyffeler [25] et al warned against too thin a cement mantle, as this may lead to an incomplete cement mantle and reduced strength of the mantle.

Should the implant be curved or flat-backed?

In an all-polyethylene component, the back of the implant bonded to the cement mantle can be curved (convex) or flat-backed. Very few studies have compared the two types of implants. Szabo et al [26] performed a clinical evaluation of the incidence of radiolucencies. Both components had a keel component and the incidence of radiolucencies at the keel was statistically different immediately

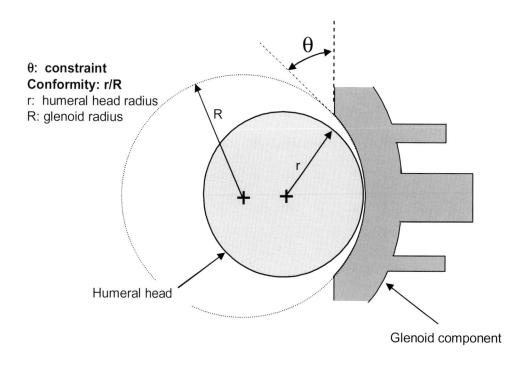

θ: **constraint**
Conformity: r/R
r: humeral head radius
R: glenoid radius

Humeral head

Glenoid component

Figure 3. Constraint is the maximum slope at the glenoid rim, which is also half the angle subtended by the glenoid. Conformity is the ratio of humeral radius over glenoid radius.

postoperatively, but there was no difference seen at the two-year follow-up. This is the only clinical study which was not randomised; in fact, separate surgeons operated with the different implants. In a non-clinical study, Anglin *et al* [18] showed that the curve-backed prosthesis performed significantly better, having half the post-rocking tensile movement. They also found that the flat-backed glenoid permanently deformed the surface of the bone substitute.

Again, there is no conclusive evidence about whether the prosthesis should be curved; however, the evidence suggests that it might be advantageous **(IIa/B)**.

How conformed and constrained should the implant be?

Conformity, defined as the ratio of humeral head radius to the glenoid radius, refers to how closely the articulating surface of the humeral component matches the surface of the glenoid. This is the main design feature affecting intra-articular joint translation. This 'fit' of the articulating surfaces is also sometimes described in terms of 'radial mismatch', being the difference between glenoid and humeral radii. The implant design feature described as 'constraint' is one of the most important implant characteristics, as it controls the force necessary to cause subluxation and dislocation of the shoulder joint. However, constraint is often used interchangeably with conformity or described in terms of the 'depth' of the glenoid. This causes confusion as, for example, a large non-conforming glenoid may have the same depth as a small conforming glenoid but will have a much smaller subluxation load. Constraint is more appropriately measured in terms of the maximum slope at the glenoid rim as shown is Figure 3. This measurement leads to a consistent relationship between constraint and subluxation forces.

Constrained or semi-constrained glenoids have a clinical history **(III/C)** of high loosening rates [27], most likely due to high fixation stresses and have been rejected as a method of replacement.

Conformity is more debatable. Common sense would indicate that an anatomical arrangement would be best. In the anatomical setting the bone is non-conforming; however, with the effect of the cartilage and labrum, the joint becomes roughly conforming and results in a flexible conformity. Anglin et al [18] showed that a conformity of 0.8 to 0.88 resulted in a natural transfer of forces and less off-centre loading, leading to a more stable joint. In a large multicentred trial, Walch et al [28] demonstrated a significant difference in the incidence of radiolucent lines with differing levels of mismatch. In fact, mismatch between 5.5-10mm was associated with less radiolucent lines at a mean follow-up of 53.5 months. Two theories might explain the better results seen with non-conforming joints; non-conforming designs offer the possibility of transferring more load to the soft tissue before reaching subluxation, thereby reducing the off-centre loads that are believed to lead to glenoid loosening [18]. The other possible explanation is that different wear particle sizes are created, and those created by a smaller humeral head are more favourable.

However, a laboratory-based Dutch study [29], indicated that exact matches between the glenoid and humeral radii led to significantly better results in terms of loosening.

So, again, there is no consensus as to whether the joint should be conforming, and, if a mismatch is present, how much there should be. Overall, however, the evidence points towards a better result if there is a mismatch in the radii **(IIa/B)**.

Which should be done, hemi or total arthroplasty?

Several studies [30-34] have compared these two operations and their outcomes. Neer's initial view, after his first hemi-arthroplasty series, was that the glenoid did not appear to be a source of pain. In these cases the articular surface was smooth and devoid of cartilage. Boyd and co-workers [30] published (in 1990) a comparative series of 64 hemi-arthroplasties and 146 total shoulders (both Neer prosthesis). Functional outcome was the same in both groups but pain relief and patient satisfaction were greater in the total shoulder group. Based on this they recommended that hemi-arthroplasties should be performed on patients with osteoarthritis, avascular necrosis, and four part fractures, and total arthroplasty should be performed on patients with inflammatory arthropathies. It was, however, neither a fair comparison nor a randomised trial.

More recent non-randomised trials comparing hemi with total arthroplasty have either found a significant difference [31] (in favour of total) or have had comparable results [32-33]. Only one truly randomised trial was found comparing the two. Gartsman et al [34] took 47 patients and randomised them into the two sub-groups. There was no statistical difference in terms of total functional score; however, the total group had greater pain relief (p=0.002) and internal rotation (p=0.003). Interestingly, they also found that the cost was $1177 greater per patient in the total arthroplasty. All the patients in this study had osteoarthritis of the shoulder.

However, these studies are short to medium-term follow-ups and it is arguably the long-term outcome which is most relevant. That is, does glenoid erosion following a hemi-arthroplasty progress to such a state, that when a conversion to a TSR would otherwise be indicated, this is no longer feasible? How does this outcome compare to loosening of the glenoid component in TSR?

So, the evidence is not conclusive, but based on the one truly randomised study, it may be that total arthroplasties are more appropriate in the setting of osteoarthritis with an intact rotator cuff **(Ib/A)**.

What to do in the cuff-deficient shoulder?

The problem of shoulder replacement is increased in the presence of an irreparable rotator cuff tear. What to do in this situation has sparked some controversy. One of the main fears is of proximal migration of the humeral component, although one study [35] did not show any correlation between migration and pain postoperatively.

Despite the centre of rotation not being restored, hemi-arthroplasty has been shown to improve pain: two studies [36, 37] have shown that hemi-arthroplasty provided marked pain relief, although slightly less relief than with an intact rotator cuff.

Total shoulder replacements seem to have problems in the presence of rotator cuff tears, and this is thought to be because of eccentric loading of the glenoid and so increased loosening. Franklin *et al* [38] compared a series of total shoulder replacements with major cuff tears, seven cases in total, to a cuff-intact group and showed increased rates of glenoid loosening of the cuff-deficient group. However, Boyd *et al* [30] did not find any association between glenoid component loosening and rotator cuff tears. In a large multicentred study [39], supraspinatus tears were not associated with a poorer outcome; however, fatty degeneration of the infraspinatus was.

One small study [40] of seven semi-constrained shoulders showed very poor results in the presence of a rotator cuff tear, six of them being reported as unsatisfactory according to the Neer classification.

None of these studies have directly compared hemi to total arthroplasty. It would seem reasonable to use a total if the tear is minor, or just involving supraspinatus, but in the presence of a massive tear, the risk of glenoid loosening is too great and a hemi-replacement should be used **(IV/C)**.

However, the current vogue in Europe is to medialise the centre of rotation using reverse shoulder replacements. Rittmeister *et al* [41] showed good results in rheumatoid cuff-deficient shoulders, using a Grammont reverse total shoulder replacement, although they still had problems with glenoid loosening, and there are worries that this method will not be successful.

Conclusions

It can be seen that there are no certain answers regarding any of the questions asked. None of the evidence is convincing, mostly due to the lack of randomised clinical trials. Based on the best current evidence it would seem reasonable to perform total shoulder arthroplasty for osteoarthritis using an unconstrained, cemented, all-polyethylene replacement. However, apart from the unconstrained characteristic, the use of design features such as a non-conforming, pegged, curved-backed prosthesis is not based on strong evidence.

So what of the future? Clearly, more research is needed. Biomechanical research in the laboratory can find future avenues of clinical research, but what is needed in the long term are large randomised trials to settle the fundamental questions of hemi versus total arthroplasty and what type of replacement to use. However, this ideal is very difficult to implement, as there are such small numbers, and many patients are lost to follow-up, often due to death in this elderly patient population. One other avenue of research that may be more practical is the use of RSA, which offers accurate measurements of migration and an early indication of loosening, but until then the evidence for glenoid replacement remains scanty at best. Arthroplasty registers in their current form cannot answer these questions.

Recommendations   **Evidence level**

The following recommendations for treatment decisions can be drawn from the literature.

- Pegs provide more secure fixation than do keels.   Ib/A
- Curve-backed glenoid components are preferred to flat-backed components.   Ib/A
- Better results have been reported for non-conforming articulations, especially   IIa/B
  where the radial mismatch is greater than 3-5mm.
- It is best not to have too much constraint in the device, so fixed-fulcrum   III/C
  prostheses should be avoided.
- Total shoulder replacement is preferred to hemi-arthroplasty in patients with   Ib/A
  osteoarthritis and an intact rotator cuff.
- For a patient with a cuff-deficient shoulder: a total shoulder replacement is   IV/C
  preferred if the cuff tear is minor; a hemi-arthroplasty is preferred if there is
  a major cuff tear; and a reversed prosthesis is suitable in the elderly with
  pseudoparalysis and anterior-superior escape of the humeral head.

Chapter 7

References

1. Neer CS II. Articular replacement of the humeral head. *J Bone Joint Surg Am* 1995; 37: 215-28.

2. Neer CS. Replacement arthroplasty for glenohumeral osteoarthritis. *J Bone Joint Surg Am* 1974; 56: 373-4.

3. Lettin AW, Copeland SA, Scales JT. The Stanmore total shoulder replacement. *J Bone Joint Surg Br* 1982; 64(1): 47-51.

4. Neer CS. Replacement arthroplasty for glenohumeral arthritis. *J Bone Joint Surg Am* 1982; 64: 319-37.

5. Severt T, Thomas BJ, Tsenter MJ, Amstutz HC, Kabo JM. The influence of conformity and constraint on translational forces and frictional torque in total shoulder arthroplasty. *Clin Orthop* 1993; 292: 151-8.

6. Torchia ME, Cofield RH, Settergren CR. Total shoulder arthroplasty with the Neer prosthesis: long-term results. *J Shoulder Elbow Surg* 1997; 6: 494-505.

7. Williams GR, Abboud JA. Total shoulder arthroplasty: glenoid component design. *J Shoulder Elbow Surg* 2005; 14(Suppl): S122-8.

8. Rahme H, Mattsson P, Larsson S. Stability of cemented all-polyethylene keeled glenoid components. A radiostereometric study with a two-year follow up. *J Bone Joint Surg Br* 2004; 86(6): 856-60.

9. Barret WP, Franklin JL, Jackins SE, Wyss CR, Matsen FA. Total shoulder arthroplasty. *J Bone Joint Surg* 1987; 69: 865-72.

10. Bell SN, Gschwend N. Clinical experience with total arthroplasty and hemiarthroplasty of the shoulder using the Neer prosthesis. *Int Orthop* 1986; 10: 217-22.

11. Cofield RH. Total shoulder arthroplasty with the Neer prosthesis. *J Bone Joint Surg Am* 1984; 99: 899-906.

12. Orr TE, Carter DR, Schurman DJ. Stress analyses of glenoid component designs. *Clin Orthop* 1988; 232: 217-24.

13. Gupta S, van der Helm FC, van Keulen F. Stress analysis of cemented glenoid prostheses in total shoulder arthroplasty. *J Biomech* 2004; 37(11): 1777-86.

14. Boileau P, Avidor C, Krishnan SG, Walch G, Kempf JF, Mole D. Cemented polyethylene versus uncemented metal-backed glenoid components in total shoulder arthroplasty: a prospective, double-blind, randomized study. *J Shoulder Elbow Surg* 2002; 11(4): 351-9.

15. Lazarus MD, Jensen KL, Southworth C, Matsen FA. The radiographic evaluation of keeled and pegged glenoid component insertion. *J Bone Joint Surg Am* 2002; 84-A(7): 1174-82.

16. Hopkins AR, Hansen UN, Amis AA, Emery RE. The effects of glenoid component alignment variation on cement mantle stresses in total shoulder arthroplasty. *J Shoulder Elbow Surg* 2004; 13: 668-75.

17. Oosterom R, Rozing PM, Bersee HE. Effect of glenoid component inclination on its fixation and humeral head subluxation in total shoulder arthroplasty. *Clin Biomech* 2004; 19(10): 1000-8.

18. Anglin C, Wyss UP, Nyffeler RW, Gerber C. Loosening performance of cemented glenoid prosthesis design pairs. *Clin Biomech* 2001; 16: 144-50.

19. Lacroix D, Murphy LA, Prendergast PJ. Three-dimensional finite element analysis of glenoid replacement prostheses: a comparison of keeled and pegged anchorage systems. *J Biomech Eng* 2000; 122(4): 430-6.

20. Gartsman GM, Elkousy HA, Warnock KM, Edwards TB, O'Connor DP. Radiographic comparison of pegged ad keeled glenoid components. *J Shoulder Elbow Surg* 2005; 14(3): 252-7.

21. Murphy LA, Prendergast PJ, Resch H. Structural analysis of an offset-keel design glenoid component compared with a center-keel design. *J Shoulder Elbow Surg* 2001; 10(6): 568-79.

22. Wallace AL, Philips RL, MacDougal GA, Walsh WR, Sonnabend DH. Resurfacing of the glenoid in total shoulder arthroplasty. A comparison, at a mean of five years, of prostheses inserted with and without cement. *J Bone Joint Surg Am* 1999; 81(4): 510-8.

23. Frich LH. Glenoidal knoglestyrke og koglestruktur. Thesis 1994; University Hospital Aarhus, Aarhus.

24. Terrier A, Buchler, P, Farron A. Bone-cement interface of the glenoid component: stress analysis for varying cement thickness. *Clin Biomech* 2005; 20: 710-7.

25. Nyffeler C, Anglin C, Sheikh R, Gerber C. Influence of peg design and cement mantle thickness on pull-out strength of glenoid component pegs. *J Bone Joint Surg Br* 2003; 85-B: 748-52.

26. Szabo BI, Buscayret F, Edwards B, Nemoz C, Boileau P, Walch G. Curve or flat back glenoid? Shoulder arthroscopy and arthroplasty, current concepts. Nice Shoulder Course, 2004: 332-43.

27. Wirth MA, Rockwood CA, Jr. Current concepts review: complications of total shoulder replacement arthroplasty. *J Bone Joint Surg Am* 1996; 78A(4): 603-16.

28. Walch G, Edwards TB, Boulahia A, Boileau P, Mole D, Adeleine P. The influence of glenohumeral prosthetic mismatch on glenoid radiolucent lines: results of a multicenter study. *J Bone Joint Surg Am* 2002; 84-A(12): 2186-91.

29. Oosterom R, Rozing PM, Verdonschot N, Bersee HE. Effect of joint conformity on glenoid component fixation in total shoulder arthroplasty. *Proc Inst Mech Eng* 2004; 218(5): 339-47.

30. Boyd AD, Thomas WH, Scott RD, Sledge CB, Thornhill TS. Total shoulder arthroplasty versus hemi-arthroplasty. Indications for glenoid resurfacing. *J Arthroplasty* 1990; 5(4): 329-36.

31. Edwards TB, Kadakia NR, Boulahia A, Kempf JF, Boileau P, Nemoz C, Walch G. A comparison of hemiarthroplasty and total shoulder arthroplasty in the treatment of primary glenohumeral osteoarthritis: results of a multicenter study. *J Shoulder Elbow Surg* 2003; 12(3): 207-13.

32. Levy O; Copeland SA. Cementless surface replacement arthroplasty (Copeland CSRA) for osteoarthritis of the shoulder. *J Shoulder Elbow Surg* 2004; 13(3): 266-71.

33. Sperling JW; Cofield RH; Rowland CM. Minimum fifteen-year follow-up of Neer hemiarthroplasty and total shoulder replacement in patients aged fifty years or younger. *J Shoulder Elbow Surg* 2004; 13(6): 604-13.

34. Gartsman GM, Roddey TS, Hammerman SM. Shoulder arthroplasty with or without resurfacing of the glenoid in patients who have osteoarthritis. *J Bone Joint Surg Am* 2000; 82(1): 26-34.

35. Boyd AD, Thornhill TS, Ewald FC, Scott RD, Sledge CB. Post-operative humeral migration in total shoulder replacement: incidence and significance. *J Arthroplasty* 1991; 6: 31-7.

36. Sanchez-Sotelo J, Cofield RH, Rowland CM. Shoulder hemiarthroplasty for glenohumeral arthritis associated with severe rotator cuff deficiency. *J Bone Joint Surg Am* 2001; 83-A(12): 1814-22.

37. Williams GR, Rockwood CA. Hemiarthroplasty in rotator cuff-deficient shoulders. *J Shoulder Elbow Surg* 1996; 5(5): 362-7.

38. Franklin JL, Barret WO, Jackins SE, Matsen FA. Glenoid loosening in total shoulder arthroplasty. Association with rotator cuff deficiency. *J Arthroplasty* 1988; 3(1): 39-46.

39. Edward TB, Boulahia A, Kempf JF, Boileau P, Nemoz C, Walch G. The influence of rotator cuff disease on the results of shoulder arthroplasty for primary osteoarthritis: results of a multicenter study. *J Bone Joint Surg Am* 2002; 84-A(12): 2240-8.

40. Nwakama AC, Cofield RH, Kavanagh BF, Loehr JF. Semiconstrained total shoulder arthroplasty for glenohumeral arthritis and massive rotator cuff tearing. *J Shoulder Elbow Surg* 2000; 9(4): 302-7.

41. Rittmeister M, Kerschbaumer F. Grammont reverse total shoulder arthroplasty in patients with rheumatoid arthritis and nonreconstructable rotator cuff lesions. *J Shoulder Elbow Surg* 2001; 10(1): 17-22.

Chapter 8

The classification of shoulder instability

Simon M Lambert BSc FRCS FRCSEd (Orth)

Consultant Orthopaedic Surgeon [1] & Honorary Senior Lecturer [2]

1 ROYAL NATIONAL ORTHOPAEDIC HOSPITAL TRUST, AND
2 INSTITUTE OF MUSCULOSKELETAL SCIENCE, UNIVERSITY COLLEGE, LONDON, UK

Introduction

Classification, by which we mean analysis and conceptual organisation, of shoulder instability is critical to accurate diagnosis and management of the wide spectrum of pathologies which constitute the disorder. This review refers to glenohumeral instability (GHI), although the system of classification described below [1] is applicable to all articulations in which the experience of symptomatic abnormal motion (the clinical syndrome of instability) is reported by the patient.

The components of stability

An articulation behaves normally if it retains structural integrity, has intact neural afferent, efferent and neuromuscular connections, and is not subject to strain in excess of the yield point for the whole system. The corollary is that glenohumeral stability depends on competent capsulolabral structures, effective muscular activity [2], intact and effective neural connections and an absence of excessive extrinsic deforming force. In the glenohumeral joint, motion about the centroid of rotation and 'containment' of the humeral head on the comparatively small glenoid is the result of concavity compression created by muscular activity (of the rotator cuff, including the tendon of the long head of biceps), the generation of negative intra-articular pressure, and conformation of the glenoid, deepened by the labrum. A congenital hypoplasia of the labrum or absence of one or more of the named ligaments of the capsule does not lead to GHI; the physical state of laxity (an alteration of the proportion of collagen types) must be distinguished from the symptom of instability. GHI can, therefore, arise if the capsulolabral architecture becomes structurally deficient, if there is abnormal muscular activation or suppression resulting in a dynamically asymmetric joint reaction force [3], or if excessive extrinsic force is applied. Any classification system has to be able to describe derangements of any or all of these three components leading to the symptom of instability: the system must include reference to structural integrity, muscular control, and trauma. Direction is less relevant as a descriptor of the presence of instability: a multidirectionally unstable shoulder dislocates in any direction according to the position of the forearm and hand at the time of displacement, under the influence of muscular activity and varying loading conditions.

The value of classification

Of great importance is the ability of a classification system to distinguish those cases of GHI in which surgical treatment is absolutely unhelpful, or even contraindicated, from those in which a variety of surgical interventions are possible and useful. Many systems for classifying GHI have been described, compounding direction, pathology, acquired characteristics, developmental anomalies, varying degrees of volition, and treatment. Until recently the failure of existing classifications to be inclusive of all pathologies has contributed to an incidence and, a misunderstanding of cause and of failure for some treatments. It is also clear that in any one individual the cause and effects of GHI do not always fit into existing schemata. For example, a shoulder which is inherently structurally unstable for capsular reasons with episodes of painful displacement, may then be subjected to trauma, with anterior dislocation. If this is complicated by palsy of subscapularis, later recurrence can then be due to inappropriate pectoralis major activity over an inadequate subscapularis. In this imaginary case there are elements of trauma, congenital collagen insufficiency, and abnormal neuromuscular sequencing. This instability is due to more than one pathology, and the reason for instability has changed over time. Other than the system described below [1] no classification of GHI to date accommodates the presence of more than one pathology, and the change in pathology with time.

Methodology

There are no prospective randomised or non-randomised evaluations of classifications of GHI. Most classifications derive from the authors' clinical experience and inevitably reflect referral or subject bias: there exist large numbers of cohort studies of various treatments, few comparing treatments, and even fewer comparing the methods of evaluating the outcome of treatment of GHI. There were no studies which set out to evaluate the validity, reliability, or reproducibility of any classification system for GHI. A search of Pubmed from 1950 to date using the search terms 'classification', 'shoulder', 'instability' produced 131 reports, of which 44 were reviews. None had a level and grade of evidence greater than III/B, and most were IV/C. Four were specific for the topic of classification [4-7]. A review of other literature [1, 8, 9] revealed further discussion of classifications and factors influential in the development of classifications, based on thoughtful analyses of the populations studied.

Classification

Glenohumeral instability has been classified according to direction, frequency, the essential pathologies present, the requirement for surgery or rehabilitation, the amount of external force (trauma) applied, the presence of congenital or acquired (microtraumatic) ligament deficiency, volition, and timing of presentation (acute or chronic). There is little agreement on what constitutes a 'chronic' dislocation.

TUBS - AMBRI [8]

The most influential descriptive system from Matsen, the TUBS-AMBRI classification (Traumatic, Unidirectional, with a Bankart lesion, often requiring Surgery - Atraumatic, often Multidirectional, commonly Bilateral, treated by Rehabilitation for a period, perhaps a year, proceeding to Inferior capsular shift if rehabilitation is insufficient for stability) [8], has emphasised the appreciation of the external applied force causing a dislocation, and the associated articular edge lesions, the traumatic Bankart or Perthe's lesion of the glenoid rim and the Hill-Sachs or Broca defect of the posterior humeral head **(IV/C)**. It also highlights the patients with no trauma in whom a capsular deficiency may exist, and is based on the earlier observations of the school of Neer [10], that some patients dislocate without trauma and appear to do so in more than one direction. These patients were treated by rehabilitation physiotherapy and some failed to gain stability; these could then be operated on using the inferior capsular shift procedure. Not all such patients gain stability; there is, therefore, a problem with definition of the indications to operate, assuming the shift procedure has been performed adequately. The classification does not, therefore, accommodate all comers, and in particular, the coexistence of traumatic and atraumatic causes of instability and the confounding existence of hyperlaxity in a single patient cannot be described.

Hyperlaxity, voluntary-ism, and prognosis [5]

In recognising these difficulties Gerber [11] proposed a system which included the concept of underlying hyperlaxity as a risk factor for instability in some individuals **(IV/C)**. Locked (chronic) dislocations (type I) were separated from unidirectional instability without (type II) and with (type III) hyperlaxity, and multidirectional instability (MDI) with (type IV) and without (type V) hyperlaxity. A sixth group (type VI) comprised the voluntary instabilities. The type II group corresponds largely to the TUBS group of the Matsen classification. The type III group comprised patients with structural abnormalities of the glenohumeral ligament complex who presented with painful recurrent subluxation, and were treated by intensive rehabilitation. It was noted that operative intervention had a poor prognosis in this group. The type IV patients presented with largely painless frequent subluxation 'without control' (but see below), and were treated as for the type III group. This group corresponded to the AMBRI group of Matsen, and shared the characteristics of the patients first labelled as having MDI, when this entity was first described. Gerber observed that most of the so-called MDI group were in fact unidirectional instabilities with multidirectional laxity (Gerber type III). The true Gerber type IV patients were considered to respond to a specific rehabilitation programme [12]. The type V group comprised a rare group of patients with two or more traumas creating a type II condition but in more than one direction, which acknowledged that more than one pathology may be present in the shoulder with GHI. It was noted that operative intervention may be difficult due to the complexity of pathology in each direction. The type VI group comprised patients who could voluntarily dislocate, commonly, both shoulders under active muscular control. In the sense that the displacement is consciously achieved on demand these can be called voluntary. Importantly, Gerber noted that when left alone these patients did not

develop degenerative or attritional structural changes, and significantly also noted that some patients with involuntary instability could acquire the ability to sublux or dislocate their shoulders. This observation again supports the concept that more than one pathology can be present in an unstable shoulder. Such a case would then be labelled, for example, a type II and type VI (perhaps: type II/VI) instability, if a unidirectional instability without hyperlaxity became complicated by acquired active glenohumeral displacement patterns.

The idea that patients could voluntarily dislocate their shoulder was identified by Rowe [6] but the psychiatric element became a dominant theme and adversely coloured thinking about this group of patients. Unpublished observations at the Royal National Orthopaedic Hospital (RNOH) by Bayley and Fisher suggest that there is no difference in the prevalence of psychiatric illness in those with so-called voluntary dislocation of the shoulder and the general population. An alternative nomenclature was used by Bayley (personal communication) at the RNOH: the term 'voluntary' implied wilful abnormality of control for gain, and as these patients were not psychiatrically different from the general population, this stigmatised such patients who were then not afforded opportunities for potentially useful treatment. The term 'habitual' was adopted to imply a regular, repeated experience or tendency to displacement in specific, predictable circumstances. However, the same term could be used to imply a learned behavioural response often associated with a particular situation; given the observation that muscular activity could create a displacement without volition or evident behavioural advantage, the term 'habitual' was dropped in favour of a description of the actual event(s) occurring during glenohumeral displacement in these cases. 'Voluntary-ism' may, therefore, be an unhelpful concept which hides some real neuromuscular disorders that have yet to be characterised, and 'habitual' is a term that may contribute to confusion about behavioural aspects of GHI.

The role of muscular activity

The concept of muscle involvement in producing instability is not new [9] and recent cohort studies suggest that muscular sequencing problems contribute more than previously understood to the overall presentation of instability [1, 6, 13, 14]. Contrary to the characterisation of the Gerber type IV as being instability 'without control', recent studies at the RNOH strongly [1, 14] indicate that such cases are influenced by abnormality of muscular sequencing or patterning during specific motions of the shoulder, i.e. there is faulty control. The observation that the shoulders of patients without hyperlaxity, but with persistent subluxation, relocated on induction of anaesthesia and redislocated on cessation of anaesthesia suggested that the displaced position was maintained by inappropriate active muscular contraction. Some of that patient group developed the cortical representation of normality for their shoulder even when the joint was clearly not located, and the located joint was perceived as being abnormal. Dynamic electromyography (DEMG) has shed light on the prevalence and relevance of abnormal muscular activity in GHI [15].

Dynamic electromyography

Bayley [1] used DEMG in latissimus dorsi (LD), pectoralis major (PM), anterior deltoid (AD) and infraspinatus (IS) to evaluate the patterns of muscular activation in patients who clearly demonstrated, visibly or by palpation, apparently abnormal muscular activation immediately before and during dislocation of the glenohumeral joint in the outpatient clinic. These muscles were chosen because they were reliably accessible. Early pilot studies were expanded into a cohort study of over 1000 cases of GHI seen at the RNOH, a tertiary referral centre, over a 22-year period (1981-2003) [16], from which DEMG data were extracted. The results can be summarised:

- 52% of the entire cohort of patients with GHI had abnormal muscle activation (muscle-patterning [MP]) during a standard set of movements;
- 47% of unidirectional GHI had MP;
- 27.6% of anterior GHI had MP, involving PM, or PM and LD coupled;
- 84.8% of posterior GHI had MP, involving LD, or AD and suppressed IS coupled;

- 83.8% of multidirectional GHI had MP, involving LD > PM > AD;
- 100% of inferior GHI had MP, involving PM and LD coupled;
- one or two muscles were implicated in 88% of unidirectional and 92% of multidirectional MP instability;
- clinical impression of MP instability was incorrect in 12% of cases;
- clinical impression was correct but the wrong muscles were identified in 33%;
- further abnormal muscles were identified by DEMG in 32.5% of cases.

DEMG provides additional information about abnormal muscle activation or suppression in subtle muscle-patterning instability in which clinical examination has a low specificity and sensitivity. DEMG was found to be most useful in patients presenting with pain, glenohumeral capsular insufficiency, and occult muscle patterning. Given that a chance of a successful outcome for rehabilitation of patients with MP instability (symptoms abolished or controlled) was diminished five-fold for anterior and ten-fold for posterior instability after inappropriate surgery in patients with MP instability, it is clear that the identification of this specific cohort is important [14]. These patients contribute to the failures of the AMBRI group after rehabilitation (if MP instability has not been recognised), and correspond to patients in the Gerber type III and IV groups. It is noteworthy that the pathology is not defined by direction but rather that the direction of instability is determined by the pathology.

Muscle-patterning instability

Muscle-patterning instability was recognised, clinically and/or electrophysiologically, in 494 shoulders (45% of the entire cohort of 1097 shoulders) in 386 patients [16]. In 44%, the MP instability affected both shoulders. The dominant arm was affected more often in right-handed patients, the non-dominant more often in left-handed patients. The central neurological basis for these differences remains obscure. There were 323 shoulders with 'pure' MP instability. One hundred and sixty-one shoulders presented a mixed picture of MP in addition to either traumatic or atraumatic structural causes for the instability. The value of recognising this form of instability is given by the success of specialist physiotherapy using biofeedback techniques versus conventional therapy for retraining abnormal muscle activity: 76% of patients had either no change or a deterioration of their condition with conventional therapy (including conventional strengthening exercises) compared to 61% of patients overall achieving improvement in their condition with specialist therapy.

Patients with abnormal muscular activation leading to 'pure' MP instability appear to present in a trimodal distribution [16] with peaks at six, 14 and 20 years. The mean age at onset of symptoms was 14 years and the mean duration of symptoms before presentation was eight years. In the under ten-year age group there were more females (71% v 47%), greater laxity (estimated with the Beighton score, 63% v 29%), and bilaterality (54% v 42%), with fewer presenting with pain (17% v 50%). As age increased laxity decreased and pain increased. Bilaterality did not appear to be associated with gender, laxity or pain. Laxity was associated with gender but not pain or bilaterality. These observations suggest different aetiologies for the MP instability in the three cohorts.

Given the limitation that only four muscles have been studied in depth, the evidence strongly suggests that these, and perhaps other muscles, are implicated in many cases of instability. Inappropriate activity in PM, LD, and AD, with suppression of IS appear either singly or as couples in the generation of instability in the shoulder with and without capsular collagen insufficiency. Whether suppression of IS reflects specific inappropriate inactivity in IS alone or reflects abnormal activation of the rotator cuff as a whole remains unknown.

Muscle-patterning and structural instability: the Stanmore classification [1]

It follows that there are three major causes of GHI: extrinsic/traumatic; intrinsic/atraumatic (collagen insufficiency or gleno-capsulo-labral) structural

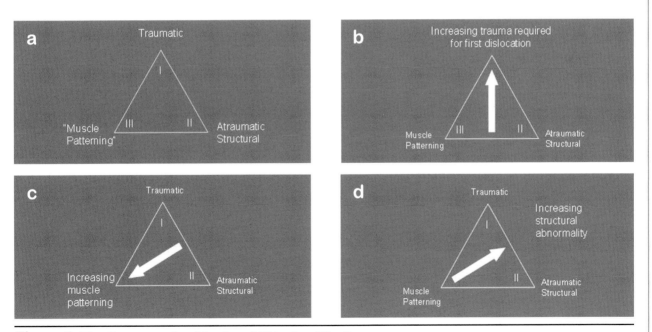

Figure 1. The Stanmore shoulder instability classification.

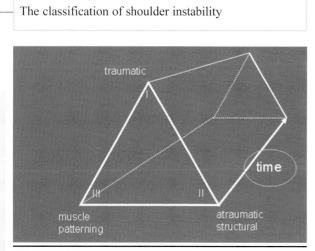

Figure 2. The aetiology of instability can change over time.

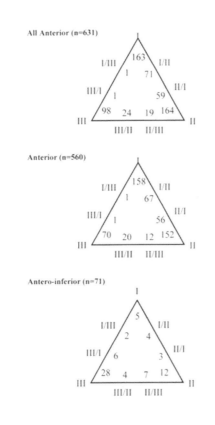

Figure 3. The distribution of diagnoses for anterior instability, distinguishing antero-inferior instability. Muscle-patterning instability (type III) predominates (39%) in this subgroup, whereas for anterior instability as a whole muscle patterning is responsible for about 15% of the presentations, and is largely due to inappropriate activity of pectoralis major. The numbers refer to numbers of shoulders studied.

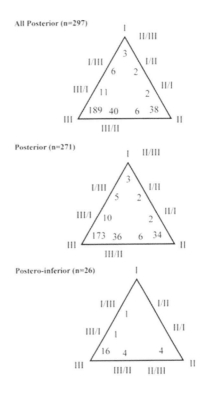

Figure 4. The distribution of diagnoses for posterior instability distinguishing postero-inferior instability. Muscle-patterning instability (type III) is as common (61%) in this subgroup as for posterior instability as a whole (63%). Latissimus dorsi, or anterior deltoid acting on a suppressed infraspinatus are the most common effectors of instability, although pectoralis major is also important. The numbers refer to numbers of shoulders studied.

abnormalities, and; muscle-patterning (inappropriate muscle activity). One, two or all three can be present in the same patient. The relationship between these elements is dynamic, and treatment should recognise the relevance of each. The current RNOH concept is that muscle patterning should be corrected before attending to the other causal factors: abnormal muscular force-couples will destroy a good capsular repair quickly unless dealt with pre-operatively.

The synthesis of the DEMG and demographic analysis of the entire instability dataset support the concept of an inter-relationship which can be defined as a triangle, with pure traumatic structural, atraumatic structural, and muscle-patterning groups represented at the apices of the triangle (Figure 1a). By convention these are labelled polar groups I, II, and III respectively. The intervening axes, joining neighbouring apices, describe the spectrum of instabilities which exist as compound conditions, i.e. trauma with atraumatic structural, atraumatic structural with muscle-patterning, and so on. These axes are labelled as subsets I/II, II/I, etc. and describe the relative proportion of the contribution of each pathology to the overall diagnosis. The space between any axis and the opposing apex represents the gradient of influence of the apical component in the instability. For instance, as we pass from the II-III axis towards the polar I apex, there is an increasing amount of trauma involved in the production of instability (Figure 1b). Similarly, as we pass from the I-II axis towards the polar III apex so increasing amounts of muscle patterning are implicated in the specific instability present (Figure 1c). As we pass from the I-III axis towards the polar II apex so increasing amounts of capsular/collagen insufficiency are implicated (Figure 1d) This schema can, therefore, be used to describe any instability, and any combination of instabilities. The utility of the schema has been demonstrated by others [17]. The evolution of instability over time (e.g. in response to treatment) can be mapped with the addition of a z-axis to represent time (Figure 2). The data for the entire set (Figures 3 and 4), and for single-diagnosis and multiple-diagnosis MDI (Figure 5), illustrate the value of the Stanmore classification as being inclusive of those cases excluded by other systems while clarifying the appropriate treatment path **(IV/C)** (Figure 6).

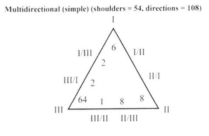

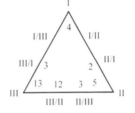

Figure 5. Multidirectional instability: single (simple) and multiple (complex) diagnoses. 'Single diagnosis' means that the pathology creating the instability in both or all directions is the same. 'Multiple diagnosis' means that the pathology of each direction of instability is different. It follows that the treatment of a case in subgroup III/II in the multiple-diagnosis MDI set is different for each direction; an inferior capsular shift might be the appropriate intervention for the II component, but the III (muscle-patterning) component should also be considered, and almost universally should be treated first. Many patients experience satisfactory return of sufficient stability with successful treatment of the III component (which is easier in the un-operated shoulder) and choose not to proceed to capsular surgery. The numbers refer to numbers of shoulders studied.

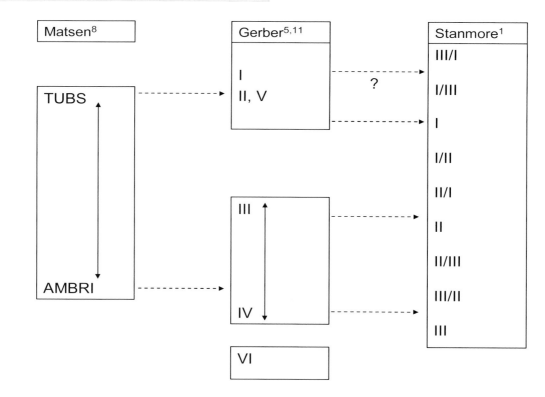

Note that the Stanmore classification includes the diagnoses of the other methods, but also allows for the inclusion of the concepts of active muscle-patterning promotion of instability, and the presence of more than one pathology, and allows for changing pathology over time.

Key:

Matsen classification

TUBS: Traumatic, Unidirectional, Bankart lesion, Surgery;
AMBRI: Atraumatic, Multidirectional, Bilateral, Rehabilitation, Inferior capsular shift;

Gerber classification

I: chronic dislocation
II: unidirectional instability without hyperlaxity
III: unidirectional instability with hyperlaxity
IV: multidirectional instability with hyperlaxity
V: multidirectional instability without hyperlaxity
VI: voluntary instability;

Stanmore classification

I: traumatic structural instability
II: atraumatic structural instability
III: muscle-patterning instability

Figure 6. A comparison of three classifications for GHI.

Conclusions

A classification system for GHI (and other joints) has to:

* accommodate more than one pathology;
* allow for a continuum of pathology;
* allow for changing pathology over time;
* allow treatment to proceed logically and evolve as the pathology changes.

The Stanmore classification encourages the clinician to consider all aspects of the specific GHI with which he is presented. The value of the classification lies in its reproducibility, reliability, inclusivity and validity in clinical practice.

Recommendations	Evidence level

The three main classification systems for shoulder instability are as follows:

* The TUBS-AMBRI classification emphasises the appreciation of the external applied force causing a dislocation, and the associated articular edge lesions, the traumatic Bankart or Perthe's lesion of the glenoid rim and the Hill-Sachs or Broca defect of the posterior humeral head. However, it does not accommodate the coexistence of traumatic and atraumatic causes of instability and the confounding existence of hyperlaxity. — IV/C
* Gerber's system includes the concept of underlying hyperlaxity as a risk factor for instability in some individuals. It was observed, however, that more than one pathology can be present in an unstable shoulder. — IV/C
* The Stanmore classification is more inclusive of those cases excluded by other systems, while clarifying the appropriate treatment path. — IV/C

References

1. Bayley JIL, Lewis A, Kitamura T. The classification of shoulder instability. New light through old windows. *Curr Orthop* 2005; 18: 97-108.
2. Kronberg M, Nemeth G, Brostrom L-A. Muscle activity and coordination in the normal shoulder. An electromyographic study. *Clin Orthop Relat Res* 1990; 257: 76-85.
3. Barden JM, Balyk R, Raso VJ, *et al*. Atypical shoulder muscle activation in multidirectional instability. *Clinical Neurophysiology* 2005; 116: 1846-57.
4. Maruyama K, Sano S, Saito K, *et al*. Trauma-instability-voluntarism classification for glenohumeral instability. *J Shoulder Elbow Surg* 1995; 4(3): 194-8.
5. Gerber C, Nyffeler RW. Classification of glenohumeral instability. *Clin Orthop Relat Res* 2002; 400: 65-76.
6. McMahon PJ, Lee TQ. Muscles may contribute to shoulder dislocation and stability. *Clin Orthop Relat Res* 2002; (403 Suppl): S18-25.
7. Cofield RH, Irving JF. Evaluation and classification of shoulder instability. With special reference to examination under anesthesia. *Clin Orthop Relat Res* 1987; 223: 32-43.
8. Thomas SC, Matsen FA III. An approach to the repair of avulsion of the glenohumeral ligaments in the management of traumatic anterior glenohumeral instability. *J Bone Joint Surg Am* 1989; 71A: 506-13.
9. Rowe CR, Pierce DS, Clark JG. Voluntary dislocation of the shoulder. A preliminary report on a clinical, electromyographic, and psychiatric study of twenty-six patients. *J Bone Joint Surg Am* 1973; 55A: 445-60.
10. Neer CS II, Foster CR. Inferior capsular shift for involuntary inferior and multidirectional instability of the shoulder: a preliminary report. *J Bone Joint Surg Am* 1980; 62A: 897-908.
11. Gerber C. Les instabilites de l'epaule. In: *Cahiers d'enseignement de la SOFCOT*, no.33. Paris: Expansion Scientifique Francaise, 1988: 51.

Chapter 8

12. Burkhead WZ Jr, Rockwood CA Jr. Treatment of instability of the shoulder with an exercise programme. *J Bone Joint Surg Am* 1992; 74A: 890.

13. Deol RS, Malone AA, Jaggi A, *et al*. Recurrent posterior shoulder instability: analysis and classification of 222 cases presenting to a tertiary referral unit. Abstract: Proceedings of the 16th Annual Scientific Meeting, The British Elbow and Shoulder Society, Cambridge, 2005.

14. Jaggi A, Malone AA, Cowan J, *et al*. The prevalence of inappropriate muscle sequencing in recurrent shoulder instability. Abstract: Proceedings of the 9th International Congress on Surgery of the Shoulder, Washington, 2004.

15. Noorani AM, Malone AA, Jaggi A. The role of dynamic electromyography in muscle patterning instability. Abstract: Proceedings of the 17th Annual Scientific Meeting, The British Elbow and Shoulder Society, Edinburgh, 2006.

16. Malone AA, Jaggi A, Lambert SM, *et al*. Demographic differences between structural and muscle-patterning instability. Abstract: Proceedings of the 17th Annual Scientific Meeting, The British Elbow and Shoulder Society, Edinburgh, 2006.

17. Gibson JC, Frostick SP, Sinopidis CS. Involuntary positional instability: when rehabilitation fails, is botulinum toxin the answer? Abstract: Proceedings of the 15th Annual Scientific Meeting, The British Elbow and Shoulder Society, Cardiff, 2004.

Chapter 9

Arthroscopic shoulder stabilisation

Jonathan J Gregory BSc MB ChB MRCS

Specialist Registrar, Orthopaedic Surgery

Stuart M Hay MB ChB FRCS FRCS (Orth)

Consultant Orthopaedic Surgeon

Specialist in Shoulder and Elbow Surgery

ROBERT JONES AND AGNES HUNT ORTHOPAEDIC HOSPITAL, OSWESTRY, UK
AND THE ROYAL SHREWSBURY HOSPITAL, SHREWSBURY, UK

Introduction

Dislocation of the glenohumeral joint is the most common large joint dislocation with an incidence of 1-2% [1] and a prevalence rate of 19.7 per 10,000 [2]. Contact sports and direct trauma to the shoulder, such as in road traffic accidents, are leading causes of anterior shoulder dislocation, but it may occur with lower energy mechanisms if the shoulder is in the 'at risk' position of abduction and external rotation. Pure anterior and antero-inferior dislocation represent 98% of shoulder dislocations.

The shoulder is stabilised by static and dynamic constraints. The static constraints include: the shape of the humeral head and glenoid, the labrum, the capsule, the coracohumeral ligament, the coraco-acromial ligament, the negative intra-articular pressure and the superior, middle and inferior glenohumeral ligaments. The dynamic stabilisers are the muscles of the rotator cuff which act to centralise the humeral head within the glenoid, the long head of biceps and the muscles stabilising the scapula.

The intra-articular pathology resulting from glenohumeral dislocation is varied. Sixty to ninety percent of traumatic shoulder dislocations will cause an antero-inferior capsulolabral avulsion (Bankart lesion). Previously, it was thought that this lesion alone was responsible for instability and redislocation. Recently, the importance of the inferior glenohumeral ligament as a humeral head restraint has been recognised and failure to address this structure at the same time as the Bankart lesion may be a cause of surgical failure.

Fractures of the posterior humeral head, known as Hill-Sachs lesions, are found in most patients after anterior dislocation, secondary to the humeral head being jammed against the anterior lip of the glenoid. Large Hill-Sachs lesions (approximately 30% of the humeral head) may engage with the anterior glenoid on external rotation and act to promote redislocation. Fractures of the antero-inferior glenoid, known as bony Bankart lesions, will often occur as a result of anterior dislocation and may predispose to recurrent dislocation. Other lesions include: avulsion of the glenohumeral ligaments from their humeral rather than glenoid attachment (HAGL lesion); superior labral tears (SLAP lesions); and anterior labral-ligamentous periosteal sleeve avulsions (ALPSA). All the intra-articular pathology must be considered when planning possible surgical intervention and in deciding between open and arthroscopic methods.

Methodology

Medline (1951-date), Embase (1974-date) and the Cochrane library were electronically searched using thesaurus headings for English language articles. Searches involved the subject headings 'shoulder', 'dislocation', 'instability', 'arthroscopy' and 'surgery'. Abstracts were appraised for their relevance and methodology. Studies were also located from the bibliographies of articles identified from the database search. The focus of this chapter will be on the evidence for arthroscopic stabilisation in the management of traumatic anterior glenohumeral dislocation.

Recurrent anterior glenohumeral instability

Instability describes an abnormal degree of translation of the humeral head relative to the glenoid, producing symptoms. Laxity, however, is normal translation of the humeral head over the glenoid surface. Instability is further classified by its aetiology (traumatic or atraumatic), direction (anterior, inferior, posterior or multidirectional), magnitude (micro-instability, subluxation or dislocation) and whether it is voluntary or involuntary.

Several studies have looked at the natural history of non-operatively managed traumatic anterior shoulder dislocation. Hovelius *et al* [3] in a ten-year study demonstrated a redislocation and instability rate of 48%. Simonet *et al* [4] had a redislocation rate of 33% and problems of painful instability in 20% in a general population study over nine years. There are many other studies in addition to these giving varying rates of redislocation from 17% to 100%. The prognosis appears to be intimately associated with the patient's age at first dislocation. In patients aged under 30, a redislocation rate of 75% is often quoted, falling to 50% in patients over 30. The rate of recurrence is greatest in patients under the age of 20 at first dislocation. The effect of age on redislocation may represent anatomical and histological differences compared to older patients. Younger patients are also more likely to return to collision sports, putting greater demands upon the shoulder. Large humeral head

defects and glenoid rim fractures are also a cause of increased rates of redislocation and instability.

The high rate of recurrent instability following non-operatively treated glenohumeral dislocation may in part be due to the position of immobilisation. Recent studies have suggested that immobilisation in internal rotation as traditionally practised may hinder the healing of Bankart lesions [5, 6]. However, placing the arm in external rotation appears to improve the chance of Bankart lesions healing in their anatomical position. External rotation splints are available to treat first-time glenohumeral dislocations and initial results with these have been promising [7], although results of larger studies are awaited **(IIb/B)**.

Open surgical treatment

When reviewing the evidence for a recent technical advance, the results must be viewed in the context of the established gold standard treatment. Prior to the development of arthroscopic shoulder stabilisation, a variety of open procedures have been used to treat instability. The Putti-Platt, Bristow, Laterjet, inferior capsular shift and Bankart procedures are amongst the most well known open procedures, with the Bankart procedure being the most widely used of these techniques. This was described by Rowe *et al* [8] and has since been modified to use suture anchors rather than curved drill holes to hold sutures to pull the avulsed capsulolabral complex onto the anterior glenoid rim. Low rates of recurrence are quoted for open Bankart procedures. Rowe *et al* [8] had a 3.5% recurrence rate in 146 shoulders with a mean follow-up of six years **(III/B)**. Similarly, Hovelius *et al* [9] had a 1.5% recurrence rate in 46 patients and Gill *et al* [10] had a 5% recurrence rate in 60 shoulders at a mean follow-up of 11.9 years. Some of these series, however, contain significant numbers of patients with only medium-term follow-up, the mean being distorted by patients with extremely long follow-up periods, e.g. Rowe *et al* had 145 patients followed-up from 1-5 years and 48 for 5-30 years giving a mean of six years. When followed-up for longer periods it has been suggested that the recurrence rate may be higher than that often quoted. Magnusson *et al* [11] reported a recurrence rate of subluxation or dislocation of 17%

with a four to nine-year follow-up of 54 shoulders. However, the redislocations (11%) all occurred within five years of surgery as did the episodes of subluxation (6%). It is noteworthy that the definitions of failure are often interpreted differently in older papers which refer to open procedures, as compared to more recent articles which refer to arthroscopic techniques.

A reduction in external rotation may be produced by open surgery, the magnitude of which depends on the procedure involved. The measured reduction in external rotation may be in the order of 7-12°, as compared to the contralateral limb [10, 11], which for high performance athletes or those involved in throwing activities may prove significant.

Arthroscopic stabilisation for recurrent instability

The benefits of arthroscopic shoulder stabilisation surgery, compared to open procedures, include reductions in: blood loss, requirement for opiate analgesia, hospital stay, time off work, operating time and complications [12]. There are also benefits in terms of reduced scarring and patient acceptability. Until recently, these benefits were felt to be at the expense of a higher rate of dislocation and subluxation after arthroscopic stabilisation.

Evolution of arthroscopic stabilisation

Several methods of arthroscopic repair have been described. Initially, staples were used to secure the detached labrum to the glenoid. This technique had a high failure rate of up to 50% [13]. Some authors were able to achieve adequate results [14, 15], but acknowledged the technical difficulty involved. Further work on the complications of using staples within the shoulder joint [16] led to this technique being discontinued.

The use of transglenoid sutures to repair the Bankart lesion then became the focus of attention [17]. This technique involved placing sutures through the avulsed labrum using a punch (Caspari punch). Drill holes were then created through the scapular neck through which the sutures were passed before being tied. They were tied superficially to the muscles on the scapula (which occasionally caused injury to the suprascapular nerve). There are many published series involving this technique with mixed results.

Two studies in patients suffering only a single dislocation (rather than recurrent instability) have recurrence rates of approximately 15% after surgery. Arciero *et al* used transglenoid sutures and reduced the redislocation rate from 80% in a non-operative group to 14% in the operative group [18]. Kirkley *et al* performed a randomised trial of transglenoid suturing versus non-operative treatment [19]. Three of 16 patients in the surgical group (18.75%) and nine of 15 patients in the non-operative group (68%) suffered redislocation.

Late failure is not uncommon with transglenoid suture techniques, as evidenced by two studies. Calvo *et al* had a failure rate of 18% as defined by recurrent instability, in 61 patients followed-up for a mean of 44.5 months [20]. The mean time of failure was 26 months (6-46). Hubbell *et al* performed a non-randomised retrospective review of 30 patients who had undergone arthroscopic transglenoid suture repair and 20 who had been treated with open capsule-labral repair [21]. At five years, 17% of patients had suffered a frank dislocation and 60% had instability after arthroscopic repair. There were no dislocations or reports of instability in the open surgery group.

Freedman *et al* performed a meta-analysis of open Bankart repair against transglenoid sutures and bio-absorbable tacks [22]. Six small studies formed the meta-analysis. Within the analysis there were 77 patients from four studies who underwent transglenoid suture repair. The rate of recurrent dislocation was 13% (confidence interval 95% 8%-21%) compared to 3% in the open surgery group (95% confidence interval 2%-6%). The total rate of recurrence (dislocation and subluxation) was even higher at 23% (95% confidence interval 13%-37%) compared to 10% in the open surgery group (95% confidence interval 8%-13%) (p<0.0001).

Transglenoid suture fixation has generally been abandoned. The causes for its failure have been explored. With both staple fixation and transglenoid suturing there is a tendency for the labrum to be medialised as it is reattached. Rather than being placed on to the anterolateral aspect of the glenoid, the labrum was fixed to the surface of the scapular neck, which reduced the ability of the labrum to resist humeral head translation. By placing the repair onto the edge of the glenoid, Savoie *et al* were able to improve their results [17].

The high failure rate of transglenoid suture repairs led to experiments with tack fixation, e.g. Suretac. The tacks were based on a cannulated system using guidewires. A guidewire was used to position the labrum onto the glenoid. The labrum and glenoid were drilled using a cannulated drill over a guidewire and an absorbable tack was then inserted over the wire. The tack had wings to lock it into the glenoid and a head that tethered the labrum in position.

Open and arthroscopic tack stabilisation were compared in a non-randomised study with a follow-up of two to six years [23]. The authors concluded that the results of the two techniques were similar. However, the numbers were small (37 arthroscopic, and 22 open) and the decision regarding the choice of arthroscopic or open repair was based on arthroscopic findings. Therefore, the two groups were not matched, with the more difficult cases receiving open repair. Karlsson *et al* [24] presented a consecutive series of 119 shoulders in randomised patients prospectively followed-up, comparing open and arthroscopic Bankart repair. The recurrence rate of subluxation and dislocation at a mean of 28 months in the arthroscopic tack fixation group was 15% (nine of 60). The open repairs had a lower rate of 10% (five of 48) recurrence over a longer period of follow-up (36 months). A prospective randomised study of 56 patients again demonstrated increased recurrence in arthroscopic tack repair, compared to open surgery (23% vs 12%) within two years of the index procedure [25]. In Freedman's meta-analysis, arthroscopic bioabsorbable tacks had a significantly higher rate of failure compared to open repair [22]. The analysis had 90 patients in the tack repair group and 156 in the open surgery group. Total rate of failure (dislocation and subluxation) was 18% (95% CI 13%-23%) in the bioabsorbable tack group, compared to 10% (95% CI 8%-13%) in the open

group ($p < 0.0001$). There was also a significantly higher rate of failure when recurrent dislocation alone is compared.

The techniques discussed all had unacceptably high rates of failure; however, these studies have each contributed to the evolution of improved techniques in arthroscopic Bankart repair.

Suture anchor repair of Bankart lesions

Wolf *et al* performed some of the early work using bone suture anchors to perform arthroscopic Bankart repair [26]. The technique involves preparation of the detached labrum by freeing it up from surrounding tissues to allow its accurate reduction on to the glenoid and then preparation of the glenoid surface including drill holes. The drill holes are at the most lateral point of the glenoid or may even just encroach onto the articular surface. Efforts are made to avoid any medialisation of the reattached labrum. Drill holes are placed at approximately 1cm intervals around the glenoid in the area of labral detachment. One of the most important aspects of arthroscopic shoulder stabilisation is the skilled technique of passing suture material through the labrum in order to facilitate accurate reconstruction of the capsulolabral tissue. Considerable research and effort has been expended by companies in the development of equipment to achieve this. Examples of such include the Linvatec Spectrum and the Caspari punch, although many others are available. Sutures are used to 'lead' the definitive suture through the labrum or indeed the definitive suture may be used initially, thereby obviating the need for a lead suture. The definitive suture is attached to a bone anchor which is then driven or screwed into the adjacent drill hole and the labrum thereby reconstructed with either a 'knotted' or a 'knotless' technique. The anchors may be either metallic or bioabsorbable. As the capsulolabral tissue is reduced to the glenoid, a 'bumper' of tissue is produced to resist humeral head translation and in the process, the anterior band of the inferior glenohumeral ligament (IGHL) is also re-tensioned. Sometimes there is no obvious Bankart lesion and the procedure will involve arthroscopic plication of the capsuloligamentous tissue alone. One of the author's own examples of this is demonstrated in Figures 1-3.

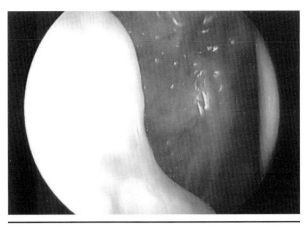

Figure 1. Showing the anterior right glenoid in the foreground, with an absent labrum and slack capsule in the background. Viewed from the posterior portal.

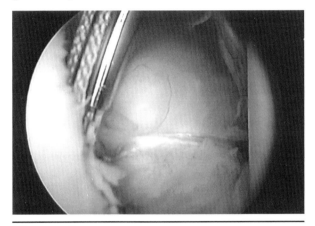

Figure 2. Showing Mitek bioknotless anchor placement into the anterior glenoid, drawing capsulolabral tissue firmly on to the glenoid. Viewed from the posterior portal.

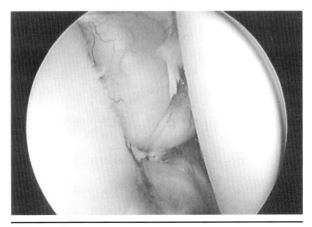

Figure 3. Showing reconstruction of the capsulo-labral 'bumper' on the antero-inferior glenoid. Viewed from the posterior portal.

In this case the labral tissue was completely detached and sitting in the inferior recess. Using a bioknotless system (Mitek) the bumper has been reconstructed.

Two of the studies with good results utilise metallic suture anchors. Burkhart and De Beer [27] retrospectively reviewed 194 consecutive arthroscopic Bankart repairs using metallic suture anchors. Their study population contained a large number of patients at high risk of recurrence due to involvement in contact sports (previously a relative contraindication to arthroscopic repair). Overall, they had 21 recurrent dislocations and subluxations in their study (10.8%) **(III/B)**. This is good considering that 101 patients were involved in contact sport. They analysed their results to try and identify risk factors for recurrence. They identified significant glenoid bone loss or engaging Hill-Sachs lesions as risk factors for failure. There were 21 patients with significant bone defects and in this subgroup there were 14 recurrences (67%). In the 173 patients without significant bone defects, there were only seven recurrences (4%). Even in the collision athletes the recurrence rate was only 6.5% when no significant bone loss had occurred.

Fabbriciani et al [28] performed one of the few prospective randomised studies in this area. They randomised 60 patients to open or arthroscopic Bankart repair utilising metallic suture anchors. The follow-up time was only 24 months in each group; however, at this time there were no episodes of dislocation in either group **(Ib/A)**. No subluxation rate is quoted but there were no significant differences in Constant and Rowe scores, except for range of motion which was significantly larger in the arthroscopic surgery group. Weaknesses of the study are that no power calculations are described and the period of follow-up is too short to detect late failure. The study only included patients with a Bankart lesion; there were no patients with capsule, tendon or glenoid injury. The exclusion of patients with capsular lesions does limit the conclusions that can be drawn from this paper.

Each of these studies provide evidence that results comparable to open surgery are achievable with arthroscopic suture anchor techniques. Unfortunately, metallic anchors have recently become less popular due to concerns expressed about the proximity of the metalwork to an articular surface. Should they be misplaced or loosen then considerable damage may be caused and in the event of secondary surgery they may be very troublesome to find and to retrieve.

Bioabsorbable suture anchors have therefore been developed, e.g. Mitek, Arthrex etc. During this development there has also been a change in operative strategy as mentioned previously. There has been a move to address other pathology within the shoulder at the time of stabilisation not just repair of the avulsed labral lesion. Cadaveric work has previously indicated that a Bankart lesion alone may be insufficient to permit humeral head dislocation [29]. The rotator interval, superior labral or 'SLAP' lesion and the capsular ligamentous complex (especially the inferior glenohumeral ligament) are often addressed. Thermal shrinkage of the capsule has also been used in some studies to augment repairs. When reviewing the results of bioabsorbable suture anchor repair and when comparing them to other arthroscopic techniques it should be remembered that the method of fixation is usually not the only difference between the techniques.

Gartsman et al [30] presented two to five-year results of bioabsorbable suture anchor repair of Bankart lesions. They systematically addressed all associated pathology in addition to the Bankart lesion: SLAP lesion, capsule, rotator interval and then undertook thermal capsulorrhaphy if they felt it was required. This was a prospective study and included all patients with a diagnosis of antero-inferior instability. It did not exclude patients with other intra-articular pathology. The 53 patients involved had a mean follow-up of 33 months. There were two patients who had frank dislocation and two with recurrent subluxation postoperatively, giving a 7.5% failure rate (III/B). An identical failure rate occurred in a prospective study of 40 patients followed-up to an average of 30 months [31]. The population involved were young, had suffered two or more dislocations and played high-risk sports. One of the failures occurred after a road traffic accident and two after sporting incidents (one of these occurred in a patient who failed to complete rehabilitation).

A case controlled study of 89 shoulders in 88 patients compared suture anchors to open surgical Bankart repair [32]. There were two patients in the open

surgery group (total 30 shoulders) and two in the arthroscopic surgery group (total 59 shoulders) who suffered postoperative redislocation (6.7% vs 3.4%). When symptoms of apprehension were also included as failure, the failure rate was almost equal between the two groups; 10% after open surgery and 10.2% after arthroscopic repair (III/B). A single-surgeon series from the same department has presented two to six-year results in 167 patients after suture anchor repair [33]. Seven patients had recurrent instability. This included four patients who had anterior apprehension on testing; one frank dislocation and two patients with subluxation, at a mean of 44 months follow-up. This gives a failure rate of 4%. Analysis of the patients who suffered failure of the index procedure found a significant association with glenoid bone defects. Where such defects were greater than 30% of the glenoid circumference this was considered a significant risk factor for failure. This supports the findings of Burkhart and De Beer discussed earlier [27].

These studies demonstrate a marked improvement in the results of arthroscopic shoulder stabilisation. Some of this is due to improvement in fixation technique, whilst some is due to the simultaneous recognition and treatment of other lesions causing instability. A consistent cause of failure of arthroscopic stabilisation is the presence of significant glenoid bone defects irrespective of the method of labral fixation [20, 27, 33]. It is generally recommended that such patients should undergo open reconstruction in the form of a Bristow-Laterjet-type procedure or bony augmentation (III/B).

Involvement in collision and contact sports is also often quoted as a relative contraindication to arthroscopic repair. However, good results have been obtained even within this population [27, 31] (III/B). Younger patients have previously had a higher rate of failure with arthroscopic stabilisation [17, 20, 30], but in more recent studies where all contributing factors leading to instability have been addressed arthroscopically, there is often no significant difference in age between the surgical failures and the successes.

First-time glenohumeral dislocation

Several studies have looked at the role of early stabilisation surgery following first-time traumatic glenohumeral dislocation. Early surgery was rarely considered when only the open techniques were available, but with the advent of arthroscopic stabilisation this is now a more common practice. Arthroscopic surgery is usually more acceptable to patients and has a recovery time similar to non-operatively managed dislocation.

We have not identified any studies comparing current best surgical technique (suture anchor repair and capsulolabral re-tensioning) against non-operative treatment, in the management of first-time anterior glenohumeral dislocation. In Arciero's series, the now superseded technique of transglenoid suture repair reduced redislocation rates from 80% in the non-operative group to 14% in the operative group [18]. Kirkley et al also reduced redislocation rates from 68% in the non-operative group to 18.75% in the operative group, treated with transglenoid sutures, at an average follow-up of 75 months [19]. On questioning, they found no difference in shoulder function between these groups. They concluded by recommending surgery for first-time dislocators, but acknowledged that 40% of patients would undergo surgery they probably did not require. The introduction of superior arthroscopic techniques since this report, with apparent lower recurrence rates, has been influential in some surgeons offering surgery for first-time dislocation, especially amongst the sporting populus.

However, the pendulum may now swing slightly in the opposite direction with the introduction of splints to be worn following first-time dislocation, designed to hold the arm in external rotation, thereby promoting healing of labral avulsions. The success of this simple, non-operative technique is the subject of intense research interest and may result in reduced rates of redislocation.

Conclusions

Arthroscopic stabilisation of the shoulder has evolved considerably since its conception and continues to do so. In our analysis of the evidence it is clear that many of the older studies present techniques which have now been superseded and distort the results, suggesting higher failure rates than is genuinely the case. In fact, with appropriate patient selection, failure rates in the order of 5% are probably achievable, even including contact sportsmen, but where the bony glenoid is deficient, an open procedure is often indicated.

It can be a technically demanding procedure but in the hands of an experienced shoulder surgeon arthroscopic stabilisation probably has results comparable to open stabilisation.

Recommendations	Evidence level
◆ Arthroscopic suture anchor fixation using metallic anchors can have results equivalent to open surgery †.	Ib/A
◆ Arthroscopic bioabsorbable suture anchors have results comparable to open surgery.	III/B
◆ Splinting the arm in external rotation after first-time traumatic anterior dislocation appears to reduce the incidence of recurrent instability.	IIb/B
◆ Collision athletes can be managed arthroscopically with bioabsorbable suture anchors.	III/B
◆ Patients with large glenoid or humeral head bony defects should be managed using open surgery due to high recurrence rates after arthroscopic procedures.	III/B

† However, concerns over possible articular surface damage or difficulty of future revision surgery or arthroplasty have led to a move away from metallic suture anchors.

References

1. Hovelius L. Incidence of shoulder dislocation in Sweden. *Clin Orthop* 1982; 166: 127-31.

2. Milgram C, Mann G, Finestone A. A prevalence study of recurrent shoulder dislocations in young adults. *J Shoulder Elbow Surg* 1998; 7: 621-4.

3. Hovelius L, Lind B, Thorling J. Primary anterior dislocation of the shoulder in young patients: a ten-year prospective study. *J Bone Joint Surg Am* 1996; 78-A: 1677-84.

4. Simonet WT, Cofield RH. Prognosis in anterior shoulder dislocation. *Am J Sports Med* 1984; 12: 19-24.

5. Itoi E, Sashi R, Minagawa H, *et al.* Position of immobilisation after dislocation of the glenohumeral joint: a study with use of magnetic resonance imaging. *J Bone Joint Surg Am* 2001; 83-A: 661-7.

6. Hart WJ, Kelly CP. Arthroscopic observation of capsulolabral reduction after shoulder dislocation. *J Shoulder Elbow Surg* 2005; 14: 134-7.

7. Itoi E, Hatakeyama Y, Kido T, *et al.* A new method of immobilisation after traumatic anterior dislocation of the shoulder: a preliminary study. *J Shoulder Elbow Surg* 2003; 12: 413-5.

8. Rowe CR, Patel D, Southmayd WW. The Bankart Procedure. A long-term end-result study. *J Bone Joint Surg* 1978; 60-A: 1-16.

9. Hovelius L, Thorling J, Fredin H. Recurrent anterior dislocation of the shoulder. Results after the Bankart and Putti-Platt operations. *J Bone Joint Surg* 1979; 61-A: 566-9.

10. Gill TJ, Micheli LJ, Gebhard F, Binder C. Bankart repair for anterior instability of the shoulder. *J Bone Joint Surg* 1997; 79-A: 850-7.

11. Magnusson L, Kartus J, Ejerhed L, *et al.* Revisiting the open Bankart experience - a four to nine-year follow-up. *Am J Sports Med* 2002; 30: 778-82.

12. Green MR, Christensen KP. Arthroscopic versus open Bankart procedures: a comparison of early morbidity and complications. *Arthroscopy* 1993; 9: 371-4.

13. Gross RM. Arthroscopic shoulder capsulorrhaphy: does it work? *Am J Sports Med* 1989; 17: 495-500.

14. Detrisac DA, Johnson LL. Arthroscopic shoulder capsulorrhaphy using metal staples. *Orthop Clin N Am* 1993; 24(1): 71-88.

15. Wheeler JH, Ryan JB, Arciero RA, *et al.* Arthroscopic versus nonoperative treatment of acute shoulder dislocations in young athletes. *Arthroscopy* 1989; 5: 213-7.

16. Zucherman JD, Matsen FA III. Complications about the glenohumeral joint related to the use of screws and staples. *J Bone Joint Surg* 1984; 66-A: 175-80.

17. Savoie FH III, Miller CD, Field LD. Arthroscopic reconstruction of traumatic anterior instability of the shoulder: the Caspari technique. *Arthroscopy* 1997; 13: 201-9.

18. Arciero RA, Wheeler JH, Ryan JB, *et al.* Arthroscopic Bankart repair versus non-operative treatment for acute, initial anterior shoulder dislocations. *Am J Sports Med* 1994; 22: 589-94.

19. Kirkley A, Werstine R, Ratjek A, Griffin S. Prospective randomized clinical trial comparing effectiveness of immediate arthroscopic stabilisation versus immobilisation and rehabilitation in first traumatic anterior dislocations of the shoulder. Long-term evaluation. *Arthroscopy* 2005; 21: 55-63.

20. Calvo E, Granizo JJ, Fernandez D, *et al.* Criteria for arthroscopic treatment of anterior instability of the shoulder. *J Bone Joint Surg Br* 2005; 87-B: 677-83.

21. Hubbell JD, Ahmad S, Bezenoff LS, *et al.* Comparison of shoulder stabilisation using arthroscopic transglenoid sutures versus open capsulolabral repairs. *Am J Sports Med* 2004; 32: 650-4.

22. Freedman KB, Smith AP, Romeo AA, *et al.* Open Bankart repair versus arthroscopic repair with transglenoid sutures or bioabsorbable tacks for recurrent anterior instability of the shoulder. *Am J Sports Med* 2004; 32: 1520-905.

23. Cole BJ, L'Insalata J, Irrgang J, Warner JP. Comparison of arthroscopic and open anterior shoulder stabilisation. *J Bone Joint Surg Am* 2000; 82-A: 1108-14.

24. Karlsson J, Magnusson L, Ejerhed L, *et al.* Comparison of open and arthroscopic stabilisation for recurrent shoulder dislocation in patients with a Bankart lesion. *Am J Sports Med* 2001; 29: 538-42.

25. Sperber A, Hamberg P, Karlsson J, *et al.* Comparison of an arthroscopic and open procedure for posttraumatic instability of the shoulder: a prospective randomized multicenter study. *J Shoulder Elbow Surg* 2001; 10: 105-8.

26. Wolf EM, Wilk RM, Richmond JC. Arthroscopic Bankart repair using suture anchors. *Op Tech Orthop* 1991; 1: 184-91.

27. Burkhart SS, De Beer JF. Traumatic glenohumeral bone defects and their relationship to failure of arthroscopic Bankart repairs: significance of the inverted-pear glenoid and humeral engaging Hill-Sachs lesion. *Arthroscopy* 2000; 16: 677-94.

28. Fabbriciani C, Milano G, Demontis A, *et al.* Arthroscopic versus open treatment of Bankart lesion of the shoulder: a prospective randomised study. *Arthroscopy* 2004; 20: 456-62.

29. Speer KP, Deng X, Borrero S, *et al.* Biomechanical evaluation of a simulated Bankart lesion. *J Bone Joint Surg Am* 1994; 76-A: 1819-25.

30. Gartsman GM, Roddey TS, Hammerman SM. Arthroscopic treatment of anterior-inferior glenohumeral instability. *J Bone Joint Surg Am* 2000; 82-A: 991-1003.

31. Bacilla P, Field LD, Savoie FH. Arthroscopic Bankart repair in a high demand patient population. *Arthroscopy* 1997; 13: 51-60.

32. Kim SH, Ha KI, Kim SH. Bankart repair in traumatic anterior instability: open versus arthroscopic technique. *Arthroscopy* 2002; 18: 755-63.

33. Kim SH, Ha KI, Cho YB, *et al.* Arthroscopic anterior stabilisation of the shoulder. *J Bone Joint Surg Am* 2003; 85-A: 1511-8.

Chapter 10

Arthroscopic rotator cuff repair

David JJ Miller MB ChB MRCS

Specialist Registrar

Stuart M Hay MB ChB FRCS FRCS (Orth)

Consultant Orthopaedic Surgeon

Specialist in Shoulder and Elbow Surgery

ROBERT JONES AND AGNES HUNT ORTHOPAEDIC HOSPITAL, OSWESTRY, UK
AND THE ROYAL SHREWSBURY HOSPITAL, SHREWSBURY, UK

Introduction

Open and mini-open techniques for rotator cuff repair are well established and still considered by many to be the gold standard. However, advances in arthroscopic surgery have allowed many experienced shoulder surgeons to treat rotator cuff tears with minimally invasive procedures. Improved surgical instrumentation, suture anchor design and the acquisition of arthroscopic skills have each contributed to the rise in popularity of the complete arthroscopic approach. Arthroscopic rotator cuff repair, although first described more than 17 years ago, remains in its infancy when compared with the open and mini-open techniques of repair.

The advantages of complete arthroscopic repair include improved postoperative pain relief, earlier and accelerated rehabilitation, improved cosmesis and minimisation of deltoid detachment or insult. However, concerns remain over the technical demands placed on the surgeon, as well as the security of repair.

Methodology

Medline (1951-date), Embase (1974-date) and the Cochrane Library were electronically searched using Thesaurus headings for English language articles. Searches involved the subject headings 'shoulder', 'rotator cuff', 'arthroscopy' and 'surgery'. Abstracts were appraised for their relevance and methodology. Studies were also located from the bibliographies of articles identified from the database search. The focus of this chapter is on the evidence for complete or all-arthroscopic rotator cuff repair in the management of full-thickness rotator cuff tears.

Natural history of rotator cuff tears

Rotator cuff tears are common and the incidence increases with age. Some studies report an incidence of 5% in patients in their fourth decade increasing to as much as 80% in the eighth decade [1]. Cadaveric studies have demonstrated a high incidence of cuff tears, from 5% to 39% [1], but in these studies no tears were reported in individuals under age 50.

There have been few reports on the natural history of rotator cuff tears, which remains poorly understood. It remains unclear why some rotator cuff tears become painful, whereas others remain asymptomatic. In fact, pain relief is observed with non-operative treatment, with improved relief over time. Indeed, non-operative management is expected to produce satisfactory pain relief in up to 50% of patients, compared to 85% using operative methods [2].

Interestingly, in a follow-up study, Yamaguchi found that 51% of previously asymptomatic patients with tears became symptomatic at a mean of 2.8 years [1] and in nine of the symptomatic patients from the original cohort of 23, 'tear progression' was identified. The consensus opinion is that cuff tears can initially be managed conservatively, and although a small number will progress over time, the process is slow and may not necessarily compromise function or become symptomatic [3, 4]. Subjecting older patients to massive cuff repairs in an attempt to prevent degenerative cuff arthropathy may be too high a risk-benefit ratio to justify.

Reports on the clinical and structural results following non-operative management of massive tears have noted both superior migration of the humeral head and an increase in tear size [5]. Fatty degeneration within the muscle bellies of the cuff muscles in this group also increased significantly and glenohumeral arthritis was more pronounced, especially with three-tendon tears. Other series have reported that 'massive' tears (i.e. tears greater than 5cm) treated non-operatively could have good clinical and functional results but the structural changes progress so that half of the previously reparable tears become irreparable within four years [5].

The indications for arthroscopic repair are similar to its open counterpart: persistent pain and reduced function impacting on the patient's activities of daily living, their work or their sport, unresponsive to 6-12 months of non-operative care. However, the surgeon's experience is perhaps the predominant factor in determining whether an arthroscopic approach is feasible.

Small to medium-size tears

Most studies report on rotator cuff tears of varying sizes. The consensus is that tears greater than 5cm are massive tears and for the purpose of this review we have included all other tear sizes in the small to medium group.

There are many controversial topics in the management of rotator cuff tears. The method of repair (open, mini-open or complete arthroscopic repair) is currently a hot topic and the evolution of arthroscopic shoulder surgery suggests that an all-arthroscopic technique will become the future gold standard.

Open repair was first described by Codman in 1911 [6]. An example of arthroscopic visualisation of a rotator cuff tear, followed by open repair is shown in Figures 1-3. Neer reported good results with anterior acromioplasty, mobilisation and repair [7] and emphasised the important principles which we still follow today, i.e. meticulous repair, adequate decompression, surgical release to allow mobile tendon units, secure fixation and closely supervised rehabilitation. Good success can certainly be achieved with this approach, but at the risk of deltoid injury with the potential devastating complication of deltoid detachment. The primary function of the rotator cuff has been studied in depth. Inman *et al* concluded that the primary function of repair is to balance force couples around the glenohumeral joint [8]. Indeed, adequate tension in the repair is now thought to be more important than a watertight closure [9].

Mini-open repair was initially described by Levy *et al* to reduce the risk of deltoid detachment [10]. It has since been validated by Paulos and Kody with 88% good to excellent clinical results, using the University of California Los Angeles (UCLA) scoring system [11]. However, mini-open repair has its limitations and is most suitable for the small to moderate-sized antero-superior tear, as the operative window is small.

Despite this limitation, another advantage of the mini-open repair was that glenohumeral arthroscopy, which is usually undertaken at the same sitting, identified a high incidence of coexistent intra-articular pathology, such as osteoarthrosis of the glenohumeral joint, a tear of the biceps tendon or glenoid labral tears [12, 13]. Indeed, up to 76% of patients were found to have additional intra-articular glenohumeral pathology, but in only 12.5% were these findings significant. In keeping with this, Gartsman *et al* found that mean pre-operative scores were better for those without intra-articular pathology than those who were

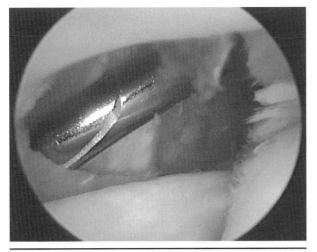

Figure 1. Shows the arthroscopic view of a rotator cuff tear. An instrument is seen within the subacromial space, through the hole in the cuff.

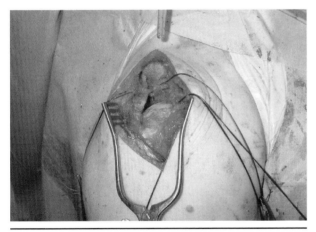

Figure 2. An open approach is made to the cuff. The humeral head is seen through the cuff tear.

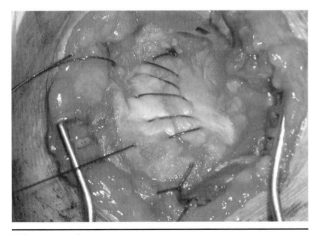

Figure 3. The cuff is repaired using a combination of continuous suture and interosseous reinforcement.

found to have additional pathology [13], although postoperative scores for the two groups were comparable once the coexistent pathology had been treated.

Furthermore, there have been reports of an increased incidence of frozen shoulder following mini-open repair, as compared to all-arthroscopic surgery [14, 15], although this is easily treated. Severud reported an improved range of motion in the all-arthroscopic group when compared to the mini-open group in a retrospective study of tears <5cm [15]. However, at final follow-up there was no significant difference in range of motion. In contrast, Youm et al reported arthrofibrosis in both treatment groups, although only two cases occurred in a cohort of 84 patients, which may have been spurious or need further investigation [16].

Complete arthroscopic repair

Complete arthroscopic repair frees the surgeon from the usual spatial constraints of a standard operative approach and allows the cuff to be approached from many different angles, in order to delineate the tear pattern more accurately, with the intention of repairing it anatomically. Early studies reported good results, but only for small to medium-size tears [17]. Other reports have also suggested less postoperative pain, accelerated rehabilitation and a good range of movement [18, 19] **(III/B)**.

Murray et al have also reported good clinical results with an all-arthroscopic technique for medium to large full-thickness tears. Indeed, 46 (95%) of a cohort of 48 had good or excellent results, with only one failed repair at medium-term follow-up [20].

Buess et al reported on a comparative study between open and arthroscopic cuff repair for all tear sizes [14]. They found that better pain relief and patient satisfaction were the main benefits of an all-arthroscopic technique, but otherwise the outcomes were similar in terms of complications and outcome scores.

Sauerbrey et al compared the clinical short-term outcomes of 26 mini-open with 28 all-arthroscopic cuff repairs and found improvement in American Shoulder Elbow Surgeon (ASES) scores in both groups, although this did not reach statistical significance [21]. Verma *et al* compared 38 patients undergoing an all-arthroscopic technique with 33 patients who had the mini-open repair for tears less than 5cm. There was no significant difference in pain or outcome scores at a two-year follow-up [22]. Interestingly, they also assessed the integrity of the cuff using ultrasound and found similar retear rates for the two groups. Not surprisingly, those who suffered retears were weaker in forward elevation and external rotation as compared to those whose repair remained intact, but they showed no difference in pain or overall outcome scores [16, 23, 24].

Recent objective evaluations using either ultrasound or MRI have demonstrated high failure rates of arthroscopic repair. Galatz *et al* reported on 18 patients that had arthroscopic repair of tears >2cm [25]. Recurrent tears were seen in 17 out of 18 patients on ultrasound at 12 months. Despite this they had ASES scores of ≥90 points in 13 patients, although this deteriorated to nine patients at 24 months. They felt that immediate rehabilitation with active-assisted pulley exercises may have contributed to early failure and recommended a more cautious rehabilitation protocol. Deterioration in outcome scores was also seen by Verma *et al* with retear rates of 24% for tears less than 5cm [22].

Jost *et al* noted that patients who suffered retears were less satisfied than patients with intact repairs [26]. They also noted that satisfaction rates for failed repairs correlated with those after arthroscopic debridement. The clinical outcomes at 7.6 years after structural failure, however, remained significantly improved over the pre-operative state in terms of pain, function, strength, and patient satisfaction.

Bishop *et al* reported on 32 patients who underwent mini-open repair and 40 patients who underwent all-arthroscopic repair, using MRI to assess cuff integrity [27] **(III/B)**. They found that retear rates were 26% for the mini-open group and 16% for the arthroscopic group for tears less than 3cm.

So far the literature suggests that arthroscopic repair of full-thickness tears produces equivalent clinical results to open and mini-open repair [15].

Reduced postoperative pain, accelerated rehabilitation and improved cosmetic appearance appear to be the main advantages, but as yet there have been no randomised studies comparing arthroscopic repair to mini-open or open repair. A group from Canada is currently setting up such a study [28]. The literature to date consists of poor quality evidence using case series to evaluate the outcome of surgical intervention. There have been studies comparing arthroscopic to mini-open repair, but these are neither blinded nor randomised and are retrospective, therefore at risk of bias [15]. The results are difficult to interpret. For instance, some of the early reports reserved arthroscopic repair for small tears whilst large and massive tears were managed by open repair. Also, different scoring systems are used throughout the literature making comparison extremely difficult.

Nevertheless, despite these limitations, the reports for complete arthroscopic rotator cuff repair have been positive, especially for the small to medium tears. High quality evidence is required to determine whether the move towards less invasive yet technically difficult procedures in cuff repair is justified. This, however, may be difficult to evaluate, given the inevitable differences in surgical ability and potential reluctance to participate.

Massive tears

Rotator cuff tears greater than 5cm are considered to be massive tears. Some reports found that pre-operative tear size is one of the major determinants of the results of rotator cuff repair. Massive cuff tears generally yield unfavourable results [29-31]. However, some authors have suggested that the clinical outcome of rotator cuff repair is independent of tear size [24, 32, 33]. Techniques such as subscapularis and latissimus dorsi tendon transfers, fascial autograft, and allograft implantation have been used to cover large defects. Several authors have now found that a watertight repair is not necessary and that balancing the force couples and restoring the function of the cuff is the primary goal [9, 34, 35].

Acromioplasty and rotator cuff debridement, as described by Rockwood, is an option in low-demand patients who are unsuitable for the demanding rehabilitation protocol [36, 37]. Several authors have reported good results with decompression and debridement without repair, with patient satisfaction rates equal to open repair [3, 37]. However, open repairs scored better for overall function and strength. Rockwood also noted that there was deterioration over time in these patients and that this was a useful technique only in selected cases. Other authors have reported inferior results with decompression and debridement alone compared with open repair [38]. Therefore, most surgeons would only resort to decompression and debridement alone after vigorous attempts at mobilisation and repair.

More recently massive tears have been repaired arthroscopically with good clinical results. Jones et al demonstrated 88% good to excellent clinical outcomes with equal results between large and massive tears at an average 32-month follow-up [35]. Indeed, they only reported one re-operation and six clinical failures (12%). These results are comparable to open repair (Bigliani 85% satisfactory results) [39]. However, objective imaging to assess cuff integrity is lacking in these studies.

A number of reports indicate a high failure rate of complete arthroscopic cuff repair identified on ultrasound or magnetic resonance imaging (MRI), especially for massive tears. Bishop et al reviewed 32 patients who underwent mini-open repair and 40 patients who underwent all-arthroscopic repair, using MRI to assess cuff integrity [27] **(III/B)**. For tears >3cm, retear rates were twice that for the arthroscopic group compared to the open group (76% arthroscopic, 38% open). Conversely, within the arthroscopic group those with intact repairs had significantly greater strength of elevation and external rotation.

Verma et al found similar retear rates for mini-open and arthroscopic repair in the larger tear group (50% mini-open, 50% arthroscopic) [22]. However, the numbers were too small to demonstrate statistical significance.

Most studies have reported higher retear rates for arthroscopic repairs than is observed after open repairs. Klepps et al had a retear rate of 31% with open repair, but this had no significant effect on clinical

outcome [40]. Harryman et al used postoperative ultrasound to demonstrate that 65% remained intact [41] and similar results were obtained by Gerber, who reported a 66% intact rate for open repair of all tears [42]. Klepps et al concluded that for open rotator cuff repair, although a retear rate of 31% was of concern, an attempt at rotator cuff repair is worthwhile and structural failure does not equate to clinical failure [40]. They also found that both those with large tears pre-operatively and those with retears postoperatively had lower outcome scores, although this was not statistically significant.

The general consensus, however, is that those suffering a retear have inferior results, despite having improved postoperative clinical outcome scores. In reality the clinical improvement could be due to the biceps tenotomy, the decompression, the debridement or due to careful rehabilitation. The distinction between these is difficult to determine.

Subscapularis tears

Subscapularis tears have largely been ignored in the literature. They constitute 3.5%-8% of rotator cuff tears. A positive Gerber's test, increased external rotation and often anterior instability may raise the index of suspicion for these lesions. Identification of these tears arthroscopically may be difficult for the inexperienced surgeon and inevitably some are overlooked. They can be identified by a comma-shaped arc of ligamentous tissue on the superolateral border of subscapularis, but are difficult to repair arthroscopically due to the confined workspace. If attempted as part of the repair of a multi-tendon tear, the subscapularis repair must be addressed first. Such tears may be accompanied by medial subluxation of the long head of biceps requiring tenotomy or tenodesis. The repair is technically demanding, but Lo and Burkhart reviewed the results of 25 consecutive arthroscopic repairs and reported that 92% of patients obtained a good or excellent result using the UCLA criteria [33].

Choice of fixation and repair technique

There have been several biomechanical studies looking at optimising the strength of rotator cuff fixation. The suture-to-tendon interface has been identified as the weak link in the repair.

Lo and Burkhart emphasised the importance of tear pattern recognition in arthroscopic repair. They identified four different pattern types: crescent, u-shape, I-shape and massive, contracted, immobile tears [33, 34]. Simple crescent types were the commonest tear pattern and can be repaired directly, without mobilisation, achieving good results. U- and I-shaped patterns require side-to-side suture to allow margin convergence, reducing the strain at the tear margin and hence reducing failure rates. Massive and retracted, immobile cuff tears require extensive mobilisation and this can now be done arthroscopically with an interval slide technique.

An optimal repair requires a doubly-loaded biodegradable polymer suture, such as No. 2 Fibrewire, six-throw arthroscopic surgeons' knots, including three reversing half hitches on alternating posts, a double-diameter knot pusher and a double row repair [34, 43-45]. Restoration of the entire rotator cuff footprint or tendon-to-bone contact area improves the chance of complete healing and failure to replicate this may lead to early failure [34, 43-45].

Previous studies have demonstrated that the modified Mason-Allen stitch, which is used in open repair techniques, leads to less gap formation and less slippage, resulting in the highest ultimate tensile load [46]. However, the massive cuff stitch is easier to perform arthroscopically than the Mason-Allen stitch.

Gerber *et al* compared single, Mason-Allen, massive cuff stitch and double-row techniques [46]. Double row and the massive stitch compared well with the Mason-Allen suture. The double-row technique has been shown to provide a stronger repair and this may lead to fewer structural failures [43]. Single-row techniques demonstrated higher failure rates at the tendon interface at lower cycles. This was also confirmed by Benjamin *et al* [44, 45] **(IIa/B)**. They found that results using the massive cuff stitch were comparable to the Mason-Allen stitch. The ultimate tensile load before failure was significantly higher than that of the simple and horizontal stitches.

Biological scaffolds

Recently, the use of biological scaffolds has been introduced to augment massive rotator cuff repairs. One such scaffold is composed of a regenerative tissue matrix made of acellular human dermal matrix and biological substrate components, including collagen types I, III, IV and VII, elastin, chondroitin sulphate and proteoglycans. The matrix functions to support the rapid revascularisation and cellular repopulation. The aims are to re-establish the important force couple provided by the rotator cuff tendons when the quality of the tissue is insufficient to restore function. This can now be done by open or arthroscopic methods. The graft acts as an interposition graft supporting the underlying tissue and reattaching the remaining tendon to a near normal position.

Previously, muscle transfers were used, but the biomechanical balance was frequently lost using these techniques. To date no studies have yet been published on the graft technique, but are eagerly awaited. Previous studies of partial arthroscopic repair alone have produced good results, so the significance of closing the defect using these biological patches is questionable and yet to be determined [47].

Complications of arthroscopic repair

So far there have been few reports of complications with an all-arthroscopic repair. Mansat reported a 10.5% overall complication rate for open repair [48]. They felt that this figure was probably an underestimate, as older patients were more prone to medical complications which may not have been identified. Deep wound infection has been reported in 1%-2% and in 15% the tendon failed to heal [48].

In comparison, Weber *et al* reported a 5.8%-9.5% complication rate for arthroscopic shoulder surgery [49]. Loosening of the anchors was seen in 0.75% of arthroscopic cuff repairs [49]. Stiffness has not been shown to be a problem, unlike after mini-open and open repairs. A difficult balance exists between early rehabilitation to avoid stiffness and protection of the repair. Various postoperative protocols have been reported. Bishop *et al* immobilised their patients with large cuff tears for four to six weeks, but noted higher rates of stiffness [27]. More early, aggressive rehabilitation was performed by Galatz *et al* with high retear rates on ultrasound [25]. Hence they recommended less aggressive rehabilitation, especially for the larger repairs. The most appropriate approach to individual rehabilitation is often difficult to determine and the decision will come down to surgical intuition rather than pure science, based on a multitude of factors.

Conclusions

Arthroscopic rotator cuff repairs are challenging to an inexperienced arthroscopic surgeon. An all-arthroscopic technique can be performed with good clinical outcomes and less peri-operative morbidity for small to moderate tears. It remains to be seen whether improved repair techniques and suture materials will allow similar results to be achieved with massive tears. The literature is still weak in this field, consisting of case series and non-randomised comparisons, but a randomised controlled study is now underway and the results are eagerly awaited.

Recommendations	Evidence level
◆ The clinical benefits of all-arthroscopic rotator cuff repair are improved postoperative pain relief, earlier rehabilitation and reduced incidence of postoperative stiffness.	III/B
◆ Double-row suture fixation provides a stronger repair with a significant higher ultimate tensile load before failure than that of simple and horizontal stitches.	IIa/B
◆ Retear rates are comparable with open and mini-open repairs for small to moderate-size tears.	III/B
◆ Most studies demonstrate higher structural failures for massive tears repaired arthroscopically compared to open repair.	III/B

References

1. Yamaguchi K, Tetro M, Blam O, *et al*. Natural history of asymptomatic rotator cuff tears: a longitudinal analysis of symptomatic tears detected sonographically. *J Shoulder Elbow Surg* 2001; 10: 199-203.

2. Ruotolo C, Nottage WM. Surgical and non-surgical management of rotator cuff tears. *Arthroscopy* 2002; 18: 527-31.

3. Burkhart SS. Arthroscopic debridement and decompression for selected rotator cuff tears. Clinical results, pathomechanics, and patient selection based on biomechanical parameters. *Orthop Clin North Am* 1993; 24: 111-23.

4. Neer CS 2nd, Craig EV, Fukuda H. Cuff-tear arthropathy. *J Bone Joint Surg Am* 1983; 65-A: 1232-44.

5. Gartsman GM, Hasan SS. What's new in shoulder and elbow surgery. *J Bone Joint Surg Am* 2006; 88-A: 230-43.

6. Codman EA. Complete rupture of the supraspinatus tendon: operative treatment with report of 2 successful cases. *Boston Med Surg J* 1911; 164: 708-10.

7. Neer CS 2nd. Anterior acromioplasty for the chronic impingement syndrome in the shoulder. A preliminary report. *J Bone Joint Surg Am* 1972; 54-A: 41-50.

8. Inman VT, Saunders JB, Abbot LC. Observations on the function of the shoulder joint. *J Bone Joint Surg Am* 1944; 26-A: 1-30.

9. Post M, Silver R, Singh M. Rotator cuff tear. Diagnosis and treatment. *Clin Orthop Relat Res* 1983; 173: 78-91.

10. Levy HJ, Uribe JW, Delaney LG. Arthroscopic assisted rotator cuff repair: preliminary results. *Arthroscopy* 1990; 6: 55-60.

11. Paulos LE, Kody MH. Arthroscopically enhanced 'miniapproach' to rotator cuff repair. *Am J Sports Med* 1994; 22: 19-25.

12. Miller C, Savoie FH. Gleno-humeral abnormalities associated with full-thickness tears of the rotator cuff. *Orthop Rev* 1994; 23: 159-62.

13. Gartsman GM, Khan M, Hammerman SM. Arthroscopic repair of full-thickness tears of the rotator cuff. *J Bone Joint Surg Am* 1998; 80-A: 832-40.

14. Buess E, Steuber KU, Waibl B. Open versus arthroscopic rotator cuff repair: a comparative view of 96 cases. *Arthroscopy* 2005; 21: 597-604.

15. Severud EL, Ruotolo C, Abbott DD. All-arthroscopic versus mini-open rotator cuff repair: a long-term retrospective outcome comparison. *Arthroscopy* 2003; 19: 234-8.

16. Youm T, Murray D, Kubiak EN, *et al.* Arthroscopic versus mini-open rotator cuff repair: a comparison of clinical outcomes and patient satisfaction. *J Shoulder Elbow Surg* 2005; 14: 455-9.

17. Ellman H, Kay SP, Wirth M. Arthroscopic treatment of full-thickness rotator cuff tears: 2 to 7 year follow-up study. *Arthroscopy* 1993; 9: 195-200.

18. Gartsman GM. All-arthroscopic rotator cuff repairs. *Orthop Clin North Am* 2001; 32: 501-10.

19. Tauro JC. Arthroscopic rotator cuff repair: analysis of technique and results at 2 and 3-year follow-up. *Arthroscopy* 1998; 14: 45-51.

20. Murray TF, Lajtai G, Mileski RM, *et al.* Arthroscopic repair of medium to large full-thickness rotator cuff tears: outcome at 2 to 6-year follow-up. *J Shoulder Elbow Surg* 2002; 11: 19-24.

21. Sauerbrey AM, Getz CL, Piancastelli M, *et al.* Arthroscopic versus mini-open rotator cuff repair: a comparison of clinical outcome. *Arthroscopy* 2005; 21: 1415-20.

22. Verma NN, Dunn W, Adler RS, *et al.* All-arthroscopic versus mini-open rotator cuff repair: a retrospective review with minimum 2-year follow-up. *Arthroscopy* 2006; 22: 587-94.

23. Kim SH, Ha KI, Park JH, *et al.* Arthroscopic versus mini-open salvage repair of the rotator cuff tear: outcome analysis at 2 to 6 years' follow-up. *Arthroscopy* 2003; 19: 746-54.

24. Warner JJ, Tetreault P, Lehtinen J. Arthroscopic versus mini-open rotator cuff repair: a cohort comparison study. *Arthroscopy* 2005; 21: 328-32.

25. Galatz LM, Ball CM, Teefey SA, *et al.* The outcome and repair integrity of completely arthroscopically repaired large and massive rotator cuff tears. *J Bone Joint Surg Am* 2004; 86-A: 219-24.

26. Jost B, Zumstein M, Pfirrmann CW. Long-term outcome after structural failure of rotator cuff repairs. *J Bone Joint Surg Am* 2006; 88-A: 472-9.

27. Bishop J, Klepps S, Lo IKY *et al.* Cuff integrity arthroscopic versus open rotator cuff repair: a prospective study. *J Shoulder Elbow Surg* 2005; 15: 290-9.

28. MacDermid JC, Holtby R, Razmjou H, JOINTS Canada, *et al.* All-arthroscopic versus mini-open repair of small or moderately-sized rotator cuff tears: a protocol for a randomised trial. *BMC Musculoskelet Disord* 2006; 7: 25.

29. Ide J, Maeda S, Takagi K. A comparison of arthroscopic and open rotator cuff repair. *Arthroscopy* 2005; 21: 1090-8.

30. Baker CL, Liu SH. Comparison of open and arthroscopically-assisted rotator cuff repairs. *Am J Sports Med* 1995; 23: 99-104.

31. Romeo AA, Hang DW, Bach RR, *et al.* Repair of full-thickness rotator cuff tears. *Clin Orthop* 1999; 367: 243-55.

32. Hersch JC, Sgaglione NA. Arthroscopically-assisted mini-open rotator cuff repairs. Functional outcome at 2 to 7-year follow-up. *Am J Sports Med* 2000; 28: 301-11.

33. Lo IKY, Burkhart SS. Current concepts in arthroscopic rotator cuff repair. *Am J Sports Med* 2003; 31: 308-24.

34. Burkhart SS, Lo IKY. Arthroscopic rotator cuff repair. *J Am Acad Orthop Surg* 2006; 14: 333-46.

35. Jones CK, Savoie FH. Arthroscopic repair of large and massive rotator cuff tears. *Arthroscopy* 2003; 19: 564-71.

36. Ogilvie-Harris DJ, Demaziere A. Arthroscopic debridement versus open repair for rotator cuff tears. A prospective cohort study. *J Bone Joint Surg Br* 1993; 75-B: 416-20.

37. Rockwood CA Jr, Burkhead WZ. Management of patients with massive rotator cuff defects by acromioplasty and rotator cuff debridement. *Orthop Trans* 1990; 12: 190-91.

38. Montgomery TJ, Yeger B, Savoie FH. Management of rotator cuff tears: a comparison of arthroscopic debridement and surgical repair. *J Shoulder Elbow Surg* 1994; 3: 70-8.

39. Bigliani LU, Cordasco FA, McIlveen SJ. Operative repair of massive rotator cuff tears: long-term results. *J Shoulder Elbow Surg* 1992; 1: 120-30.

40. Klepps S, Bishop J, Lin J, *et al.* Prospective evaluation of the effect of rotator cuff integrity on the outcome of open rotator cuff repairs. *Am J Sports Med* 2004; 32: 1716-22.

41. Harryman DT 2nd, Mack LA, Wang KY, *et al.* Repairs of the rotator cuff. Correlation of functional results with integrity of the cuff. *J Bone Joint Surg Am* 1991; 73-A: 982-9.

42. Gerber C, Fuchs B, Hodler J. The results of repair of massive tears of the rotator cuff. *J Bone Joint Surg Am* 2000; 82-A: 505-15.

43. Waltrip RL, Zheng N, Dugas JR. Rotator cuff repair. A biomechanical comparison of three techniques. *Am J Sports Med* 2003; 31: 493-7.

44. Benjamin C, MacGillivray JD, Clabeaux J, *et al.* Biomechanical evaluation of arthroscopic rotator cuff stitches. *J Bone Joint Surg Am* 2004; 86-A: 1211-6.

45. Benjamin C, Comerford L, Wilson J. Biomechanical evaluation of arthroscopic rotator cuff repairs: double-row compared with single-row fixation. *J Bone Joint Surg Am* 2006; 88-A: 403-10.

46. Gerber C, Schneeberger AG, Beck M. Mechanical strength of repairs of the rotator cuff. *J Bone Joint Surg Br* 1994; 76-B: 371-80.

47. Burkhart SS. Partial repair of massive rotator cuff tears: the evolution of a concept. *Orthop Clin North Am* 1997; 28: 125-32.

48. Mansat P, Cofield RH, Kersten TE. Complications of rotator cuff repair. *Orthop Clin North Am* 1997; 28: 205-13.

49. Weber SC, Abrams JS, Nottage WM. Complications associated with arthroscopic shoulder surgery. *Arthroscopy* 2002; 18(2 Suppl 1): 88-95.

Chapter 11

Rehabilitation of the shoulder

Joanna C Gibson MCSP

Clinical Specialist Physiotherapist

LIVERPOOL UPPER LIMB UNIT, ROYAL LIVERPOOL UNIVERSITY HOSPITAL, LIVERPOOL, UK

Introduction

Physiotherapy is often the first line of management for shoulder pain, although to date there is a general lack of evidence regarding its efficacy. A recent Cochrane report [1] reviewing physiotherapy interventions for shoulder pain, stiffness and/or disability concluded that there is little evidence to support or refute the efficacy of common interventions. Unfortunately many of the published reviews include a spectrum of shoulder pathology, lack specificity of diagnosis and are generally too heterogeneous with respect to treatments and follow-up. They are, therefore, of limited use for clinical practice; in the absence of accurate and well-defined clinical diagnoses there is insufficient guidance for the development of treatment programmes.

Methodology

Electronic searches were performed for all rehabilitation interventions in key clinical conditions including shoulder impingement, rotator cuff disease, tendinopathy, tendinosis, stiff shoulder, frozen shoulder, adhesive capsulitis and instability. The bibliographic databases of Medline, Cumulative Index to Nursing and Allied Health Literature (CINAHL), Embase, PEDro, Cochrane Database and Pubmed were utilised. In addition, hand-searching of relevant conference proceedings, textbooks and journals not included in the databases were undertaken. Eight relevant systematic reviews were identified and considered [1-8].

The findings were considered by clinical diagnosis, identifying significant factors that might influence treatment selection and the current evidence relating to specific treatment modalities.

Impingement syndrome

Subacromial impingement syndrome (SAIS) is a symptomatic diagnosis that may be the result of several patho-anatomical processes. It is perhaps the most widely researched clinical diagnosis with respect to the effectiveness of physiotherapy and conservative management options, which reflects the fact that it is the most common disorder of the shoulder (accounting for 44%-65% of all complaints of shoulder pain) [9]. The primary management of SAIS is usually conservative and is often undertaken in the primary care sector by general practitioners or physiotherapists [2].

Evidence suggests that subacromial impingement has a multifactorial aetiology. Authors propose inflammation of the bursa, degeneration or overuse of the rotator cuff tendons, weak or dysfunctional rotator cuff and/or scapula musculature, posterior capsular tightness, postural dysfunctions of the spinal column and bony or soft tissue anomalies, as contributory factors [10]. The role of each is unclear. However, it is important to note that most published research has focused on the role of pain-relieving modalities aimed at a proposed inflammatory element rather than specific manual therapy or exercise therapy addressing the mechanical aspects.

Clinical factors

Modern research provides good evidence that there are abnormalities in normal function of the dynamic stabilisers of the glenohumeral joint [11-13] in SAIS. Tyler et al [14] demonstrated a 28% deficit in external rotation strength using a hand-held dynamometer ($p < 0.01$) in patients with SAIS. Dynamic imaging studies [15] have demonstrated increased humeral head superior translation of 1-1.5mm and increased anterior translation of approximately 3mm during active elevation in patients with SAIS. These findings suggest that effective physiotherapy should address the rotator cuff and translational control of the glenohumeral joint.

Altered scapula kinematics have been consistently demonstrated in patients with SAIS [11, 16, 17]. Three-dimensional kinematic analysis has demonstrated decreased posterior tilt, upward rotation and external rotation of the scapula during glenohumeral elevation in patients with SAIS. Electromyographic analysis has further demonstrated a consistent deficit in serratus anterior activity and abnormalities in normal timing of activation in the upper and lower fibres of trapezius during elevation of the glenohumeral joint [17-19].

Posture and mobility of the thoracic spine can directly influence scapulothoracic and glenohumeral kinematics [20, 21]. A relatively small increase in thoracic spine flexion results in a more anteriorly tilted and elevated scapula at rest. Kebaetse et al [20] demonstrated that this small increase in thoracic spine flexion decreased the amount of force generated at 90° of glenohumeral scapular plane abduction.

Harryman et al [22] showed that surgically increasing tightness of the posterior capsule of cadavers resulted in increased superior and anterior translation during passive glenohumeral joint flexion. Tightness of the posterior capsular structures has been demonstrated in patients with SAIS when compared to healthy controls [11, 23].

These findings suggest that effective physiotherapy management should incorporate rotator cuff rehabilitation specifically addressing translational control, scapula muscle rehabilitation, mobilisation of the posterior capsule and postural correction.

Treatment

Desmeules' systematic review of manual and physical therapy in SAIS revealed only seven randomised controlled trials that met their criteria for review [2]. There was a consistent lack of uniformity in defining, evaluating and treating SAIS. The few trials that were well designed offered limited evidence to support the efficacy of physical therapy. Michener et al [6] identified 12 randomised clinical trials investigating the efficacy of physical interventions for the treatment of patients with SAIS. Bigliani et al's review [24] of the literature indicated that most patients who have impingement syndrome eventually recover with non-operative intervention.

Exercise

Conservative management outcomes are encouraging. Morrison et al's [25] retrospective study of 616 patients who had SAIS reported excellent or satisfactory results in 67% of patients undergoing conservative treatment. All patients were managed with NSAIDs and a specific supervised physical therapy regime consisting of isotonic exercises for strengthening of the rotator cuff. Haahr et al [26] compared the effect of exercise with graded physiotherapy training to arthroscopic subacromial decompression in 90 patients with subacromial impingement. The physiotherapy programme was carried out over a 12-week period after which patients were expected to continue their exercises at home two to three times a week until follow-up. At 12-month review there was no statistically significant difference in pain or functional scores. It is of note that the greatest improvement occurred in the first three months of treatment. There is good evidence that those patients who are likely to respond to this type of approach will show some evidence of improvement within the first 12 weeks of treatment, although improvement can continue for up to 12 months [27, 28] **(Ib/A)**.

Rahme *et al* [29] conducted a randomised prospective study to compare open anterior acromioplasty with a physiotherapy regime. Criteria for a successful outcome were a reduction of the initial pain score by more than 50% judged by a visual analogue scale. At six-month follow-up, success was reported in 57% of the surgically treated patients and in 33% of the physiotherapy group. However, in this study it is possible that patients may have been biased towards surgery, as most (88%) stated that previous injection treatment or therapy had not been effective before the start of the study. These findings suggest that surgery may be best indicated in patients who have failed exercise or injection treatment **(IIb/B)**. Dickens *et al* [30] showed that even in patients who had failed injection treatment and were listed for surgery, 26% still benefited from physiotherapy to the point that they no longer required surgery.

Exercise and mobilisation

Two RCTs [31, 32] show that the effects of education and an exercise programme may be enhanced with respect to decreasing the pain of SAIS by adding mobilisation **(Ib/A)**. Conroy and Hayes [31] examined whether subjects receiving joint mobilisations and comprehensive treatment (hot packs, active range of motion, physiological stretching, muscle strengthening, soft tissue mobilisation and patient education) would have improved pain, function and mobility compared with similar patients receiving comprehensive treatment alone. They concluded that mobilisation decreased 24-hour pain and pain on specific testing in patients with primary shoulder impingement. Both groups showed improvements in mobility and function. Bang and Deyle [32] demonstrated greater short-term improvement in pain and self-reported shoulder function when therapeutic exercise was combined with manual therapy.

Supervised vs home exercise programme

There is a lack of evidence to identify whether a supervised programme is preferable to a home exercise programme. Walther *et al* [33] performed a randomised prospective trial to compare the results of treating subacromial impingement by a guided self-training programme with treatment by conventional physiotherapy or a functional brace. Sixty patients were randomised into one of the three groups. The Constant-Murley score was assessed after six and 12 weeks. Shoulder pain was monitored with a visual analogue scale. All three groups showed a significant improvement in shoulder function as well as a significant reduction in pain. There were no statistically significant differences among the groups. The comparable effect of the functional brace remains unclear but the authors postulate that this may be explained by an influence on proprioception. Interestingly, Machner *et al* [34] demonstrated that patients with impingement syndrome stage II demonstrated reduced kinaesthetic sense.

Current evidence suggests that therapeutic exercise is more beneficial to patients with SAIS than no treatment or placebo treatment **(Ib/A)**. It remains unclear what the optimal exercise regime is, the frequency and intensity of an exercise programme or which patients are most likely to benefit from an exercise-based approach.

Ultrasound

Green *et al*'s [1] meta-analysis of two RCTs showed no evidence that ultrasound is effective in the management of shoulder pain, except in the case of calcific tendinitis. Gursel *et al* [35] performed a randomised placebo-controlled trial comparing the use of true and sham ultrasound combined with other physiotherapy modalities. Their results showed no additional benefit of combining true or sham ultrasound in the management of soft tissue disorders of the shoulder. This is consistent with most studies of ultrasound which have found no evidence of its efficacy. In fact, on the contrary, there is tentative evidence for a lack of efficacy in patients defined as having SAIS [36] **(Ib/A)**.

Cold therapy

The Philadelphia Panel [7] found insufficient evidence to support or refute the use of cold therapy in the management of SAIS. This is mirrored in the findings of Green et al [1]. This treatment modality is widely advocated in the literature, although van der Heijden et al [8] reported one RCT which showed it to be ineffective for the management of shoulder pain.

Acupuncture

Studies looking at the effectiveness of acupuncture in the treatment of SAIS have provided equivocal evidence. Johansson et al [37] compared the use of acupuncture and continuous ultrasound in addition to home exercises in the management of 85 patients with impingement, randomised into two groups. Whilst both groups improved, the acupuncture group had a larger improvement in disability scores over the course of 12 months. Their results suggest that acupuncture is more efficacious than ultrasound when applied to supplement home exercises. Currently, there is insufficient evidence to support or refute the use of acupuncture as a single intervention in the treatment of SAIS.

Rotator cuff disease

Diseases of the rotator cuff cover a spectrum of disorders encompassing tendinosis, tendonitis, tendinopathy and tears. Interpretation of the available literature about this patient group can be challenging because of a lack of consensus, once more, regarding terminology and classification. Our

increased understanding of rotator cuff pathology has challenged the rationale for some physiotherapy modalities. Electrotherapy is often prescribed to address an inflammatory component but current evidence regarding tendinosis and tendinopathy questions whether an inflammatory component exists.

It is still unclear why some patients with rotator cuff tears are asymptomatic and others have disabling pain. Kelly et al [38] evaluated the differential firing patterns of the rotator cuff, deltoid and scapula stabiliser muscle groups in normal control subjects and in patients with symptomatic and asymptomatic two-tendon rotator cuff tears. Electromyographic activity from 12 muscles and kinematic data were collected simultaneously during ten functional tasks. Both symptomatic and asymptomatic subjects showed a trend towards increased muscle activation during all tasks compared with the normal subjects, suggesting compensatory strategies. They concluded that differential shoulder muscle-firing patterns in patients with rotator cuff pathology may play a role in the generation or absence of symptoms. Asymptomatic subjects demonstrated increased firing of the intact subscapularis, whereas symptomatic subjects appeared to rely on torn rotator cuff tendons and periscapular muscle substitution, resulting in compromised function. The findings of these authors are reflected in other studies and suggest a basis for specific exercise prescription.

Treatment

Grant et al's [4] systematic review of interventions for rotator cuff pathology concluded that generally the methodological quality of currently available studies was low. They concluded that currently there is insufficient evidence to strongly support or negate the effectiveness of any available treatment intervention for rotator cuff disorders.

Exercise and tendinopathy

Wies et al [39] performed a randomised controlled trial of physiotherapy for rotator cuff tendinopathies to assess the efficacy of physiotherapy approaches. Ninety shoulders were randomised to one of four groups: therapeutic exercise (TE), manual therapy (MT), combined TE/MT, or placebo. Final assessments were done one week following the last treatment session. Their results showed a statistically significant reduction in the Shoulder Pain and Disability Index for the therapeutic exercise group alone. The addition of manual therapy and the manual therapy group alone did not improve significantly. Their conclusion was that the best practice for treatment of rotator cuff tendinopathies should centre on therapeutic exercise **(Ib/A)**.

Davenport et al [40] proposed the EdUReP model for non-surgical management of tendinopathy. This theoretical model was informed by evidence from basic and clinical science. The model comprises Education, Unloading, Reloading and Prevention but has not been subjected to a rigorous clinical trial to assess its effectiveness. The majority of work regarding tendinopathy has to date concentrated on the achilles and patella tendons [41, 42]. Due to the functional differences between these tendons and the rotator cuff it is not yet clear to what extent it is possible to extrapolate management strategies based on this research to the rotator cuff tendon [43]. Unloading strategies have been proposed to reduce tendon forces in the painful stage, but there is limited evidence to indicate that this can be applied to the rotator cuff. Eccentric exercise is well described in the management of lower limb tendinopathies [42]. Clinical studies point to the efficacy of an eccentric strengthening regime but this has yet to be demonstrated in the rotator cuff.

Exercise and rotator cuff tears

Heers et al's [44] series of 30 patients (38 shoulders) with rotator cuff tears, confirmed by ultrasonography, were included in a prospective study of exercise therapy. Patients were grouped according to the size of their tear: partial defects, full-thickness defects of the supraspinatus and massive rotator cuff defects. The home exercise programme consisted of stretching and strengthening exercises that were performed by the patients daily for a period of 12 weeks and monitored by a physician every two weeks. All groups showed improvement in range of movement. The Constant score improved significantly ($p < 0.05$) in

all groups. The results of this study show that patients with rotator cuff defects do benefit from simple home exercises, independent from the size of the defect **(IIb/B)**. Bartolozzi et al [45] reported their results of conservative management in 136 patients with rotator cuff disease, reporting good to excellent results in 66% of the patients at six months. Improvement continued for up to one year. This is an important factor and has been demonstrated by other authors [46, 47]. Patients with rotator cuff pathology can take up to six months to show significant improvement and will continue to improve for up to two years **(Ib/A)**. Restrictions imposed by waiting lists and pressure for early discharge may limit the effectiveness of an exercise-based approach to treatment of these patients if not administered for an adequate time period.

Adhesive capsulitis

Adhesive capsulitis, or frozen shoulder, is a condition characterised by global restriction in the range of movement of the glenohumeral joint. Its aetiology is poorly understood. Authors classify patients into primary and secondary groups [48]. Currently, there is no robust evidence on the superiority of any one treatment compared to another. Modern literature commonly recommends the use of multiple modalities, which precludes assessment of the effectiveness of individual treatments. Three stages of the disease are recognised and one of the problems in interpreting the literature is the failure of authors to clarify the stage of the disease at treatment and the diagnostic criteria used.

Research into abnormalities of muscle control in adhesive capsulitis consistently demonstrates compensatory strategies involving excessive activation of the upper fibres of trapezius and inhibition of the lower fibres of trapezius, both compensating for capsular restriction [49, 50].

Treatment options

There does not appear to be any definitive agreement on the most effective form of treatment for this condition. Most studies have focused primarily on restoring the range of movement with adjunctive modalities to address pain.

Exercise

Diercks et al[51] performed a randomised prospective study of 77 patients with idiopathic frozen shoulder to compare the effect of intensive physical rehabilitation treatment, including passive stretching and manual mobilisation (stretching group) with supportive therapy and exercises within the pain limits (supervised neglect group). All patients were followed-up for 24 months after the start of treatment. In the patients treated with supervised neglect, 89% had normal or near-normal painless shoulder function (Constant score >80) at the end of the observation programme. Sixty-four percent reached this result within 12 months. In contrast, in the group receiving intensive physical therapy treatment only 63% reached a score of 80 or more after 24 months. The authors concluded that supervised neglect yields better outcomes than intensive physical therapy and passive stretching in patients with frozen shoulder. One of the key findings was that intensive stretching succeeded in prolonging the course of the disease and increased pain levels **(Ib/A)**. The success of an essentially home-based exercise programme is consistent with the findings of other authors [52, 53] **(IIa/B)**.

Exercise and injection

Ryans et al [54] studied 80 patients with frozen shoulder of less than six months' duration and randomised them into one of four groups. Patients had either injection of triamcinolone and eight sessions of 'standard physiotherapy', injection alone, placebo injection plus physiotherapy or placebo injection alone. All patients were required to undertake a home exercise programme. Their results showed that shoulder disability scores improved significantly more in the group having a corticosteroid injection, although the range of movement improved more in the physiotherapy group. The treatment effect was significant at six weeks but at 16 weeks the effect was no longer significant. Ryans et al [54] concluded that there was no interaction effect between injection and physiotherapy. This is in contrast to the findings of Carette et al [55] who performed a similar study in 93 patients with adhesive capsulitis of less than one year's duration. They concluded that a single intra-articular injection of corticosteroid administered under fluoroscopy, combined with a simple home exercise

programme, is effective in improving pain and disability in patients with adhesive capsulitis **(Ib/A)**. Adding supervised physiotherapy provided faster improvement in shoulder range of motion. At one year they reported no significant difference in improvement with respect to all outcome measures in all four groups.

Acupuncture

Sun et al[56] undertook a randomised controlled trial to evaluate the effectiveness of acupuncture as a treatment for idiopathic frozen shoulder. Thirty-five patients with a diagnosis of frozen shoulder were randomly allocated to an exercise group or an exercise plus acupuncture group and treated for a period of six weeks. Results showed that the exercise plus acupuncture group experienced significantly greater improvement with treatment than the exercise only group. The authors conclude that the combination of acupuncture with exercises may offer effective treatment for frozen shoulder **(Ib/A)**.

The debate on the effectiveness of physiotherapy in treatment of frozen shoulder continues. The length and type of intervention and the stage at which it may be appropriate need further work. Currently recognised treatment strategies such as hydrotherapy, mirror visual feedback and the Swiss ball are not represented in the current literature.

Instability

Shoulder instability continues to provide a challenge to the physiotherapist. Classification systems are often confusing and a lack of uniformity and poorly defined diagnostic criteria makes comparison of treatment modalities for different subgroups difficult [57]. McFarland et al [58] demonstrated that variations in the criteria used for the diagnosis of multidirectional instability affected the distribution of patients with this condition. The accurate diagnosis of instability is critical in determining appropriate management [59].

Several authors have demonstrated alterations in muscle activity after both traumatic and atraumatic instability [60-62]. Morris et al [63] demonstrated altered patterns of shoulder girdle muscle activity and imbalances in muscle forces in patients with multidirectional instability (MDI), thus supporting the theory that impaired co-ordination of shoulder muscle activity and inefficiency of the dynamic stabilisers of the glenohumeral joint are involved in the aetiology of MDI. Warner et al [11] demonstrated a relative deficit in the strength of the internal rotators in patients with anterior instability. In later work, Warner et al [64] used Moire topography to assess scapula dynamics in an asymptomatic population and patients with instability and found asymmetry and an abnormal pattern in 18% of the asymptomatic population and 64% of the instability group.

Barden et al [65] demonstrated that patients with MDI may have a reduced capacity to use proprioception to refine and control the motor output of the upper limb as a consequence of proprioceptive deficits. The presence of proprioceptive deficits in patients following traumatic dislocation is well documented [66].

The spinal stretch reflex has been used to evaluate elements of dynamic joint stability and function. Auge et al [67] showed that patients with atraumatic instability demonstrate a prominent reflex response, which indicates decreased supraspinal reflex control processes. In contrast, the asymptomatic athletic population demonstrated a quiescent reflex response indicating enhanced reflex control mechanisms. This indicates an alteration in central processing as a result of developmental factors.

These findings suggest that an effective rehabilitation programme for patients with instability should comprise proprioceptive re-education, re-education of dynamic stability of the glenohumeral joint (glenohumeral and scapula musculature) together with re-education of optimal muscle activation patterns. There is also clear evidence that the subgroups of instability may demonstrate specific patho-aetiological differences which change the bias of the initial treatment approach.

Treatment

Gibson's systematic review of non-operative management of shoulder instability concluded that in the case of non-operative management of shoulder instability the quantity and quality of evidence are low. A period of immobilisation of three to four weeks followed by a structured rehabilitation programme of 12 weeks' duration maximised return to premorbid activity level in traumatic dislocations; this was supported by weak evidence. Handoll et al (2004) concluded in their Cochrane Review that the limited evidence available supports primary surgery for young adults, usually male, engaged in highly demanding physical activities who have sustained their first acute traumatic dislocation. They concluded that current evidence suggests non-surgical treatment should remain the primary treatment option for other categories of patient.

Exercise

Burkhead and Rockwood [68] looked at 140 shoulders in 115 patients with a diagnosis of traumatic or atraumatic, recurrent anterior, posterior or multidirectional subluxation. Patients were treated with a specific set of graduated muscle strengthening exercises based on the use of elastic tubing. Only 16% (12) of the patients with traumatic subluxation (74 shoulders) had a good or excellent result from the exercises compared with 53 (80%) of the 66 shoulders that had atraumatic subluxation.

Kiss et al [69] assessed the results of non-operative treatment in 62 patients with atraumatic instability at 3.7 years. All patients underwent a programme incorporating visual biofeedback, proprioceptive training, scapulothoracic and glenohumeral muscle pattern correction. Ultimately, 61% of patients had no symptoms of instability following the programme. Takwale et al [70] diagnosed 50 patients with a mean age at presentation of 17.3 years, as having involuntary positional instability of the shoulder. They were managed by a programme of careful explanation, analysis of abnormal force couples and then muscle retraining carried out by a specialist physiotherapist. The mean follow-up was two years. Six shoulders had a poor result, but 52 were graded as good to excellent. Nine patients relapsed and required further episodes of retraining.

Authors agree that in the case of atraumatic instability a rehabilitation programme addressing proprioception and re-education of the scapulothoracic and glenohumeral musculature is successful in up to 88% of patients [59, 68-70] **(IIa/B)**.

Exercise plus electromyography biofeedback

Reid's randomised controlled trial [71] of 20 subjects compared isokinetic resistance exercises (designed to improve muscle strength and endurance) and an EMG biofeedback re-education programme (designed to improve motor control) in athletes with anterior instability. The two groups were compared with respect to function and strength at 8, 26 and 52 weeks. Results showed that the functional endurance programme was more effective than the isokinetic resistance programme for improving function at work and in sport at eight and 52 weeks of follow-up and improving pain at 26 and 52 weeks. The Stanmore group [59] report symptomatic improvement in up to 88% of patients with muscle patterning instability using a rehabilitation programme incorporating electromyography biofeedback. However, they report that only 34% of patients achieved a stable shoulder. Importantly, they report that those patients with muscle patterning instability who have had surgical intervention are up to five times less likely to respond to appropriate rehabilitation. Other authors have described similar results in patients with instability, but lack a control group and report only small case series [72].

Electromyographic biofeedback may offer a means of enhancing the results of non-operative treatment **(IIb/B)**.

Exercise plus orthosis

Ide *et al* [73] evaluated the results of shoulder strengthening exercises with a novel shoulder orthosis to stabilise the scapula in 46 patients with MDI.

Patients performed the prescribed exercise programme for a period of eight weeks. Rotator cuff strength and functional scores significantly improved following the programme. The lack of a control group limits the validity of this study but in view of the accepted proprioceptive deficits in this patient group, an orthosis that enhances proprioception would seem an appropriate adjunct to exercise **(IIb/B)**.

It is clear that the lack of a commonly accepted classification system limits comparison of results and meaningful conclusions. The value of any classification system lies in its ability to predict a response to a specific form of treatment [68]. For future research to have optimum validity there must be a consensus regarding the classification system used.

Conclusions

Johannson *et al* [74] looked at the evidence available from systematic review of the scientific literature and compared it to clinicians' (GPs and physiotherapists) trusted treatment approaches. They found that the clinicians' trust in treatments has a weak association with available scientific evidence. It is apparent from this review that there needs to be more high quality, sound methodological studies evaluating rehabilitation strategies based on our increased understanding of the aetiological factors in shoulder disorders [75, 76]. There is an urgent need for further well-designed clinical trials and more research regarding physiotherapy intervention. However, there is also a need to establish a uniform method of defining shoulder disorders and reach consensus in outcome measures used. Currently, trial selection criteria vary widely, even for the same diagnostic groups, and there is a diversity of outcome measures used, making comparison and interpretation of results difficult.

Recommendations	Evidence level

Impingement syndrome

- Patients with SAIS should undergo a trial of therapeutic exercise before surgical measures are considered. — Ia/A
- An exercise programme aimed at restoring range (particularly the posterior capsule), strength and dynamic control of the rotator cuff and scapula musculature is beneficial in the treatment of SAIS. — Ia/A
- Patients who are likely to respond to an exercise-based approach for SAIS will show some evidence of improvement within the first 12 weeks of treatment. — Ib/A
- Passive mobilisation techniques of the upper quadrant enhance the beneficial effects of exercise in the management of SAIS. — Ib/A
- Ultrasound is not recommended for the treatment of SAIS. — IIa/B
- Cold therapy does not appear to have a role in the management of SAIS. — IIa/B
- Acupuncture as a single intervention is of limited benefit; however, it may be of some benefit when applied in conjunction with a home exercise programme. — Ib/A

Rotator cuff disease

- Chronic rotator cuff tears should undergo a six-month period of therapeutic exercise irrespective of size before surgical options are considered. — Ib/A
- Rotator cuff tendinopathy should be treated with therapeutic exercise; current evidence suggests this should be performed within the pain-free range. — Ib/A
- There is no evidence to suggest that electrotherapy or cold therapy have a role to play in the management of rotator cuff tears. — Ia/A

Adhesive capsulitis

- Aggressive stretching and manual therapy are contraindicated in the painful stages of frozen shoulder. — Ib/A
- A home exercise programme with regular monitoring is successful with respect to improving pain and sagittal plane movements in patients with symptoms of <1 year duration. — IIa/B
- Injection combined with a home exercise programme may improve pain levels and function in the short term in frozen shoulder. — Ib/A
- Acupuncture may be of some benefit when applied in conjunction with a home exercise programme. — Ib/A

Instability

- A rehabilitation programme comprising visual biofeedback proprioceptive training, scapulothoracic and glenohumeral muscle pattern correction is successful in up to 88% of patients with atraumatic instability. — IIa/B
- Electromyographic biofeedback may enhance the results of conservative treatment. — IIb/B
- There may be a role for orthoses that reinforces optimal scapula position and enhances proprioception in the management of atraumatic instability. — IIb/B

Chapter 11

References

1. Green S, Buchbinder R, Hetrick S. Physiotherapy interventions for shoulder pain. *The Cochrane Database of Systematic Reviews*, 2003; 2.

2. Desmeules F, Cote CH, Fremont P. Therapeutic exercise and orthopaedic manual therapy for impingement syndrome: a systematic review. *Clinical Journal of Sport Medicine* 2003; 13: 176-82.

3. Gibson K, Growe A, Korda L, *et al*. The effectiveness of rehabilitation for non-operative management of shoulder instability: a systematic review. *J Hand Ther* 2004; 17(2): 229-42.

4. Grant HJ, Arthur A, Pichora DR. Evaluation of interventions for rotator cuff pathology: a systematic review. *J Hand Ther* 2004; 17(2): 274-99.

5. Handoll HGG, Almaiyah MA, Rangan A. Surgical versus non-surgical treatment for acute anterior shoulder dislocation (review). *The Cochrane Database of Systematic Reviews*, 2004; 1.

6. Michener LA, Kalsworth MK, Burnet EN. Effectiveness of rehabilitation for patients with subacromial impingement syndrome: a systematic review. *J Hand Ther* 2004; 17(2): 152-64.

7. Philadelphia Panel. Evidence-based clinical practice guidelines on selected rehabilitation interventions for shoulder pain. *Phys Ther* 2001; 81: 1719-30.

8. Van der Heijden GJ, Van der Windt DA, De Winter AF. Physiotherapy for patients with soft tissue disorders: a systematic review of randomised clinical trials. *Br Med J* 1997; 315: 25-30.

9. Van der Windt DA, Koes BW, de Jong BA, *et al*. Shoulder disorders in general practice: incidence, patient characteristics, and management. *Ann Rheum Dis* 1995; 54: 959-64.

10. Michener LA, McClure PW, Karduna AR. Anatomical and biomechanical mechanisms of subacromial impingement syndrome. *Clinical Biomechanics* 2003; 18: 369-79.

11. Warner J, Micheli L, Arslanian L, *et al*. Patterns of flexibility, laxity and strength in normal shoulders and shoulders with instability and impingement. *Am J Sports Med* 1990; 18(4): 366-75.

12. Reddy AS, Mohr KJ, Pink MM, *et al*. Electromyographic analysis of the deltoid and rotator cuff muscles in persons with subacromial impingement. *J Shoulder Elbow Surgery* 2000; 9(6): 519-23.

13. Leroux JL, Codine P, Thomas E, *et al*. Isokinetic evaluation of rotational strength in normal shoulders and shoulders with impingement syndrome. *Clin Orthop Relat Res* 1994; 304: 108-15.

14. Tyler TF, Nahow RC, Nicholas SJ, *et al*. Quantifying shoulder rotation weakness in patients with shoulder impingement. *J Shoulder Elbow Surgery* 2005; 14(6): 570-4.

15. Ludewig PM, Cook TM. Translations of the humerus in persons with shoulder impingement symptoms. *J Orthop Sports Phys Ther* 2002; 32(6): 248-57.

16. Ludewig PM, Cook TM. Alterations in shoulder kinematics and associated activity in people with symptoms of shoulder impingement. *Phys Ther* 2000; 80: 276-92.

17. Lukasiewicz AC, McClure P, Michener L, Pratt N, Sennett B. Comparison of 3-dimensional scapular position and orientation between subjects with and without shoulder impingement. *J Orthop Sports Phys Ther* 1999; 29: 574-86.

18. Cools AM, *et al*. Isokinetic scapular muscle performance in overhead athletes with and without impingement symptoms. *Journal of Athletic Training* 2005; 40(2): 104-10.

19. Cools A, Witvrouw E, Declerq G, *et al*. Scapular muscle recruitment pattern: trapezius muscle latency in overhead athletes with and without impingement symptoms. *Am J Sports Med* 2003; 31: 542-9.

20. Kebaetse M, McClure P, Pratt NA. Thoracic position effect on shoulder range of motion, strength and three dimensional scapular kinematics. *Arch Phys Med Rehabil* 1999; 80: 945-50.

21. Lewis JS, Wright C, Green A. Subacromial impingement syndrome: the effect of changing posture on shoulder range of movement. *J Orthop Sports Phys Ther* 2005; 35(2); 72-87.

22. Harryman DT, Sidles JA, Clark JM, *et al*. Translation of the humeral head on the glenoid with passive glenohumeral movement. *J Bone Joint Surg Am* 1990; 72(9): 1334-43.

23. Tyler TF, Nicholas SJ, Roy T, *et al*. Quantification of posterior capsule tightness and motion loss in patients with shoulder impingement. *Am J Sports Med* 2000; 28(5): 668-73.

24. Bigliani LU, Levine WN. Subacromial impingement syndrome. *J Bone Joint Surg* 1997; 79-A(12): 1854-68.

25. Morrison DS, Frogameni AD, Woodworth P. Non-operative treatment of subacromial impingement syndrome. *J Bone Joint Surg* 1997; 79-A(5): 732-7.

26. Haahr JP, Ostergaard S, Dalsgaard J, *et al*. Exercises versus arthroscopic decompression in patients with subacromial impingement: a randomised, controlled study in 90 cases with a one-year follow-up. *Ann Rheum Dis* 2005; 64: 760-4.

27. Brox JI, Gjengedal E, Uppheim G, *et al*. Arthroscopic surgery versus supervised exercises in patients with rotator cuff disease (stage II impingement): a prospective, randomised, controlled study in 125 patients with a 2 1/2 year follow-up. *J Shoulder Elbow Surgery* 1999; 8: 102-11.

28. McClure PW, Bialker J, Neff N, *et al*. Shoulder function and 3-dimensional kinematics in people with shoulder impingement syndrome before and after a six-week exercise programme. *Phys Ther* 2004; 84(9): 832-48.

29. Rahme H, Solem-Bertoft E, Westerberg CE, *et al*. The subacromial impingement syndrome: a study of results of treatment with special emphasis on predictive factors and pain generating mechanisms. *Scand J Rehab Med* 1998; 30: 253-62.

30. Dickens VA, Williams JL, Bhamra MS. Role of physiotherapy in the treatment of subacromial impingement syndrome: a prospective study. *Physiotherapy* 2005; 91: 159-64.

31. Conroy DE, Hayes KW. The effect of joint mobilisation as a component of comprehensive treatment for primary shoulder impingement syndrome. *J Orthop Sports Phys Ther* 1998; 28(1): 3-14.

32. Bang MD, Deyle GD. Comparison of supervised exercise with and without manual physical therapy for patients with shoulder impingement syndrome. *J Orthop Sports Phys Ther* 2000; 30: 126-37.

33. Walther M, Werner A, Stahlschmidt T, *et al*. The subacromial impingement syndrome of the shoulder treated by

conventional physiotherapy, self-training, and a shoulder brace: results of a prospective, randomised study. *J Shoulder Elbow Surgery* 2005; 14(4): 385-92.

34. Machner A, Merk H, Becker R, *et al*. Kinaesthetic sense of the shoulder in patients with impingement syndrome. *Acta Orthop Scand* 2003; 74(1): 85-8.

35. Gursel YK, Ulus Y, Bilgic A, *et al*. Adding ultrasound in the management of soft tissue disorders: a randomised controlled trial. *Phys Ther* 2004; 84: 336-43.

36. Nykanen M. Pulsed ultrasound treatment of the painful shoulder: a randomised, double blinded study. *Scand J Rehabil Med* 1995; 27: 105-8.

37. Johansson KM, Adolfsson LE, Foldevi MOM. Effects of acupuncture versus ultrasound in patients with impingement syndrome: randomised clinical trial. *Phys Ther* 2005; 85(6): 490-501.

38. Kelly BT, Williams RJ, Cordasco FA, *et al*. Differential patterns of muscle activation in patients with symptomatic and asymptomatic rotator cuff tears. *J Shoulder Elbow Surg* 2005; 14(2): 165-71.

39. Wies J, Humphreys H, Latham M, *et al*. A randomised placebo-controlled trial of physiotherapy for rotator cuff tendinopathies. British Elbow and Shoulder Society, 16th Annual Scientific Meeting, 2005.

40. Davenport TE, Kulig K, Matharu Y, *et al*. The EdUReP model for non-surgical management of tendinopathy. *Phys Ther* 2005; 85: 1093-103.

41. Cook JL, Khan KM, Purdam C. Achilles tendiopathy. *Man Ther* 2002; 7(3): 121-30.

42. Khan K, Cook JL, Bonar F, *et al*. Histopathology of common tendinopathies. *Sport Med* 1999; 27(6): 393-408.

43. Ashe MC, McCaulaey T, Khan K. Tendinopathies in the upper extremity: a paradigm shift. *J Hand Therapy* 2004; 17(3): 329-34.

44. Heers G, Anders S, Werther M, *et al*. Efficacy of home exercises for symptomatic rotator cuff tears in correlation to the size of the defect. *Sportverletz Sportschaden* 2005; 19(1): 22-7.

45. Bartolozzi A, Andreychik D, Ahmad S. Determinants of outcome in the treatment of rotator cuff disease. *Clin Orthop Relat Res* 1994; 308: 90-7.

46. Goldberg B, Nowinski R, Matsen F. Outcome of non-operative management of full-thickness rotator cuff tears. *Clin Orthop Relat Res* 2000; 382: 99-107.

47. Brox JI, Staff PH, Ljunggren A, *et al*. Arthroscopic surgery compared with supervised exercises in patients with rotator cuff disease (stage II impingement syndrome). *Br Med J* 1993; 307: 899-903.

48. Dudkiewicz I, Oran A, Salai M, *et al*. Idiopathic adhesive capsulitis: long-term results of conservative treatment. *Isr Med Assoc Journal* 2004; 6(9): 524-6.

49. Lin JJ, Wu YT *et al*. Trapezius muscle imbalance in individuals suffering from frozen shoulder syndrome. *Clin Rheumatology* 2005; 24(6): 569-75.

50. Rundquist PJ, Anderson DD, Guanche CA, *et al*. Shoulder kinematics in subjects with frozen shoulder. *Arch Phys Med Rehabil* 2003; 84(10): 1473-9.

51. Diercks RL, Stevens M. Gentle thawing of the frozen shoulder: a prospective study of supervised neglect versus intensive physical therapy in seventy-seven patients with frozen shoulder syndrome followed-up for two years. *J Shoulder Elbow Surgery* 2004; 13(5): 499-502.

52. Griggs SM, Ahn A, Green A. Idiopathic adhesive capsulitis: a prospective functional outcome study of non-operative treatment. *J Bone Joint Surg* 2000; 82-A(10): 1398-407.

53. Jurgel J, Rannama L, Gapeyeva H, *et al*. Shoulder function in patients with frozen shoulder before and after 4-week rehabilitation. *Medina* (Kaunas) 2005; 41(1): 30-8.

54. Ryans I, Montgomery A, Galway R, *et al*. A randomized controlled trial of intra-articular triamcinolone and/or physiotherapy in shoulder capsulitis. *Rheumatology* (Oxford) 2005; 44: 529-35.

55. Carette S, Moffet H, Tardif J, *et al*. Intraarticular corticosteroids, supervised physiotherapy, or a combination of the two in the treatment of adhesive capsulitis of the shoulder. *Arthritis Rheumatology* 2003; 48(3): 829-38.

56. Sun KO, *et al*. Acupuncture for frozen shoulder. *Hong Kong Med J* 2001; 7(4): 381-91.

57. Gerber C, Nyffeler RW. Classification of glenohumeral joint instability. *Clin Orthop Relat Res* 2002; 400: 65-76.

58. McFarland EG, Kim TK, Park HB. The effect of variation in definition of diagnosis of mulitdirectional instability of the shoulder. *J Bone Joint Surg Am* 2003; 85-A(11): 2138-44.

59. Lewis A, Kitamura T, Bayley JIL. The classification of shoulder instability: new light through old windows. *Curr Orthop* 2004; 18: 97-108.

60. Barden JM, Balyk R, Raso VJ, *et al*. Atypical muscle activation in multidirectional instability. *Clinica Neurophysiology* 2005; 116: 1846-57.

61. Kronberg M, Bronstrom LA, Nemeth G. Differences in shoulder muscle activity between patients with generalised joint laxity and normal controls. *Clin Orthop Relat Res* 1991; 269: 182-92.

62. Myers JB, Ju YY, Hwanh JG, *et al*. Reflexive muscle activation alterations in shoulders with anterior glenohumeral joint instability. *Am J Sports Med* 2004; 32(4): 1013-21.

63. Morris AD, kemp GJ, Frostick SP. Shoulder electromyography in multidirectional instability. *J Shoulder Elbow Surg* 2004; 13(1): 24-9.

64. Warner J, Micheli L, Arslanian L, *et al*. Scapulothoracic motion in normal shoulders and shoulders with glenohumeral instability and impingement syndrome: a study using Moiré topography analysis. *Clin Orthop* 1992; 285: 191-9.

65. Barden JM, Balyk R, Raso VJ, *et al*. Dynamic upper limb proprioception in multidirectional shoulder instability. *Clin Orthop* 2004; 420: 181-9.

66. Myers JB, Lephart SM. Sensorimotor deficits contributing to glenohumeral joint instability. *Clin Orthop Relat Res* 2002; 400: 98-104.

67. Auge WK, Morrison DS. Assessment of the infraspinatus spinal stretch reflex in the normal, athletic, and multidirectionally unstable shoulder. *Am J Sport Med* 2000; 28(2): 206-13.

68. Burkhead WZ Jr, Rockwood CA Jr. Treatment of instability of the shoulder with an exercise programme. *J Bone Joint Surg* 1992; 74-A: 890-6.

Chapter 11

69. Kiss J, Damrel D, Mackie A, *et al.* Non-operative treatment of multidirectional instability. *Int Orthop* 2001; 24: 354-7.

70. Takwale VJ, Calvert P, Rattue H. Involuntary positional instability of the shoulder in adolescents. Is there any benefit from treatment? *Am J Sports Med* 2000; 82: 719-23.

71. Reid DC, Saboe LA, Chepeha JC. Anterior shoulder instability in athletes: comparison of isokinetic resistance exercises and an electromyographic biofeedback re-education program - a pilot program. *Physiotherapy Canada* 1996; Fall: 251-6.

72. Beall MS, Diefenbach G, Allen A. Electromyographic biofeedback in the treatment of voluntary posterior instability of the shoulder. *Am J Sports Med* 1987; 15: 175-8.

73. Ide J, Maeda S, Yantaga M, *et al.* Shoulder-strengthening exercise with an orthosis for multidirectional shoulder instability: quantative evaluation of rotational shoulder strength before and after the exercise programme. *J Shoulder Elbow Surgery* 2003; 12(4): 342-5.

74. Johansson K, Oberg B, Adolfsson L, *et al.* A combination of systematic review and clinicians' beliefs in interventions for subacromial pain. *Br J General Practice* 2002; 52: 145-52.

75. Van der Heijden GJ. Shoulder disorders: a state of the art review. *Ballieres Clin Rheumatol* 1999; 13: 287-309.

76. Mitchell C, Adebajo A, Hay E, Carr A. Shoulder pain: diagnosis and management in primary care. *Br Med J* 2005; 331: 1124-8.

Chapter 11

Chapter 12

Radial head replacement

Kalpesh Shah MS Orthopaedics MRCS
Specialist Registrar, Trauma & Orthopaedics
Lech Rymaszewski FRCS (Ed) FRCS (Eng) MSc
Consultant Orthopaedic Surgeon

GLASGOW ROYAL INFIRMARY, GLASGOW, UK

Introduction

Radial head replacement has become increasingly popular over the last few years with a choice of at least 13 different designs of prosthesis. Some may assume that although simple radial head excision usually gives good clinical outcomes, replacement will ensure consistently superior clinical results. In theory, radial head replacement should prevent the problems seen after radial head excision: valgus elbow instability, restriction of elbow and forearm movement, proximal radial migration and degenerative changes in the elbow and wrist, giving rise to chronic pain, loss of strength and function. However, the evidence to support radial head replacement relies heavily on laboratory studies and there are no published laboratory or clinical results for the majority of prostheses that are commercially available.

Removal of the radial head in an elbow with undamaged ligaments or ulna has a minor effect on stability in laboratory experiments, as the coronoid is the most important articular stabiliser of the elbow joint [1]. Radial head excision performed acutely for displaced fractures, or for pain and stiffness due to arthritis / deformity is, therefore, usually a simple and effective procedure. However, the radial head has a critical role as a secondary stabiliser if the collateral ligaments or interosseous membrane have been disrupted or the coronoid process fractured, in which case radial head excision will exacerbate the instability.

The main indication for radial head replacement is therefore to aid stability following acute trauma allowing early mobilisation, when the radial head fracture cannot be reliably fixed internally [2]. The decision whether to fix, excise or replace is still controversial and depends on the comminution of the fracture, the quality of the bone, the surgeon's training / experience and the availability of implants. Irrespective of the method of management, it is essential to ensure that the joint remains congruent in the early recovery phase, whilst the elbow is being mobilised in the first few weeks after injury.

The aim of this chapter is to examine the evidence to support radial head replacement.

Methodology

A broad search of the English literature on radial head replacement was carried out, using Pubmed, Medline and Ovid databases. In total, 40 publications were identified, with 17 being cadaveric/laboratory biomechanical experiments and only 12 clinical papers reporting metal replacements since 1975, usually with small numbers of patients.

Anatomy / biomechanics (Table 1)

The radial head contributes to the stability of the elbow and transfers significant load to the capitellum during normal elbow movements: up to three times body weight during strenuous activities, due to the lever arm of the forearm [3] (Figure 1a).

Radial head excision produces:

- increased tension in the medial ligament and compression on the lateral aspect of the coronoid with the lateral part of the trochlea (Figure 1b). The elbow remains stable to a valgus stress, provided that the medial collateral ligament (MCL) complex is intact, i.e.

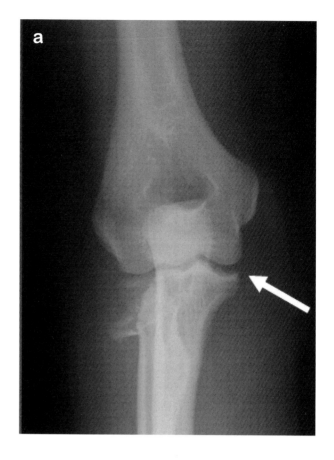

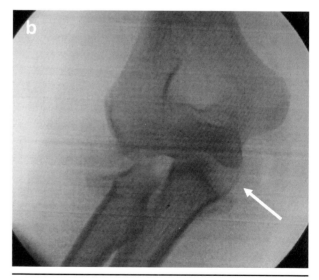

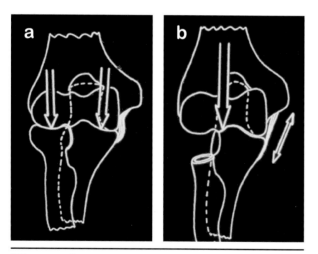

Figure 1. a) Compression forces transmitted equally to the distal humerus on grasping an object, due to contraction of the forearm muscles. b) Forearm prevented from going into valgus after radial head excision by tension in the medial collateral ligament (MCL) with compression at the lateral lip of the trochlea.

Figure 2. a) Acute radial head fracture with grossly depressed fragments, marked soft tissue swelling on the medial aspect and slight widening of the medial joint line (arrow). b) Stress view demonstrating gross valgus instability due to medial ligament disruption (the primary stabiliser) and a depressed radial head fracture (the secondary stabiliser).

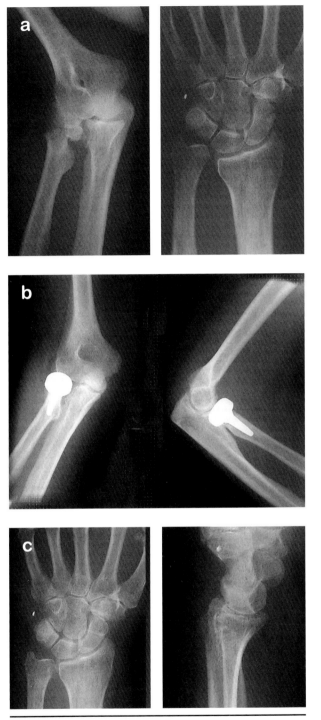

the medial ligament is the primary stabiliser [4]. However, if the medial ligament is disrupted the elbow will sublux under load if the radial head is absent (Figure 2) **(IIb/C)**;

♦ mild varus and external rotatory laxity by losing the capture of the radial head articulation with the capitellum and removing tension in the lateral collateral ligament (LCL) complex. This complex is the most important constraint to varus and external rotatory stresses. Radial head excision in the presence of LCL disruption significantly aggravates varus and external rotatory laxity of the elbow joint [5, 6] **(IIb/C)**;

♦ proximal migration of the radius by a few millimetres [7, 8], as the central band of the interosseous membrane is largely responsible for preventing any further movement. If the central band and distal radio-ulnar joint are disrupted then radial head excision will produce very significant proximal translation, i.e. an Essex-Lopresti lesion (Figure 3) **(IIb/C)**;

♦ posterior subluxation if the coronoid is deficient [9], due to the posteriorly direct forearm muscles crossing the elbow joint (Figure 4) **(IIb/C)**.

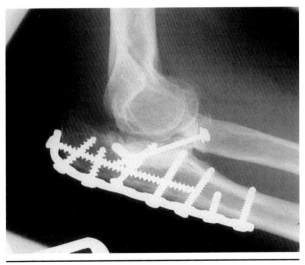

Figure 3. a) Radio-ulnar dissociation with proximal migration due to a comminuted radial head fracture, rupture of the central band of the interosseous membrane and distal radio-ulnar joint ligaments - the Essex-Lopresti lesion. b) Metal radial head replacement has restored the anatomy at the elbow. c) Metal radial head replacement has restored radial length and the wrist anatomy.

Figure 4. Posterior subluxation of the humero-ulnar joint due to failure of fixation of the coronoid process, resulted in pain, stiffness and early degenerative changes. Insertion of a metal radial head spacer at the time of the initial surgery could have averted this complication by preventing posterior subluxation, thereby protecting the fixation of the coronoid.

Chapter 12

Table 1. Biomechanical studies on radial head replacement.

Author	No	Measurement	Experimental condition	Conclusion
Tejwani et al 2005 [8]	12 cadavers	Forces at distal ulna	1. Radial Head Replacement (RHR) 2. Excision of Interosseous Membrane (IOM) 3. Reconstruction of IOM + RHR	IOM reconstruction + RHR reduces distal ulnar force to a level below that for an intact forearm
Johnson et al 2005 [13]	Osseous model & elbow specimen	Elbow kinematics and stability	1. Radial head fracture 2. Radial head excision 3. RHR All with/without integrity of collateral ligaments	Radial head secondary stabilizer to collateral ligaments
Jensen et al 2005 [6]	6 cadavers	Elbow laxity	1. Intact elbow 2. Radial head excision 3. LCL division 4. RHR 5. LCL repair	RHR + LCL repair or LCL repair alone restores stability
Beingessner et al 2004 [14]	8 cadavers	Kinematics and stability	1. Radial head excision + disrupted ligaments 2. RHR + intact ligaments 3. RHR + disrupted ligaments	RHR=native radial head in a stable elbow Radial head fracture with disrupted ligaments RHR alone may be insufficient for stability
Deutch et al 2003 [5]	12 cadavers	Elbow laxity	1. RHR 2. +/- LCL reconstruction 3. Coronoid fracture	RHR + LCL reconstruction or LCL reconstruction alone restores stability
Pomianowski et al 2001 [15]	9 cadavers	Valgus stability	1. Monopolar RHR 2. Bipolar RHR 3. MCL insufficiency	RHR if ORIF not possible
King et al 1999 [16]	8 cadavers	Valgus stability	1. MCL transection 2. RHR (silastic or metallic)	Metal RHR provides valgus stability equal to an intact radial head Silastic RHR conferred no increase in elbow stability
Gupta et al 1997 [17]	Finite element analysis method	Force transmitted across radio-capitellar joint	1. RHR 2. MCL insufficiency	Silicone biomechanically unsatisfactory Metal/ceramic transmit force but strain shielded radial cortex Polyethylene uniform load distribution
Pribyl et al 1986 [18]	5 cadavers	Valgus stress	1. Native radial head 2. RHR 3. Radial head excision	Radial head acts as a stabiliser to valgus stress

In theory, radial head replacement should improve stability if ligaments have been disrupted, and restore normal biomechanical loading after excision, thus preventing the development of osteoarthrosis. However, the anatomy of the radial head and neck is complex and variable, and, therefore, it is very unlikely that its shape can be accurately reproduced with a prosthesis. There are significant differences between individuals with regard to the usually elliptical shape of the radial head, the offset from the axis of the radial neck and neck-shaft angle. Accurate positioning of the implant to transmit normal loads whilst ensuring congruent tracking with the capitellum and lesser sigmoid notch of the ulna is therefore very difficult to achieve [10-12].

There is, therefore, good evidence from the laboratory that metal radial head replacements improve stability, often approaching that of the normal elbow, in cadaveric studies when the relevant soft tissues have been disrupted. There is considerable evidence that silicone rubber is an inadequate material, as it deforms easily under load with little increase in elbow stability. However, it has also been demonstrated that in complex injuries radial head replacement forms only part of the solution, as other procedures may also be required: MCL repair, LCL repair, coronoid and proximal ulnar fracture fixation [5, 19, 20].

Clinical evidence

Morrey classified radial head fractures as simple and complex, i.e. with or without associated injury [21]. A radial head fracture in isolation is a relatively benign problem, but complications are likely to arise if it is associated with concomitant injuries, i.e. medial / lateral collateral ligament or interosseous membrane disruption, coronoid / proximal ulnar fracture and elbow dislocation.

Approximately 10% of patients with a radial head fracture have an obvious elbow dislocation with disruption of the lateral as well as medial ligamentous complexes [22, 23]. Radial head excision in this situation carries a significant risk of re-dislocation, and this is even greater if the coronoid has been fractured: 'the terrible triad' (Figure 4). A significant number of patients with radial head fractures have unrecognised ligamentous injuries that will be aggravated by radial head excision [24, 25]. Early subluxation of the humero-ulnar articulation may then occur leading to pain, stiffness and loss of function. Less frequently, valgus instability due to inadequate medial collateral ligament healing, axial instability due to interosseous membrane injury (Essex-Lopresti) or posterolateral rotatory instability [26] may result.

Although small series [27, 28] (Table 2) have reported excellent results of reduction and internal fixation of comminuted radial head fractures, larger studies have noted a high incidence of unsatisfactory results with increasing comminution, especially if associated with dislocation. Ring *et al* [29] reported on 56 radial head fractures and recommended that open reduction and internal fixation (ORIF) should be reserved for relatively simple fracture patterns, and comminuted fractures, especially if associated with dislocation, are probably better treated with excision +/- prosthesis.

Table 2. Open reduction internal fixation of radial head fracture studies.

Author	Mason type 3	Mason type 4/ other injuries	Comminution	Follow-up	Elbow score/outcome
Ikeda *et al* 2003 [27]	3	7	B2.3- 7 B2.2-3 (AO classification)	28.5 months	90.7
Ring *et al* 2002 [29]	26	27	14/26 Mason 3 had >3 fragments	4 years	Unsatisfactory if associated dislocation/comminuted fracture
Esser *et al* 1995 [28]	9	6	-	7 years 4 months	Good/excellent

Table 3. Satisfactory long-term results after radial head excision for fractures.

Author	Mason type 2 & 3	Mason type 4	Follow-up	Results/ conclusion
Herbertsson et al 2004 [30]	49	12	18 years	Majority had good results. Mason type 4 had tendency to poorer outcomes - 4 out of 12 had daily pain
Eren et al 2002 [31]	16	4	7 years	Majority had good results. Excision justified
Janssen et al 1998 [32]	0	21	16-30 years	Arthroplasty after excision only if elbow unstable
Coleman et al 1987 [33]	17	-	8-46 years	Majority had excellent results
Broberg et al 1987 [34]	21	8	15 years	Delayed excision justified

Good long-term results of radial head excision after trauma have been reported (Table 3), even if associated with dislocation, indicating that the soft tissues usually heal well if the joint remains congruent and is then capable of withstanding the loads applied during strenuous activities.

Poor results have been reported mainly after radial head fractures with associated injuries (Table 4).

Table 4. Poor long-term results after radial head excision.

Author	No	Follow-up	Results
Hall et al 2005 [26]	42 All had associated elbow dislocation	44 months	17% posterolateral instability
Leppilahti et al 2000 [35]	23	5 years	High complication rate: proximal migration of radius, limited elbow movement
Josefsson et al 1989 [23]	18 All had associated elbow dislocation	3-34 years	Stiffness - 14 Pain on effort - 8 Weakness - 7
Mikic et al 1983 [36]	69	Late	50% poor results

Radial head arthroplasty

There is good evidence that a metal radial head replacement acts as a spacer to aid stability in acute injuries, allowing early active movement while bony and soft tissue healing occurs [9, 42]. Implants are usually well tolerated and relatively few have to be removed. There have been no reports of instability or other problems after removal, once adequate healing has taken place.

The aim of inserting a replacement, even as a spacer, is to maintain normal kinematics and loading of the capitellum, at least initially. There is a lack of good instrumentation to ensure that the correct length and orientation of the radial head is restored. Van Glabbeek *et al* [12] demonstrated on cadavers that axial understuffing or overstuffing the radiohumeral joint by greater than 2.5mm alters both elbow kinematics and radiocapitellar pressure (Figure 5). The results of radial head replacement are shown in Tables 5 and 6.

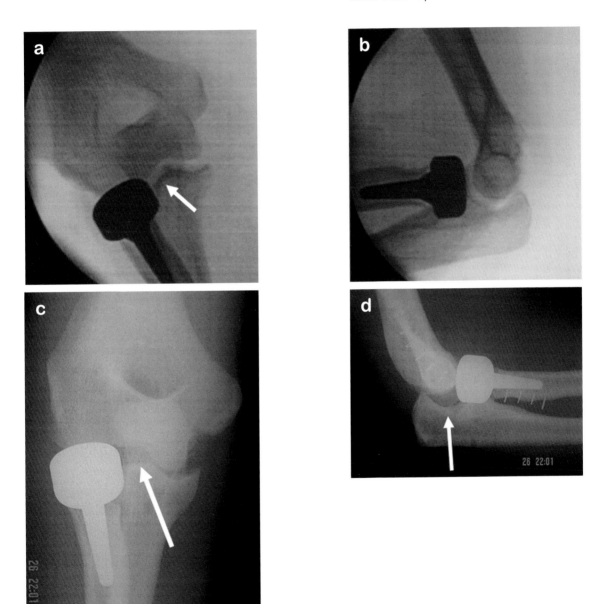

Figure 5. a) & b) It is essential to check intra-operatively with image intensification to ensure the correct size of prosthesis has been inserted. Special care must be paid to ensure that the lateral humero-ulnar joint is not widened due to 'over-stuffing'. c) & d) Gross overstuffing of the radial head prosthesis. There is an increased humero-ulnar joint space (arrow) seen on anteroposterior and lateral views.

Table 5. Clinical studies showing outcome after radial head replacement.

Author	Mason Type 4 i.e. associated elbow dislocation	Olecranon/ proximal ulna/ significant coronoid fracture	Medial collateral ligament tear	Prosthesis/ treatment	Follow-up	Outcome (Mayo performance elbow index)
Ashwood et al 2004 [37]	0	0	16 (and 16 Mason Type 3 fracture)	Titanium + medial collateral repair/ reconstruction	2.8 years	8 - Excellent 5 - Good 3 - Fair
Pugh et al 2004 [38]	20 terrible triad	-	-	Titanium	34 months	15 - Excellent 13 - Good 7 - Fair 1 - Poor
Moro et al 2001 [39]	15	1	1	Titanium	39 months	17 - Excellent or good 5 - Fair 3 - Poor
Harrington et al 2001 [40]	14	4	2	Titanium	12.1 years	12 - Excellent 4 - Good 2 - Fair 2 - Poor
Popovic et al 2000 [41]	8	3	0	Bipolar Judet	32 months	4 - Excellent 4 - Good 2 - Fair 1 - Poor
Knight et al 1993 [42]	13	8	0	Vitallium	4.5 years	No dislocations or prosthetic failures 2 implants removed due to loosening
Harrington et al 1981 [9]	4	8	5	Titanium (+2 silastic)	4 years	Good

Currently available designs include metal monoblock and modular implants, with variable stem lengths of up to 6cm (Figure 6). The stem may be press-fit, have surface ongrowth treatments or be fixed with cement, but this can cause problems if a well fixed stem has to be removed. Abnormal tracking may be responsible for pain and stiffness due to impingement with capitellar damage. Bipolar designs are likely to improve tracking by maintaining good contact at the radio-capitellar and superior radio-ulnar joints during movement, but more of the radial neck needs to be resected to accommodate the bipolar mechanism.

There are no studies comparing clinical results after implantation of different designs and there is a paucity of long-term studies after replacement.

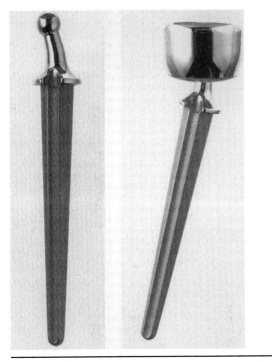

Figure 6. A Judet bipolar prosthesis with a stem length of 5/6 cm.

Table 6. Radial head replacement in acute/chronic Essex-Lopresti injury and laboratory experiments.

Author	No	Clinical/experimental condition	Treatment	Follow-up	Results
Tejwani et al 2005 [8]	12 cadavers	Interosseous membrane (IOM) section + radial head excision	IOM reconstruction + RHR	-	IOM reconstruction + RHR better than RHR alone to reduce forces at distal ulna
Moro et al 2001 [39]	3 patients	Acute Essex-Lopresti injury	Metal RHR	39 months	Good - 1 Fair - 1 Poor - 1
Ruch et al 1999 [43]	1 patient	Chronic Essex-Lopresti injury secondary to failed radial head replacement (silastic)	Metal RHR IOM reconstruction TFCC repair	2 years	Good
Judet et al 1996 [44]	2 patients	Chronic Essex-Lopresti injury after radial head excision	Bipolar RHR + arthrolysis	31 months	No complications with good correction of radio-ulnar index
Sellman et al 1995 [45]	9 cadavers	IOM section + radial head excision	IOM reconstruction + RHR	-	Gross axial stiffness restored with metal RHR

TFCC=Triangular fibro-cartilaginous complex

Conclusions

Treatment of acute, displaced radial head fractures is controversial. The radial head acts as a secondary stabiliser if there is disruption of the collateral ligaments or interosseous membrane, or a fracture of the coronoid, and radial head excision in such situations exacerbates the instability. There is good clinical and biomechanical evidence that a metal replacement for a radial head fracture that cannot be reliably fixed in an unstable elbow will act as a spacer to aid stability and allow early active motion while soft tissue/bony healing occurs. In theory, metal radial head replacement should be effective in preventing/treating significant proximal radial migration due to tearing of the interosseous membrane, although there are few detailed clinical reports.

Recommendations	Evidence level
◆ There is little evidence that the results of radial head excision are improved by insertion of a prosthesis if the soft tissues and humero-ulnar joint are intact.	IIb/B
◆ There is good clinical/biomechanical evidence that a metal replacement for a radial head fracture that cannot be reliably fixed in an unstable elbow will act as a spacer to aid stability and allow early active motion while soft tissue/bony healing occurs.	IIb/B
◆ Silicone rubber is a poor material for a spacer: it deforms easily under load and may break or cause soft tissue inflammatory reactions.	IIb/C
◆ In theory, metal radial head replacement should be effective in preventing/treating proximal radial migration in an Essex-Lopresti lesion, although few successful cases have been reported.	IIb/C

References

1. Morrey BF, Ann KN. Stability of the elbow: osseous constraints. *J Shoulder Elbow Surg* 2005; 14(1 Suppl S): 174S-178S.
2. King GJW. Management of comminuted radial head fractures with replacement arthroplasty. *Hand Clin* 2004; 20: 429-41.
3. Amis AA, Dowson D, Wright V. Analysis of elbow forces due to high-speed forearm movements. *J Biomech* 1980; 13(10): 825-31.
4. Morrey BF, Tanaka S, Ann KN. Valgus stability of the elbow. A definition of primary and secondary constraints. *Clin Orthop Relat Res* 1991; 265: 187-95.
5. Deutch SR, Jensen SL, Tyrdal S, *et al*. Elbow joint stability following experimental osteoligamentous injury and reconstruction. *J Shoulder Elbow Surg* 2003; 12(5): 466-71.
6. Jensen SL, Olsen BS, Tyrdal S, *et al*. Elbow joint laxity after experimental radial head excision and lateral collateral ligament rupture: efficacy of prosthetic replacement and ligament repair. *J Shoulder Elbow Surg* 2005; 14(1): 78-84.
7. Hotchkiss RN, An KN, Sowa DT, *et al*. An anatomic and mechanical study of the interosseous membrane of the forearm: pathomechanics of proximal migration of the radius. *J Hand Surg Am* 1989; 14 (2 Pt 1): 256-61.
8. Tejwani SG, Markolf KL, Benhaim P. Reconstruction of the interosseous membrane of the forearm with a graft substitute: a cadaveric study. *J Hand Surg Am* 2005; 30(2): 326-34.
9. Harrington IJ, Tountas AA. Replacement of the radial head in the treatment of unstable elbow fractures. *Injury* 1981; 12(5): 405-12.
10. van Riet RP, Van Glabbeek F, Baumfeld JA, *et al*. The effect of the orientation of the noncircular radial head on elbow kinematics. *Clin Biomech* (Bristol, Avon) 2004; 19(6): 595-9.
11. Birkedal JP, Deal DN, Ruch DS. Loss of flexion after radial head replacement. *J Shoulder Elbow Surg* 2004; 13(2): 208-13.
12. Van Glabbeek F, van Riet RP, Baumfeld JA, *et al*. Detrimental effects of overstuffing or understuffing with a radial head replacement in the medial collateral ligament-deficient elbow. *J Bone Joint Surg Am* 2004; 86-A (12): 2629-35.

13. Johnson JA, Beingessner DM, Gordon KD, et al. Kinematics and stability of the fractured and implant-reconstructed radial head. J Shoulder Elbow Surg 2005; 14(1 Suppl S): 195S-201S.

14. Beingessner DM, Dunning CE, Gordon KD, et al. The effect of radial head excision and arthroplasty on elbow kinematics and stability. J Bone Joint Surg Am 2004; 86-A (8): 1730-9.

15. Pomianowski S, Morrey BF, Neale PG, et al. Contribution of monoblock and bipolar radial head prostheses to valgus stability of the elbow. J Bone Joint Surg Am 2001; 83-A (12): 1829-34.

16. King GJ, Zarzour ZD, Rath DA, et al. Metallic radial head arthroplasty improves valgus stability of the elbow. Clin Orthop Relat Res 1999; 368: 114-25.

17. Gupta GG, Lucas G, Hahn DL. Biomechanical and computer analysis of radial head prostheses. J Shoulder Elbow Surg 1997; 6(1): 37-48.

18. Pribyl CR, Kester MA, Cook SD, et al. The effect of the radial head and prosthetic radial head replacement on resisting valgus stress at the elbow. Orthopaedics 1986; 9(5): 723-6.

19. Jensen SL, Deutch SR, Olsen BS, et al. Laxity of the elbow after experimental excision of the radial head and division of the medial collateral ligament. Efficacy of ligament repair and radial head prosthetic replacement: a cadaver study. J Bone Joint Surg Br 2003; 85 (7): 1006-10.

20. Ring D, Jupiter JB, Zilberfarb J. Posterior dislocation of the elbow with fractures of the radial head and coronoid. J Bone Joint Surg Am 2002; 84-A (4): 547-51.

21. Morrey BF. The Elbow and its Disorders, 3rd ed. Philadelphia: W.B. Saunders, 2000.

22. McKee MD, Schemitsch EH, Sala MJ, et al. The pathoanatomy of lateral ligamentous disruption in complex elbow instability. J Shoulder Elbow Surg 2003; 12(4): 391-6.

23. Josefsson PO, Gentz CF, Johnell O, et al. Dislocations of the elbow and intraarticular fractures. Clin Orthop Relat Res 1989; 246: 126-30.

24. Itamura J, Roidis N, Mirzayan R, et al. Radial head fractures: MRI evaluation of associated injuries. J Shoulder Elbow Surg 2005; 14(4): 421-4.

25. Davidson PA, Moseley JB Jr, Tullos HS. Radial head fracture. A potentially complex injury. Clin Orthop Relat Res 1993; 297: 224-30.

26. Hall JA, McKee MD. Posterolateral rotatory instability of the elbow following radial head resection. J Bone Joint Surg Am 2005; 87(7): 1571-9.

27. Ikeda M, Yamashina Y, Kamimoto M, et al. Open reduction and internal fixation of comminuted fractures of the radial head using low-profile mini-plates. J Bone Joint Surg Br 2003; 85: 1040-4.

28. Esser RD, Davis S, Taavao T. Fractures of the radial head treated by internal fixation: late results in 26 cases. J Orthop Trauma 1995; 9(4): 318-23.

29. Ring D, Quintero J, Jupiter JB. Open reduction and internal fixation of fractures of the radial head. J Bone Joint Surg Am 2002; 84-A (10): 1811-5.

30. Herbertsson P, Josefsson PO, Hasserius R, et al. Uncomplicated Mason type-II and III fractures of the radial head and neck in adults. A long-term follow-up study. J Bone Joint Surg Am 2004; 86-A (3): 569-74

31. Eren OT, Tezer M, Armagan R, et al. Results of excision of the radial head in comminuted fractures. Acta Orthop Traumatol Turc 2002; 36(1): 12-6.

32. Janssen RP, Vegter J. Resection of the radial head after Mason type-III fractures of the elbow: follow-up at 16 to 30 years. J Bone Joint Surg Br 1998; 80(2): 231-3.

33. Coleman DA, Blair WF, Shurr D. Resection of the radial head for fracture of the radial head. Long-term follow-up of seventeen cases. J Bone Joint Surg Am 1987; 69(3): 385-92.

34. Broberg MA, Morrey BF. Results of treatment of fracture-dislocations of the elbow. Clin Orthop Relat Res 1987; 216: 109-19.

35. Leppilahti J, Jalovaara P. Early excision of the radial head for fracture. Int Orthop 2000; 24(3): 160-2.

36. Mikic ZD, Vukadinovic SM. Late results in fractures of the radial head treated by excision. Clin Orthop Relat Res 1983; 181: 220-8.

37. Ashwood N, Bain GI, Baird R, et al. Management of Mason type-III radial head fractures with a titanium prosthesis, ligament repair, and early mobilization. J Bone Joint Surg Am 2004; 86-A (2): 274-80.

38. Pugh DM, Wild LM, Schemitsch EH, et al. Standard surgical protocol to treat elbow dislocations with radial head and coronoid fractures. J Bone Joint Surg Am 2004; 86: 1122-30.

39. Moro JK, Werier J, MacDermid JC, et al. Arthroplasty with a metal radial head for unreconstructable fractures of the radial head. J Bone Joint Surg Am 2001; 83-A (8): 1201-11.

40. Harrington IJ, Sekyi-Out A, Barrington TW, et al. The functional outcome with metallic radial head implants in the treatment of unstable elbow fractures: a long-term review. J Trauma 2001; 50(1): 46-52.

41. Popovic N, Gillet P, Rodriguez A, et al. Fracture of the radial head with associated elbow dislocation: results of treatment using floating radial head prosthesis. J Orthop Trauma 2000; 14(3): 171-7.

42. Knight DJ, Rymaszewski LA, Amis AA, et al. Primary replacement of the fractured radial head with a metal prosthesis. J Bone Joint Surg Br 1993; 75(4): 572-6.

43. Ruch DS, Change DS, Koman LA. Reconstruction of longitudinal stability of the forearm after disruption of interosseous ligament and radial head excision (Essex-Lopresti lesion). J South Orthop Assoc 1999; 8: 47-52.

44. Judet T, Garreau de Loubresse C, Piriou P, et al. A floating prosthesis for radial head fractures. J Bone Joint Surg 1996; 78B: 244-9.

45. Sellman DC, Seitz WH, Postak PD, et al. Reconstructive strategies for radioulnar dissociation a biomechanical study. J Orthop Trauma 1995; 9: 516-22.

Radial head replacement

Chapter 13

Total elbow arthroplasty in elective and trauma surgery

Andreas Hinsche FRCSEd (Tr & Orth)
Consultant Orthopaedic Surgeon [1]
David Stanley MB BS BSc (Hons) FRCS
Consultant Upper Limb Surgeon [2]

1 QUEEN ELIZABETH HOSPITAL, GATESHEAD, UK
2 THE ELBOW AND SHOULDER UNIT, THE NORTHERN GENERAL HOSPITAL, SHEFFIELD, UK

Introduction

Total elbow arthroplasty began in the early 1940s when Boerema and de Waard [1] reported their experience of using a single-axis metallic hinge replacement for elbow reconstruction. This was followed by other hinge arthroplasties [2-4], all of which were noted to give excellent early results but then failed, due primarily to loosening of the humeral component [5]. The typical failure mode resulted in the axis of the prosthesis being displaced posteriorly whilst the tip of the humeral component moved anteriorly, sometimes breaching the anterior cortex.

In an attempt to overcome this problem, implants were designed with supplementary plates that were screwed either to the posterior or anterior humeral surfaces [6] (Figure 1). Unfortunately, these also became loose and failed to give satisfactory long-term results.

The next generation of hinge arthroplasties is perhaps best exemplified by the Stanmore implant designed by Lettin and Scales [7]. This was a slim metal prosthesis with a high-density polyethylene bushing between the two components. It was inserted with preservation of the collateral ligaments. Although this

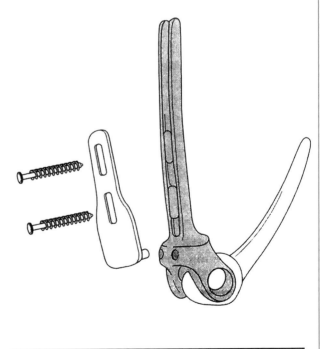

Figure 1. Nederpelt's prosthesis. This is a fully constrained prosthesis with a posterior plate to try and prevent loosening.

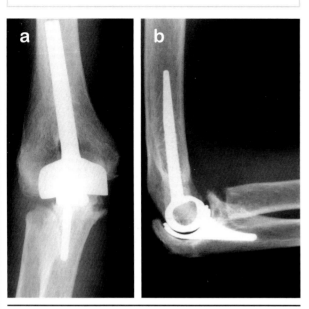

Figure 2. The Kudo implant. a) Anteroposterior view. b) Lateral view.

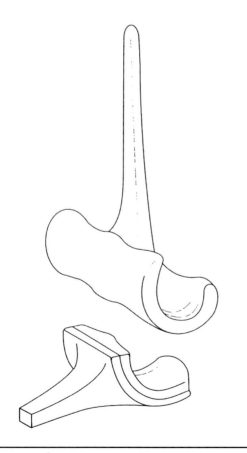

Figure 3. The capitello-condylar implant designed by Ewald.

produced better results than the original hinges, loosening rates of up to 20% still occurred [8] **(IIb/B)**.

Modern total elbow arthroplasties fall into three categories:

* unlinked or resurfacing implants;
* linked implants;
* convertible implants.

Methodology

A comprehensive search of the current literature for the period 1995 to 2005 was carried out electronically using the Medline database. In addition, the Cochrane database identified a few additional papers. The search focused particularly on the indications for total elbow arthroplasty. In addition, since total elbow arthroplasty is relatively infrequently performed, the papers were analysed for the length of follow-up in order to determine the effectiveness of the procedure. Particular emphasis was placed on more recent publications in order to reflect the current views of elbow specialists throughout the world.

Unlinked or resurfacing implants

Although these implants are unlinked they vary in their degree of constraint. The Kudo arthroplasty [9] (Figure 2) is relatively unconstrained with a saddle-shaped humeral articulation and reciprocal ulnar component. The capitello-condylar implant designed by Ewald [10] (Figure 3) and the Souter-Strathclyde arthroplasty [11] (Figure 4) have an axis articular surface more closely resembling the normal elbow joint anatomy. These implants have significantly greater constraint. All elbow arthroplasties of this type are dependent for stability on soft tissue balance at the time of insertion **(IIb/B)**.

Linked implants

Linked implants differ markedly from the original hinge prostheses since, although the humeral and ulnar components are joined, the design incorporates valgus and varus laxity. This, in theory, should reduce

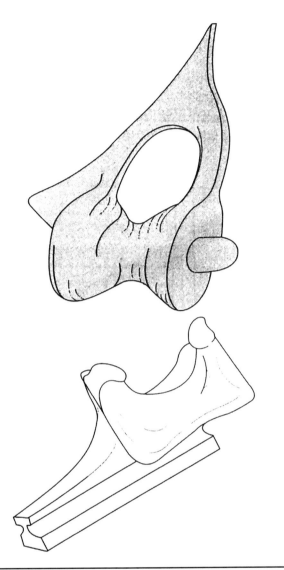

Figure 4. The Souter-Strathclyde prosthesis. It closely resembles the normal anatomy of the elbow.

the stress forces at the bone/cement interface and therefore reduce the rate of loosening. Elbow arthroplasties of this type include the Coonrad-Morrey prosthesis [12] (Figure 5) and the more recently developed Discovery **(IIb/B)**.

Convertible implants

These implants have the advantage of being able to be used as unlinked prostheses but can also be inserted as linked implants when additional stability is

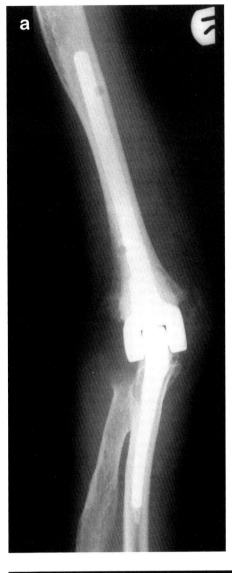

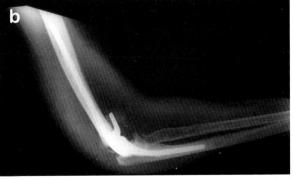

Figure 5. The Coonrad-Morrey prosthesis. It is a linked implant with valgus and varus laxity. a) Anteroposterior view. b) Lateral view.

required. Arthroplasties with these features include the Acclaim and the new Latitude arthroplasty.

Indications for total elbow arthroplasty

The primary indication for total elbow arthroplasty is advanced inflammatory arthritis of the elbow [13-27] **(IIb/B)**.

Other indications include:

- acute distal humeral fractures in the elderly [28-30];
- flail or unstable elbows [31, 32];
- osteoarthritis [33];
- distal humeral fracture non-union [34];
- post-traumatic arthritis [35];
- elbow ankylosis [36].

Choice of prosthesis

The choice of prosthesis for the different clinical scenarios does not follow rigid guidelines. It depends on the degree of joint destruction, the bone stock and the soft tissue support. In patients with severe bone loss it may be impossible to insert an unlinked prosthesis and maintain stability. Similarly, in elderly patients with comminuted distal humeral fractures, a linked implant is normally necessary in order to achieve adequate humeral fixation. On the other hand, patients with inflammatory arthritis and a stable joint would be expected to achieve an acceptable outcome with an unlinked arthroplasty.

Within the UK the four implant types which have more than a 10% market share are the Coonrad-Morrey (Zimmer), Capitello-condylar (Johnson & Johnson), Kudo (Biomet) and Souter-Strathclyde (Stryker Howmedica) [37].

Assessment of outcome

In order to be able to assess different prostheses it would clearly be advantageous for all published data on total elbow arthroplasties to use one outcome score. This, unfortunately, is not the case and a recent review by Little, Graham and Carr [37] identified that most authors use their own scoring systems. This, as

Turchin *et al* have shown, makes the interpretation of results difficult [38]. It is not possible to directly compare one scoring system with another, although it has been shown that the individual components (pain, range of movement, function etc.) can be compared [38].

Another difficulty when assessing outcome relates to the observation that 44% of the published data is from the implant designers' institutions [37]. As such, the results obtained may not be representative of what might be expected from a non-designer surgeon.

The length of follow-up is another important factor when assessing outcome. The original implant designs were very successful in the short term, but then failed, most frequently due to loosening. As such, when the results of a particular prosthesis are being evaluated it is important to consider the length of follow-up. Although there are now many publications with short to medium-term follow-up [8-36], we have been able to identify only two with a minimum ten-year follow-up [39, 40] **(IIb/B)**.

Results of total elbow arthroplasty

Pain

A reduction in pain is almost invariably achieved following total elbow arthroplasty. However, with time it has been shown that pain at rest, pain at night, pain with movement, and pain with loading or stress all tend to increase the longer the follow-up period [41].

Range of movement

Improvement in motion is normally expected following total elbow arthroplasty irrespective of the indication for surgery. In their long-term follow-up of the GSB III arthroplasty, Gschwend *et al* identified a greater improvement in movement postoperatively in patients who had undergone a total elbow replacement for post-traumatic osteoarthritis than in those treated for rheumatoid arthritis (Table 1) [40]. The greater improvement in movement in patients with post-traumatic osteoarthritis compared to those with rheumatoid arthritis was also one of the findings noted by Little, Graham, and Carr in their review of the English language literature on total elbow

Table 1. The mean range of movement pre and postoperatively following total elbow replacement in rheumatoid patients and those with post-traumatic osteoarthritis. Adapted from [40].

	Rheumatoid arthritis		Post-traumatic osteoarthritis	
	Pre-op	Post-op	Pre-op	Post-op
Fixed flexion deformity	40.3°	27.8°	58°	44°
Flexion	120.0°	144.2°	88°	141°
Total	79.7°	116.3°	30°	97°

arthroplasty [37]. These authors also noted that linked implants restored a better range of movement than was achieved with unlinked prostheses [37].

Function

Wright et al [42], in a study comparing functional outcome in patients undergoing linked and unlinked arthroplasties primarily for rheumatoid arthritis, found no difference in outcome (Table 2). This is in contrast to the literature review by Little et al [37] where a higher proportion of excellent and good results were found with the use of linked implants (82%) compared to unlinked prostheses (78%).

Age

In a survivorship analysis of the Souter-Strathclyde elbow arthroplasty, Talwalkar et al [43] showed that age did not affect outcome. Rheumatoid patients with a

mean age of 42 years at the time of surgery had no significant difference in the incidence of loosening when compared to patients with a mean age of 64 years.

Complications

In a recent review of the literature [37] the complication rate of total elbow arthroplasty is quoted as being between 14% and 80% with a median rate of 33%. This figure is similar to that reported by Gschwend et al [44] (43%) following their review of the literature for the period 1986-1992 **(IIb/B)**.

Intra-operative complications

Bone fracture

Intra-operative bone fractures occur in less than 3% of patients undergoing total elbow arthroplasties. If this happens during the surgical procedure it may

Table 2. The functional outcome in patients treated with unlinked and linked prostheses. The functional score is from 0-4, with 4 indicating excellent function. Adapted from [42].

Function	Unlinked prostheses (average)	Linked protheses (average)
Reach back pocket	2.73	3.00
Rise from chair	2.82	3.15
Perineal care	3.27	3.15
Wash axilla	3.15	3.31
Eat with utensil	3.18	3.31
Comb hair	2.64	3.31
Dress	2.64	2.62

not be possible to insert an unlinked implant and in this situation the surgeon must be prepared to use a linked prosthesis. It may also be necessary to internally fix the fracture.

Ulnar nerve problems

Ulnar nerve problems following total elbow arthroplasty have been reported in 1.7% to 26% [44, 37]. Although the majority are temporary and fully recover, 5% will have a permanent sensory and/or motor deficit [37]. Damage to the nerve may result from compromise of its blood supply during mobilisation, traction or incomplete release of the nerve, direct surgical trauma, haematoma formation around the nerve or thermal injury from the methylmethacrylate cement **(IIb/B)**.

Postoperative complications

Loosening

The rate of loosening of linked implants (5%) is lower than unlinked devices (10%) over a similar follow-up period [37]. If radiolucent lines on radiographs are studied, however, these are noted to be more common in linked implants (15%) than unlinked prostheses (11%) [37] (Figure 6).

The causes of loosening are undoubtedly multi-factorial and include the posterior pull of the elbow flexors when the elbow is at 90°, the cyclical loading of the distal humerus, distraction forces during full elbow flexion, and lateral rotation stresses during supination and pronation [45]. Souter suggested that the main cause of loosening was the transfer of rotational forces across the elbow to the humeral cement/bone interface rather than via the collateral ligaments [5] **(IIb/B)**.

Infection

Little *et al* [37] have shown that since 1989 the rate of infection of total elbow arthroplasties has remained fairly constant at about 4%. Both Gschwend *et al* [44] and Morrey [46], however, have stated that their own infection rates are less than 3% **(IIb/B)**.

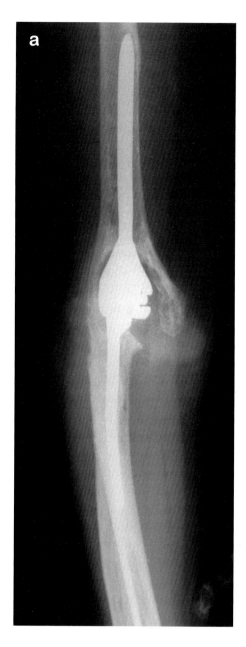

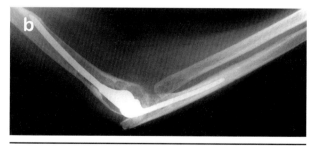

Figure 6. Radiolucent lines are seen around this prosthesis indicating loosening of the implant. a) Anteroposterior view. b) Lateral view.

The treatment options for an infected total elbow arthroplasty usually involve removal of the prosthesis with a thorough debridement of the soft tissues. The patient may be left with an excision arthroplasty or alternatively, if the infection can be successfully treated with antibiotics, a re-implantation can be performed at a later date. Occasionally, if the infection is diagnosed early, it may be possible to perform a debridement of the joint and prescribe antibiotics rather than remove the implant.

Instability and implant disassembly

Gschwend, in an analysis of the world literature between 1986 and 1992, identified an elbow arthroplasty instability rate of 6.5% [44]. It is a complication of unlinked prostheses and results from inaccurate implant alignment or inadequate soft tissue reconstruction [47] (Figure 7) **(IIb/B)**.

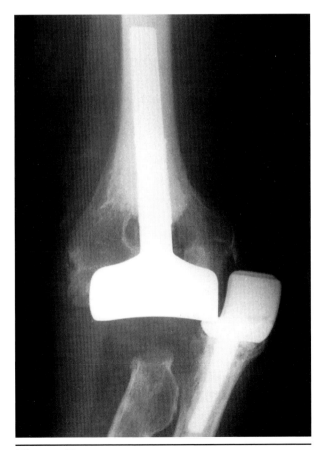

Figure 7. A dislocated Kudo prosthesis.

Implant disassembly occurs with linked or convertible arthroplasties and results from failure or breakage of the linkage mechanism, or disassociation of the components. It has a reported rate of 6% [37].

Extensor mechanism insufficiency

Postoperative extensor mechanism insufficiency can be divided into two types. Total avulsion of the triceps will affect the stability of the arthroplasty and will result in an increased risk of aseptic loosening. It is reported in 3% of total elbow replacements [37]. The literature would suggest it is a feature of the surgical approach. It is seen in 0.56% where a triceps turndown is used, 2.8% where the triceps is kept in continuity with the periosteum of the ulna, and 11% when the triceps is fully released from the ulna [37] **(IIb/B)**.

The second type of insufficiency relates to postoperative weakness of the triceps. This almost certainly is a common sequel of all posterior approaches for total elbow arthroplasty. Unfortunately, there is no information on this within the literature, as it is currently an under-appreciated complication.

Implant failure

Prosthetic fractures account for less than 1% of all total elbow arthroplasty complications [44]. They are usually associated with implant loosening and most often occur at the junction between the stable and loosened parts of the prosthesis.

Conclusions

The overall revision rate following total elbow arthroplasty is 13%. As such it is essential that the surgeon undertaking the primary total elbow arthroplasty is well trained in the operative technique, aware of the pros and cons of the different prostheses, and capable of dealing with any difficulties that might be encountered during the surgical procedure. Providing these criteria are met it is to be hoped that we will continue to see improvements in the outcome of total elbow arthroplasty with fewer complications and greater patient satisfaction.

Recommendations	Evidence level
Condition and implant type	

- Inflammatory arthritis/good bone preservation: unlinked implant, linked implant, convertible implant.   IIb/B
- Inflammatory arthritis/bone loss: linked implant, convertible implant.   IIb/B
- Flail or unstable elbow instability: linked implant, convertible implant.   IIb/B
- Distal humeral fracture in the elderly: linked implant, convertible implant.   IIb/B
- Osteoarthritis: unlinked implant, linked implant, convertible implant.   IIb/B
- Distal humeral fracture non-union: linked implant, convertible implant.   IIb/B
- Post-traumatic arthritis: unlinked implant, linked implant, convertible implant.   IIb/B
- Elbow ankylosis: unlinked implant, linked implant, convertible implant.   IIb/B

References

1. Boerema I, de Waard DJ. Osteoplastische Verakening von Metall prosthesen bei Pseudarthrose and bei Orthoplastik. *Acta Chir Scand* 1942; 86: 511-24.

2. Dee R, Sweetnam DR. Total replacement arthroplasty of the elbow joint for rheumatoid arthritis: two cases. *Proc R Soc Med* 1969; 63: 653-5.

3. McKee GT. Total replacement of the elbow joint. Proceedings of 12th Sicot Congress, Amsterdam. *Excerpta Medica* 1973: 891-3.

4. Shiers LGP. Replacing the shot-out joint. *Roy Naval Med Serv* 1976; 62: 149-51.

5. Souter WA. The evolution of total replacement arthroplasty of the elbow. In: *Elbow joint.* Kashiwagi D, Ed. Amsterdam: Elsevier Science Publishers (Biomedical Division), 1985: 255-6.

6. Nederpelt KJ. Eight years experience with endoprostheses for the elbow joint. *Acta Orthopaedica Belgica* 1975; 41: 499-504.

7. Scales JT, Lettin AWF, Bayley I. The evolution of the Stanmore hinged total elbow replacement 1967-1976. In: *Joint replacement in the upper limb.* London: Institute of Mechanical Engineers Conference Publications, 1977: 53-62.

8. Johnson JR, Getty CJM, Lettin AWF, Glasgow MMS. The Stanmore total elbow replacement for rheumatoid arthritis. *J Bone Joint Surg* 1984; 66B: 732-6.

9. Kudo H, Iwano K, Watanabe S. Total replacement of the rheumatoid elbow with a hingeless prosthesis. *J Bone Joint Surg* 1980; 62A: 277-85.

10. Ewald FC, Scheinberg RD, Poss R, *et al.* Capitello-condylar total elbow arthroplasty two to five-year follow-up in rheumatoid arthritis. *J Bone Joint Surg* 1980; 62A: 1259-63.

11. Souter WA. A new approach to elbow arthroplasty. *Engineering Med* 1981; 10: 59-64.

12. Morrey BF, Adams RA. Semi-constrained elbow replacement for rheumatoid arthritis of the elbow. *J Bone Joint Surg* 1992; 74A: 479-90.

13. Kudo H, Iwano K. Total elbow arthroplasty with a non-constrained surface replacement prosthesis in patients who have rheumatoid arthritis: a long-term follow-up study. *J Bone Joint Surg* 1990; 72A: 355-62.

14. Trail IA, Nuttall D, Stanley JK. Survivorship and radiological analysis of the standard Souter-Strathclyde total elbow arthroplasty. *J Bone Joint Surg* 1999; 81B: 80-4.

15. Morrey BF, Bryan RS, Dobyns JH, Lincheid RL. Total elbow arthroplasty a five-year experience at the Mayo clinic. *J Bone Joint Surg* 1981; 63A: 1050-63.

16. Harder DH, Beauchamp RD. Total replacement arthroplasty of elbow in rheumatoid arthritis. *Can J Surg* 1977; 20: 234-6.

17. Souter WA. Arthroplasty of the elbow with particular reference to metallic hinge arthroplasty in rheumatoid patients. *Orthop Clin North Am* 1973; 4: 395-413.

18. Ewald FC, Simmons ED Jr, Sullivan JA, *et al.* Capitello-condylar total elbow replacement in rheumatoid arthritis: long-term results. *J Bone Joint Surg* 1993; 75A: 498-507.

19. Connor PM, Morrey BF. Total elbow arthroplasty in patients who have juvenile rheumatoid arthritis. *J Bone Joint Surg* 1998; 80A: 678-88.

20. Kudo H, Iwano K, Nishino J. Total elbow arthroplasty with use of non-constrained humeral component inserted without cement in patients who have rheumatoid arthritis. *J Bone Joint Surg* 1999; 81A: 1268-80.

21. Rozing P. Souter-Strathclyde total elbow arthroplasty. *J Bone Joint Surg* 2000; 82B: 1129-34.

22. Schneeberger AG, Hertel R, Gerber C. Total elbow replacement with the GSB III prosthesis. *J Shoulder Elbow Surg* 2000; 9: 135-9.

23. Dainton JN, Hutchins PM. A medium-term follow-up study of 44 Souter-Strathclyde elbow arthroplasties carried out for rheumatoid arthritis. *J Shoulder Elbow Surg* 2002; 11: 486-92.

24. Ikavalko M, Lehto MU, Repo A, *et al.* The Souter-Strathclyde elbow arthroplasty: a clinical and radiological study of 525 consecutive cases. *J Bone Joint Surg* 2002; 84B: 77-82.

25. Potter D, Claydon P, Stanley D. Total elbow replacement using the Kudo prosthesis: clinical and radiological review with five to seven-year follow-up. *J Bone Joint Surg* 2003; 85B: 354-7.

26. Kudo H. Non-constrained elbow arthroplasty for mutilans deformity in rheumatoid arthritis: a report of six cases. *J Bone Joint Surg* 1998; 80B: 234-9.

27. Canovas F, Ledoux D, Bonnel F. Total elbow arthroplasty in rheumatoid arthritis: 20 GSB lll prostheses followed 2-5 years. *Acta Orthop Scand* 1999; 70: 564-8.

28. Cobb TK, Morrey BF. Total elbow arthroplasty as primary treatment for distal humeral fractures in elderly patients. *J Bone Joint Surg* 1997; 79A: 826-32.

29. Garcia JA, Mykula R, Stanley D. Complex fractures of the distal humerus in the elderly: the role of total elbow replacement as primary treatment. *J Bone Joint Surg* 2002; 84B: 812-6.

30. Kamineni S, Morrey BF. Distal humeral fractures treated with noncustom total elbow replacement. *J Bone Joint Surg* 2004; 86A: 940-6.

31. Ramsey ML, Adams RA, Morrey BF. Instability of the elbow treated with semiconstrained total elbow arthroplasty. *J Bone Joint Surg* 1999; 81A: 38-47.

32. Mighell MA, Dunham RC, Rommel EA, Frankle MA. Primary semiconstrained arthroplasty for chronic fracture-dislocations of the elbow. *J Bone Joint Surg* 2005; 87B: 191-5.

33. Espag MP, Back DL, Clark DI, Lunn PG. Early results of the Souter-Strathclyde unlinked total elbow arthroplasty in patients with osteoarthritis. *J Bone Joint Surg* 2003; 85B: 351-3.

34. Gallay SH, Mckee MD. Operative treatment of nonunions about the elbow. *Clin Orthop* 2000; 37O: 87-101.

35. Morrey BF, Adams RA, Bryan RS. Total replacement for post-traumatic arthritis of the elbow. *J Bone Joint Surg* 1991; 73B: 607-12.

36. Baksi DP. Sloppy hinge prosthetic elbow replacement for post-traumatic ankylosis or instability. *J Bone Joint Surg* 1998; 80B: 614-9.

37. Little CP, Graham AJ, Carr AJ. Total elbow arthroplasty. *J Bone Joint Surg* 2005; 87B: 437-44.

38. Turchin DC, Beaton DE, Richards RR. Validity of observer-based aggregate scoring systems as descriptors of elbow pain, function and disability. *J Bone Joint Surg* 1998; 80A: 154-62.

39. Gill DRJ, Morrey BF. The Coonrad-Morrey total elbow arthroplasty in patients with rheumatoid arthritis: 10-15 year follow-up study. *J Bone Joint Surg* 1998; 80A:1327-35.

40. Gschwend N, Scheier NH, Baehler AR. Long-term results of the GSB 111 elbow arthroplasty. *J Bone Joint Surg* 1999; 81B: 1005-12.

41. Van Der Lugt JCT, Geskus RB, Rozing PM. Primary Souter-Strathclyde total elbow prosthesis in rheumatoid arthritis. *J Bone Joint Surg* 2004; 86A: 465-73.

42. Wright TW, Wong AM, Jaffe R. Functional outcome comparison of semiconstrained and unconstrained total elbow arthroplasties. *J Shoulder Elbow Surg* 2000; 9: 524-30.

43. Talwalkar SC, Givissis PK, Trail IA, *et al.* Survivorship of the Souter-Strathclyde elbow replacement in the young inflammatory arthritis elbow. *J Bone Joint Surg* 2005; 87B: 946-9.

44. Gschwend N, Simmen BR, Matejovsky Z. Late complications in elbow arthroplasty. *J Shoulder Elbow Surg* 1996; 5: 86-96.

45. Souter WA. Total replacement arthroplasty of the elbow. In: *Joint replacement in the upper limb.* London: Institute of Mechanical Engineers Conference Publications, 1977: 99-106.

46. Morrey BF. Complications of elbow replacement surgery. In: *The elbow and its disorders.* Morrey BF, Ed. Philadelphia: WB Saunders Co, 1993: 665-75.

47. Figgie HE, Inglis AE. Current concepts in total elbow arthroplasty. *Adv Orthop* 1986; 9: 195-212.

Chapter 13

Chapter 13

Chapter 14

Distal radius fractures

Graham Cheung MRCS

Specialist Registrar, Orthopaedic Surgery

Simon Pickard FRCS (Orth)

Consultant Orthopaedic Surgeon and Specialist in Hand Surgery

David Ford FRCS (Orth)

Consultant Orthopaedic Surgeon and Specialist in Hand Surgery

ROBERT JONES AND AGNES HUNT ORTHOPAEDIC HOSPITAL, OSWESTRY, UK
AND THE ROYAL SHREWSBURY HOSPITAL, SHREWSBURY, UK

Introduction

Fractures of the distal radius remain one of the most common injuries facing orthopaedic surgeons today. O'Neill *et al* suggested an incidence of 36.8/10,000 person-years in women and 9.0/10,000 person-years in men who are aged 35 years and over [1]. In a population of 500,000 this equates to 20 new distal radius fractures per week. Despite this, the best method of treatment remains controversial.

Methodology

A Pubmed search from 2000 to 2006 was performed, looking primarily for well-designed comparative studies published in English. The paucity of such studies led to an extension to include case series. Supplemental references were obtained from review articles and also from expert knowledge of the literature.

Indications for surgery

Instability

Instability has been defined as the inability of a fracture to resist displacement after it has been manipulated into an anatomic position. Lafontaine *et al*, after reviewing a series of 167 cases, suggested five factors predictive of instability: initial dorsal angulation greater than 20°, dorsal comminution, radiocarpal intra-articular involvement, associated ulnar fractures and age greater than 60 years [2]. They concluded that fractures presenting with three or more of these factors were much more likely to lose position with cast immobilisation.

Leone *et al* performed an observational study to see if they could find predictors of early and late displacement. They followed-up 71 patients, 50 with displaced fractures that were reduced and put into a cast and 21 that were undisplaced, which were simply treated in a cast. The mean age was 64.9 years. They found that radial inclination, age, radial shortening and volar tilt were predictive for loss of position [3]. Unexpectedly, they showed that one third of undisplaced fractures in patients over the age of 65 subsequently collapsed.

Nesbitt *et al*, on reviewing 50 patients with at least three of Lafontaine's instability factors, reported that on follow-up patients greater than 58 years of age were at 50% risk for secondary displacement. The risk of an unacceptable radiological result was found to increase with age [4].

The value of remanipulating a Colles' fracture that has redisplaced after primary reduction and plaster immobilisation was assessed in 50 patients by McQueen *et al*. In those over 60 years old, remanipulation failed to achieve a lasting improvement in position, while the majority of those less than 60 years maintained a significant improvement in dorsal angulation [5].

Joint congruency

Knirk and Jupiter reviewed 43 intra-articular wrist fractures in young adults in 1986 and found that joint congruency in this group was the most critical factor in predicting outcome. At a mean follow-up of 6.7 years, 91% of those that had healed with joint incongruency of more than 2mm went on to develop radiological evidence of arthrosis, compared with 11% of those with a congruent joint [6].

Catalano *et al* retrospectively reviewed 26 intra-articular fractures in patients less than 45 years old that had been treated operatively, at a minimum of 5.5 years. They found a positive correlation between the amount of residual displacement and the development of arthrosis. However, the functional status at the time of the most recent follow-up, as determined by physical examination and on the basis of the responses on the questionnaire, did not correlate with the magnitude of the residual step and gap displacement at the time of fracture healing. All patients had a good or excellent functional outcome, irrespective of radiographic evidence of osteoarthrosis of the radiocarpal or the distal radio-ulnar joint, or non-union of the ulnar styloid process [7]. Fernandez *et al*, on the other hand, reviewed 50 adults (mean age 49.6 years) and found that intra-articular incongruence of 1mm or greater correlated with a lower Short-Form 36 score and with the development of arthrosis. Interestingly, those injured while working were more than four times less likely to

return to work than those injured while away from work [8].

Does the anatomical result affect the final function?

McQueen and Caspers reviewed 30 patients at a minimum of four years after injury (mean age 69 years). All fractures were treated by reduction and plaster immobilisation. They assessed strength, dexterity, activities of daily living, median nerve function, range of movement, cosmesis and pain. They found malunion of a Colles' fracture was more likely to result in a weak, deformed, stiff and probably painful wrist [9]. However, Beumer and McQueen assessed 60 fractures in 59 patients. The mean patient age was 82 years. In 44 dorsally displaced fractures, reduction failed in seven cases initially and 37 subsequently lost reduction during plaster immobilisation. In nine wrists with volar displaced fractures, reduction was achieved in six; all subsequently became malunited. Therefore, a total of 53/60 fractures healed in a malunited position. They found no correlation between fracture classification, initial displacement, and final radiographical outcome. On the basis of these observations they concluded that reduction of fractures of the distal radius was of minimal value in the very old and frail, dependent or demented patient [10].

Gartland and Werley reviewed 60 cases of distal radius fractures treated with reduction and plaster immobilisation, 60% of which "healed in a position typical of a fresh unreduced Colles' fracture". Functionally, 32% of this series had unsatisfactory results that correlated with a loss of volar tilt [11].

Batra and Gupta retrospectively reviewed 69 patients following various treatments including plaster immobilisation, external fixation, open reduction and internal fixation (ORIF) and percutaneous pinning. Functional assessment was made one year after the injury. The most important factor affecting the functional outcome was radial length, followed by volar tilt. Carpal instability was an indicator of poor functional results. The relative movement of the lunate with respect to the distal radial articular surface, when defined as an effective radio lunate flexion of more than 25°, was also associated with poor functional results [12].

This compares with Young *et al*, who reviewed 85 patients, randomised to plaster or external fixation. They used the Gartland and Werley score to show that most patients in each group had an excellent or good outcome and patient satisfaction was comparable and high in both groups. Despite a high level of radiographic malunion (50%), overall function, range of movement and activities of daily living were not limited [13].

Fujii *et al* reviewed the results of 22 severely deformed distal radius fractures in elderly patients. Although most of the patients had satisfactory outcomes and the functional results did not correlate with radiographic evidence of minor deformities, the functional results of the patients with radial shortening of 6mm or more were poor. Also, grip power was found to be the most significant factor affecting subjective evaluation and did not improve significantly in patients with injuries of the non-dominant hand [14].

MacDermid prospectively studied 120 patients with distal radius fractures. They completed a baseline evaluation that determined their age, sex, education level, injury compensation status, AO fracture type, pre-reduction radial shortening and post-reduction radial shortening. Six months later, patients self-reported pain and disability using the Patient-Rated Wrist Evaluation (PRWE) and were tested for physical impairment (grip, wrist range of motion and dexterity). The most influential predictor of pain and disability at six months was the pursuit of injury compensation. Patient education level and pre-reduction radial shortening also contributed predictive information. Wrist impairment was moderately correlated with patient-reported pain and disability [15].

Kirschner wiring

Willenegger and Guggenbühl in 1959 described closed reduction and stabilisation with two Kirschner wires (K-wires) through the radial styloid, anchoring into the opposite cortex [16]. Kapandji in 1976 suggested inserting the K-wires 'intrafocally', i.e. into the fracture gap [17].

Walton *et al* reviewed 102 patients that were treated with an intrafocal, blunt-ended 1.6mm K-wire

through Lister's tubercle and a second wire through the radial styloid. A third volar wire was used, if necessary, through the bed of flexor carpi radialis between the tendon and the artery. All were done through mini-open incisions and none engaged the opposite cortex. Forty-three percent of the fractures treated were extra-articular. Twenty-two patients were lost to follow-up. According to the modified Lindstrom classification, 93% obtained good or excellent radiological results and 95% were good or excellent functionally. Complications included two malunions in high-energy injuries and six had mild pin-track infections, all of which settled with oral antibiotics and K-wire removal. One further patient had skin abrasions from a tight plaster rubbing on a wire. There were three carpal tunnel decompressions (CTD). Three patients developed scar adherence and one patient had a wire migrate into the medullary canal, which was left, as it was asymptomatic. There were no episodes of superficial radial nerve injury, neuroma formation or tendon injury [18].

Strohm *et al*, in a randomised controlled trial, compared two K-wires inserted through the radial styloid, as described by Willenegger and Guggenbühl, with a modified Kapandji technique previously described by Fritz *et al* [19]. This technique employs two intrafocal wires with the addition of a wire through the radial styloid, inserted through a stab incision. The wires were buried and the skin closed. Those treated with the Willenegger procedure were immobilised for six weeks in a position of function, while those treated using the Kapandji procedure were left in a volar slab for just three weeks. All the wires were removed under local anaesthesia after six weeks. There was a fairly even split in A2, A3 and C1 AO classification. The distribution of fracture types between the two groups was fairly even. Although the results were good overall, the Kapandji technique was found to give significantly better results, both functionally and radiologically. How much of this was due to the differing immobilisation regimes is uncertain. Complications did not differ significantly between the Willenegger and Kapandji techniques: 17% and 13% nerve irritation, 12% and 8% wire migration and one case each of reflex sympathetic dystrophy (RSD) and carpal tunnel syndrome (CTS) were observed [20].

Complications of K-wiring

Various studies have discussed the complications of K-wiring. In a review of 40 patients, Singh *et al* found a 20% rate of injury to sensory branches of the superficial radial nerve, but no cases of infection or wire migration [21]. Hochwald *et al*, in a cadaveric study, compared percutaneous fixation with a limited open technique using a soft tissue protector. They found that in the percutaneous group, the superficial radial nerve was touching the K-wires in 8/22 cases, compared to 1/22 with the limited open technique [22]. Habernek *et al* reported on 80 patients treated with radial styloid pinning. Although no tendon ruptures occurred, 12 patients had paraesthesia in the distribution of the radial sensory nerve [23]. Harrison *et al* reported two cases of extensor pollicis longus (EPL) tethering following K-wiring, using ultrasound scanning to detect its presence [24].

External fixation

Dicpinigaitis *et al* reported on the radiological results of 70 cases treated with bridging external fixation and supplementary K-wires. These were followed-up for six months. The average age of the patient was 51 years and 30% had supplementary cancellous allograft. Fixators were removed at six to eight weeks. No comment was made on the classification of the fractures. Although dorsal displacement, radial inclination, radial height, radial shift, and ulnar variance were in the main maintained, over the follow-up period, there was continual loss of volar tilt to an average of 4.2°. Cases with ≥20° of initial dorsal tilt showed a slightly higher chance of subsequent loss of reduction than those with ≤10°. In this series bone grafting was associated with a higher risk of subsequent loss of position, although this may have been due to selection bias; the more comminuted the fracture, the more likely the authors were to bone graft. There was a slightly increased loss of reduction if the fixators were removed at six rather than eight weeks, although this was not statistically significant. No comments on function or complications were made [25].

Kapoor *et al* found that although external fixation was excellent in maintaining restored length, it did not prevent late dorsal collapse. There was a 14% rate of increased dorsal tilt due to collapse compared with 7% with plate fixation [26].

With or without K-wires?

Lin *et al* reviewed 20 patients with external fixation alone and compared them with 36 patients treated with supplementary intramedullary K-wires. They retrospectively assessed radiological and functional data. Subjective outcomes were also measured. All types of distal radius fracture were included in the study. They found that surgical correction of radial height and inclination was achieved in both groups, but volar tilt was only improved in the wired group. All three corrections were gradually lost in the unwired group. Clinical examination at six months revealed significantly better findings in the wired group. Where grip strength was 76% of the contralateral side in the wired group, it was only 50% in the unwired group. No mention was made of any complications [27].

Four or five pins?

Werber *et al* performed a prospective randomised study of 59 patients, with unstable, intra-articular and extra-articular fractures. In both groups a bridging external fixator was used between the radius and second metacarpal, but in the five-pin group, an extra pin was inserted into the distal fracture fragment(s). No bone graft was used in either group. The two metacarpal pins were allowed to articulate at three weeks and the fifth pin (where applicable) was removed seven weeks after surgery. All fixators were removed at nine weeks. The five-pin group had significantly better radial inclination, radial length and volar tilt. Range of movement in all directions and grip strength were also significantly better in the five-pin group, although neither side was as good as the uninjured side (74% and 44% of normal). In terms of complications, four in the four-pin group and two in the five-pin group had discharge from pin sites. Six in each group had pain and swelling in their hands, lasting on average 59 days. There were no cases of RSD, tendon rupture, nerve compression syndrome, or fixator failure [28].

Bridging or non-bridging?

Krishnan *et al* performed a prospective randomised trial comparing bridging and non-bridging external fixators, with 30 patients in each group. Most were complex intra-articular fractures (AO type C). The non-bridging group was allowed to mobilise their wrist at two weeks, whereas the bridging group was immobilised for six weeks. Even at one year, the grip strength for both groups was less than 50% of the uninjured side. In terms of movement, there was more flexion in the non-bridging group. Otherwise by the end of the review there was little to choose between the two groups. Thirty-nine complications (65%!) occurred in 33 patients, 21 in the non-bridging group and 18 in the bridging group. Thirty-two percent of patients had pin-site infections; most were treated with oral antibiotics. Two patients required hospital admission, one requiring incision and drainage and early removal of the fixator. This patient developed superficial radial nerve irritation, RSD and suffered a fracture during manipulation. Also, there were three EPL ruptures, two other nerve injuries, four fixation failures and some scar tethering [29].

Atroshi *et al* also compared bridging and non-bridging fixators. They included both intra- and extra-articular fractures (19 patients in each group) which were followed-up for one year. The mean operating time was shorter for wrist-bridging fixation by ten minutes (95% CI 3-17). There was no significant difference in Disabilities of the Arm, Shoulder, and Hand (DASH) scores between the groups. No statistically significant differences in pain score, range of motion, grip strength, or patient satisfaction were found. The non-bridging group had a significantly better radial length at 52 weeks; mean difference in change in ulnar variance from baseline was 1.4mm (95% CI 0.1-2.7) (p=0.04). Volar tilt and radial inclination were similar in both groups. Complications included two re-fractures, one after a fall and another during fixator removal. One fracture displaced and was treated by a further reduction and percutaneous wire. There were 15 (39%) pin-site infections, although none were deep, and all were diagnosed within two weeks of surgery. One with a bridging fixator had transient numbness in the radial nerve distribution. Although both groups of patients were said to have a similar number of patients with median nerve symptoms, this was not quantified [30].

McQueen performed a randomised, prospective study on 60 patients (30 in each group) with unstable fractures of the distal radius (both intra- and extra-articular), comparing bridging with non-bridging external fixation using pins placed in the distal fragment of the radius. The average age was 61 years and they were followed-up for one year. The radiological results showed significant improvement in the non-bridging group at all stages of review. In particular, normal volar tilt and carpal alignment were regained and maintained, whereas in the bridging group, 30% lost more than 10° of volar tilt and 57% no longer had normal carpal alignment. The functional results at six weeks, three months, six months and one year showed statistically better grip strength and flexion in the non-bridging group at all stages of review. Other ranges of movement showed an early advantage in the non-bridging group. Complications affected 42% of patients, including pin-track infections (15%) for both groups and two EPL ruptures in the non-bridging group. Two patients in the bridging group suffered RSD and 14 in the bridging group went on to malunion. The author concluded that this showed non-bridging external fixation is the treatment of choice for unstable fractures of the distal radius, which have sufficient space for the placement of pins in the distal fragment [31]. In fact, this study showed non-bridging external fixation to be superior to bridging where possible, rather than it being the treatment of choice.

Plating

Dorsal

Carter *et al* reported a case series of 73 fractures in 71 patients using a low-profile dorsal plate. The average age of patients included was 45 years. Many had comminuted and intra-articular fractures; all were unstable. A satisfactory reduction was achieved in 86% and, in 88% of these, the position was maintained. Eighty-two percent were rated using the Gartland and Werley scale as being excellent, 14% good and 4% were poor. There were no wound infections, no tendon ruptures and no nerve injuries. There were two cases of RSD and 19% of patients required metalwork removal, most frequently for extensor tendon irritation [32].

This extensor irritation is also identified in the study by Ring *et al*. Twenty-two cases of AO type C2 and C3 were treated using a Pi plate (Figure 1). Five of the cases reported developed tenosynovitis [33]. Kambouroglou and Axelrod described one late fracture fixation and one osteotomy for malunion, which resulted in extensor tendon ruptures [34].

Simic *et al* reviewed 51 fractures in 50 patients that had a low-profile dorsal (LoCon-T) plate. Most were extra-articular and were assessed at a minimum of one year, both clinically and radiologically. According to the Gartland and Werley score, 31 patients were rated as excellent and 19 were good. The average DASH score was 11.9 (on a scale of 0-100, where 0 is normal function). There were no wound infections, haematomas, extensor tendon ruptures or irritation, or cases of complex regional pain syndrome [35].

Rozental *et al* compared a regular dorsal Pi plate with various other low-profile plates in a total of 28 patients with a mean age of 42 years. The mean duration of follow-up was 21 months. Nineteen patients had been treated with a Synthes Pi plate and nine had been treated with another low-profile plate. There were no instances of loss of reduction, malunion, or non-union. The mean score on the DASH questionnaire was 14.5 points. Nineteen were rated as excellent and nine were good, according to the scoring system of Gartland and Werley. Nine patients had postoperative complications requiring repeat surgical treatment for hardware removal or extensor tendon reconstruction. All nine re-operations were performed in patients who had been treated with a Synthes Pi plate, while none were performed in patients who had been treated with a low-profile plate (p<0.025) [36].

Volar

Kamano *et al* reviewed 33 patients that had acute dorsally displaced distal radius fractures. Most included an intra-articular component. The mean age was 54 years and although some (the exact number is not quoted), required a cancellous, iliac crest

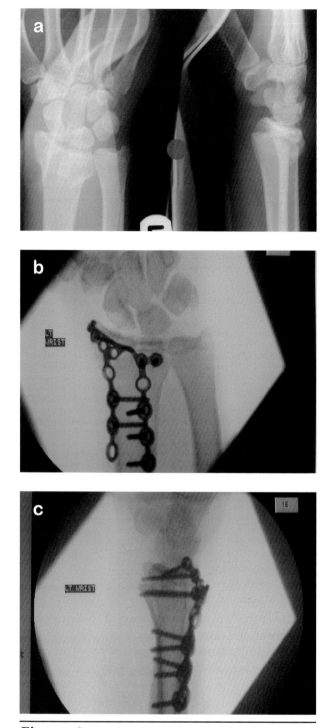

Figure 1. a) Pre-operative and b) & c) intra-operative X-rays of a patient with a Pi plate.

autograft, this was done through the same approach. Non-locking plates were used. Twelve patients had excellent results, 20 had good results and one, who

Chapter 14

had a concurrent scaphoid fracture and subsequent finger stiffness, was rated as fair, according to the Gartland and Werley scale. There were no extensor tendon or radial artery injuries and no patients required removal of metal [37].

Kamano *et al* in 2005 went on to report on 40 patients with a mean age of 57 years treated using a different make of non-locking volar plate (Biotechni Co., Ltd., Ciotat, France). On the Gartland and Werley scoring system there were 12 excellent and 28 good results. Grip strength recovered to an average of 78% of the uninjured side. One patient developed complex regional pain syndrome and one diabetic patient had a mild skin infection. There were no problems with extensor tendon injury [38].

Fixed-angled devices and locking plates, where screws or pegs are inserted into the plate (effectively creating a fixed-angled device), are designed to provide subchondral support in the distal fragment. This means the fragment can be approached from the volar side and this avoids the need to disrupt and irritate the extensor tendons.

Rozental went on to review 41 patients, 18 type A fractures, four type B fractures, and 19 type C AO fractures that were treated with either the Synthes (Figure 2) or Hand Innovations volar locking plates. The mean age was 53 years and although most were falls from a standing height, three were involved in road accidents, two were involved in falls of greater than 20 feet and three were sporting injuries. Bone grafting was used in an undefined number of patients. The average score on the DASH questionnaire was 14 and all patients achieved excellent and good results on the Gartland and Werley scoring system, indicating minimal impairment in activities of daily living. Nine patients experienced postoperative complications. There were four instances of loss of reduction with fracture collapse, three patients required hardware removal for tendon irritation, one patient developed a wound dehiscence, and one patient had metacarpophalangeal joint stiffness. When compared with previous reports on dorsal plating, volar plates were felt to have a higher incidence of fracture collapse but a lower rate of hardware-related complications [39].

Orbay, the founder of the Hand Innovations company, published two studies on their distal volar radius (DVR) plate (Figure 3) [40, 41]. The first in 2002 reviewed 29 patients with 31 dorsally displaced, unstable distal radial fractures using a new fixed-angle internal fixation device. At a minimal follow-up time of 12 months the fractures had healed with highly satisfactory radiographic and functional results. The final volar tilt averaged 5°; radial inclination, 21°; radial shortening, 1mm; and articular incongruity, 0mm. Grip strength was 79% of the contralateral side. The overall outcome according to the Gartland and Werley scales showed 19 excellent and 12 good results. The series included a mixture of intra- and extra-articular fractures. Two fractures had additional fixation of a volar marginal articular fragment, which were removed at six weeks. Complications included one hardware removal for extensor irritation because one peg was too long. Nine patients that had pre-operative carpal tunnel syndrome had releases with complete resolution. In 2004, he went on to describe 24 fractures in elderly patients (older than 75 years), which were retrospectively reviewed. There were no plate failures or significant loss of reduction, although there was settling of the distal fragment in three patients (1-2mm). This settling stopped once the support pegs came in contact with the subchondral bone. There was one case of complex regional pain syndrome, but no report of tendon irritation and all plates were left *in situ*.

Wong *et al* retrospectively reviewed 30 distal radius fractures (mean age 58.6 years); twenty-nine were intra-articular. According to Gartland and Werley scoring, 24 were excellent, five were good and one was fair. Radiologically, 22 were excellent and eight had good outcomes. Four patients had hypertrophic scars and one had an EPL attrition rupture, which was not attributed to the hardware [42].

Musgrave and Idler performed a retrospective review of 32 distal radius fractures fixed with a Synthes Locking Compression Plate (LCP). Nine fractures had an additional radial styloid plate. Eleven fractures were extra-articular (AO type A) and 21 fractures were complete intra-articular (AO type C). There were 11 complications in nine patients. Two patients developed a complex regional pain syndrome. There was one asymptomatic volar carpal ganglion, one case of cellulitis that responded to oral antibiotics, one subsequent trigger finger, one delayed

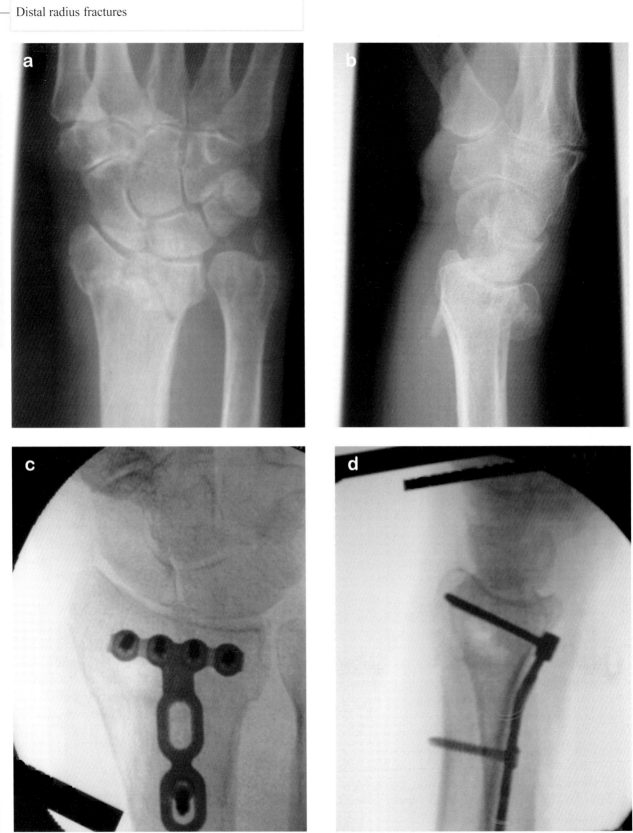

Figure 2. a) & b) Pre-operative and c) & d) intra-operative X-rays of a patient with a Synthes plate.

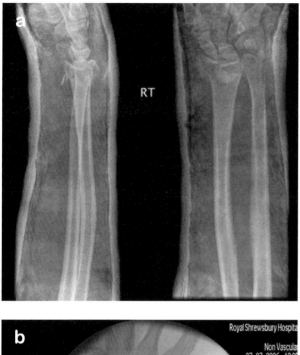

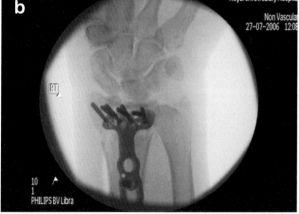

Figure 3. a) Pre-operative and b) & c) intra-operative X-rays of a patient with a DVR plate.

union, one mildly symptomatic volar bursa and one case of arthrofibrosis requiring capsulectomy. The delayed union occurred in a 71-year-old patient with an AO C2.3 fracture and a comminuted distal ulnar fracture. Allograft bone was used in the radius fracture. Two volar plates were removed, neither of which was symptomatic. One volar plate was removed from the patient having capsulectomy for arthrofibrosis and the other volar plate was removed from a patient who had carpal tunnel release 15 months after the distal radius fracture. There was one other case of carpal tunnel syndrome, which developed in a patient five months after fixation of the distal radius fracture. One radial styloid plate was believed to be symptomatic and was removed [43].

Ruch and Papadonikolakis retrospectively compared 20 patients that were treated with a dorsal plate and 14 patients that were treated with a volar non-locking plate. There were no differences between the two groups in grip strength, DASH scores, and percentage of wrist range of motion, except in wrist pronation. Volar plating, however, resulted in significantly better Gartland and Werley scores than dorsal plating. Volar collapse (volar tilt >18°) was noted in five of the 20 patients in the dorsal plating group. In one patient volar collapse was related to a loose screw. No collapse was noticed in any of the patients in the volar plating group. There were no statistically significant differences in the radiographic measurements between the dorsal and volar plates. The rate of complications was significantly higher in the dorsal plating group (six of 20 patients) compared with the volar plating group (four of 14 patients) [44].

Letsch *et al* also retrospectively compared dorsal and volar (non-locking) plating. They found that although the radiological outcome was significantly better amongst the dorsal-plated group and the functional outcome showed a trend towards a better result amongst the dorsal group, this difference wasn't significant [45].

Arthroscopic assistance

Edwards *et al* assessed 15 patients arthroscopically that had been percutaneously pinned under fluoroscopic control. They found that some gaps of greater than 1mm were visible in the articular surface that were not seen using a C-arm [46].

Kamano *et al* reviewed the results of 15 comminuted intra-articular high-energy fractures that were treated with arthroscopically-assisted volar plating and autologous bone graft. Minimum follow-up was 24 months. According to the Gartland and Werley system, five patients had excellent results and ten had good results. Grade 1 arthritic changes were found in ten patients even though with no step-off on radiographs [47].

Ruch *et al* performed a prospective case-matched comparison of the functional and radiologic outcomes of arthroscopically-assisted (AA) versus fluoroscopically-assisted (FA) reduction and external fixation of distal radius fractures. There were 15 patients in each group. Those who had arthroscopically-assisted surgery had significantly better range of movement in terms of flexion, extension and supination. The authors felt that arthroscopy would identify pathology that was not visible radiologically, so injuries such as triangular fibrocartilage complex (TFCC) tears could be treated simultaneously. Although there was a difference in the DASH scores, (19 in the FA group and 11 in the AA group), this was not significant [48].

Comparative studies

Plaster or external fixation?

Young *et al* used the Gartland and Werley score to show that most patients in each group had an excellent or good outcome and patient satisfaction was comparable and high in both groups. The fixator group had significantly less radial shortening ($p<0.05$). Despite a high level of radiographic malunion (50%), overall function, range of movement and activities of daily living were not limited. Twenty-five percent of patients had minor radiological signs of post-traumatic arthritis, although only one patient was symptomatic. They felt that, in the long term, external fixation of distal radius fractures did not confer an improved outcome when compared to plaster immobilisation [13].

Kreder *et al* performed a randomised controlled trial comparing plaster immobilisation with external fixation using optional K-wires for extra-articular metaphyseal fractures. There were 59 patients in the casting group and 54 in the fixator group. Although there was a trend towards better function amongst the fixator group, at two years this was not significant. Two patients in the external fixator group developed a deep infection that required debridement and antibiotics, while one patient in each group developed RSD [49].

External fixation or K-wiring?

Harley *et al* performed a prospective randomised controlled trial involving a total of 50 patients, all less than 65 years old, with predominantly comminuted intra-articular fractures. The use of augmented external fixation did not improve the mean radiographic parameters of radial length, radial angulation, or volar tilt. Restoration of volar tilt of highly comminuted fractures was difficult to achieve regardless of the technique. Improved articular surface reduction was realised with the use of an external fixator but overall, only three patients were noted to have steps or gaps greater than 2mm. No significant differences in mean DASH scores, total range of motion, grip strength, or health-related quality of life were observed between the groups. All three patients diagnosed with RSD had had external fixation. There were two pin infections amongst the pinning group and four in the external fixator group [50].

External fixation or plating

Grewal *et al* performed a prospective randomised trial comparing dorsal plating with mini-open reduction, percutaneous fixation, and external fixation. All fractures were AO type C in patients less than 70 years old, followed-up for a mean of 18 months. The external fixator group showed an average grip strength of 97% compared with the normal side and 86% in the dorsal plate group, but no significant difference was found in the DASH scores. The plate group had significantly longer tourniquet times when compared with the external fixator group. The plate group also had higher levels of pain at one year when compared with the external fixator group; however, this equalised after hardware removal. The dorsal plate group, showed a higher complication rate (72.4%) when compared with the external fixator group (24.2%). The fixator group had two patients who developed complex regional pain syndromes, one had distal radio-ulnar joint instability, one had sensory loss, one had a stiff hand, one had pin-tract infections and one required an ulnar shortening. This compared with the plating group that had three cases of complex regional pain syndrome, one compartment syndrome, five cases of tendinitis, three cases of sensory impairment and one required an ulnar shortening osteotomy. Eight patients required removal of hardware [51].

Wright *et al* compared the volar fixed-angle Tine plate with external fixation. This study included patients with comminuted unstable intra-articular and extra-articular fractures. Eleven patients treated with external fixation were followed-up for an average of 47 months and retrospectively reviewed. Prospective data were gathered on 21 patients who were treated with ORIF through a volar approach using a fixed-angle implant. Follow-up evaluation for this group averaged 17 months. The mean passive wrist range of movement at final follow-up evaluation in patients treated with external fixation was 59° extension and 57° flexion, compared with 63° extension and 64° flexion in patients treated with ORIF. The use of ORIF with a volar fixed-angle implant resulted in stable fixation of the distal articular fragments, allowing early post-surgical wrist motion. The PRWE and DASH scores for the groups were equivalent, whereas intra-articular step-off, volar tilt, and radial length were better in the ORIF group. There were few complications, implant removal was not necessary, and early post-surgical wrist range of movement was initiated without loss of reduction [52].

Conclusions

It is very difficult to draw any hard and fast rules concerning the treatment of distal radius fractures. This overview of the literature has shown that the majority of the studies available are small and include a disparate group of patients. There is little in the way of large well-designed prospective randomised controlled trials with long-term follow-up. Even those studies that focus on a particular type of fracture are weakened because such injuries are very difficult to classify, with high levels of intra- and inter-observer error [53, 54]. Intra-articular fractures in particular, also commonly have associated soft tissue injuries which cannot be recognised on plain radiographs alone, the bearing for which, in terms of outcome, remains unclear [55, 56].

Three or more of the following factors are associated with loss of position and should be considered for intervention other than plaster immobilisation alone: dorsal angulation >20°, dorsal comminution, radiocarpal involvement, concomitant ulnar fracture, and age >60 years old. The exception is very frail, elderly, low-demand patients who do not suffer from loss of position despite malunion. In general though radial shortening of >6mm and loss of volar tilt are associated with loss of function **(III/B)**.

Greater than 1-2mm of joint incongruency will lead to the development of radiological arthrosis and should be treated where possible, although the functional benefit of treating such lesions remains unclear **(III/B)**.

Most infections resulting from K-wires seem to be superficial and easily treated with oral antibiotics and wire removal. It is interesting that the one study in which the wires were buried and the wounds closed did not have any infections [20]. This should be balanced against the need for a second procedure to remove the wires.

External fixation seems to be associated with high rates of complication including infection, stiffness and loss of position **(III/B)**.

Volar and low-profile dorsal plates are associated with fewer problems in terms of hardware morbidity than dorsal plating **(Ib/A)**. Volar fixed-angled devices, such as locking plates, have shown promising early results and by providing subchondral support may negate the need to use bone graft in the presence of bone loss. Fixed-angled devices allow for a more anatomical reduction than external fixation **(III/B)**.

Recommendations	Evidence level
◆ Unstable fractures other than in low-demand patients should be treated with more definitive fixation than plaster alone.	III/B
◆ If K-wires are to be used they should be performed in a mini-open modified intra-focal technique with supplementary wires.	III/B, Ib/A
◆ If external fixation is to be performed, it should be done with a supplementary technique to stabilise the distal fragment(s).	Ib/A
◆ Internal fixation with a fixed-angled device has been shown to allow early mobilisation without loss of reduction and has a low complication rate with very satisfactory functional and radiological results.	III/B

Chapter 14

References

1. O'Neill TW, Cooper C, Fin JD, Lunt M, Purdie D, Reid DM, Rowe R, Woolf AD, Wallace W; UK Colles' Fracture Study Group. Incidence of distal forearm fracture in British men and women. *Osteoporos Int* 2001; 12(7): 555-8.

2. Lafontaine M, Delince P, Hardy D, Simons M. Instability of fractures of the lower end of radius: apropos of a series of 167 cases. *Acta Orthop Belg* 1989; 55: 203-16.

3. Leone J, Bhandari M, Adili A, Mckenzie S, Moro JK, Dunlop RB. Predictors of early and late stability following conservative treatment of extra-articular distal radius fractures. *Arch Orthop Trauma Surg* 2004; 124(1): 38-41.

4. Nesbitt KS, Failla JM, Les C. Assessment of instability factors in adult distal radius fractures. *J Hand Surg Am* 2004; 29: 1128-38.

5. McQueen MM, MacLaren A, Chalmers J. The value of remanipulating Colles' fractures. *J Bone Joint Surg Br* 1986; 68(2): 232-3.

6. Knirk JL, Jupiter JB. Intraarticular fractures of the distal end of the radius in young adults. *J Bone Joint Surg Am* 1986; 68: 647-59.

7. Catalano LW 3rd, Cole RJ, Gelberman RH, Evanoff BA, Gilula LA, Borrelli J Jr. Displaced intra-articular fractures of the distal aspect of the radius. Long-term results in young adults after open reduction and internal fixation. *J Bone Joint Surg Am* 1997; 79(9): 1290-302.

8. Fernandez JJ, Gruen GS, Hrndon JH. Outcome of distal radius fractures using the Short-Form 36 health survey. *Clin Orthop Relat Res* 1997; 341: 36-41.

9. McQueen M, Caspers J. Colles' fracture: does the anatomical result affect the final function? *J Bone Joint Surg Br* 1988; 70(4): 649-51.

10. Beumer A, McQueen MM. Fractures of the distal radius in low-demand elderly patients: closed reduction of no value in 53 of 60 wrists. *Acta Orthop Scand* 2003; 74(1): 98-100.

11. Gartland JJ Jr, Werley CW. Evaluation of healed Colles' fractures. *J Bone Joint Surg Am* 1951; 33-A(4): 895-907.

12. Batra S, Gupta A. The effect of fracture-related factors on the functional outcome at 1 year in distal radius fractures. *Injury* 2002; 33(6): 499-502.

13. Young CF, Nanu AM, Checketts RG. Seven-year outcome following Colles' type distal radial fracture. A comparison of two treatment methods. *J Hand Surg Br* 2003; 28(5): 422-6.

14. Fujii K, Henmi T, Kanematsu Y, Mishiro T, Sakai T, Terai T. Fractures of the distal end of radius in elderly patients: a comparative study of anatomical and functional results. *J Orthop Surg* (Hong Kong) 2002; 10(1): 9-15.

15. MacDermid JC, Donner A, Richards RS, Roth JH. Patient versus injury factors as predictors of pain and disability six months after a distal radius fracture. *J Clin Epidemiol* 2002; 55(9): 849-54.

16. Willenegger H, Guggenbühl A. Operative treatment of certain cases of distal radius fracture. *Helv Chir Acta* 1959; 26: 81-94.

17. Kapandji A. Internal fixation by double intrafocal plate. Functional treatment of non-articular fractures of the lower end of radius. *Ann Chir* 1976; 30: 903-8.

18. Walton NP, Brammar TJ, Hutchinson J, Raj D, Coleman NP. Treatment of unstable distal radial fractures by intrafocal, intramedullary K-wires. *Injury* 2001; 32: 383-9.

19. Fritz T, Werching D, Klavora R, Kireglstein C, Friedl W. Combined Kirschner wire fixation in the treatment of Colles' fracture. A prospective, controlled trial. *Arch Orthop Trauma Surg* 1999; 119: 171-8.

20. Strohm PC, Müller CA, Boll T, Pfister U. Two procedures for Kirschner wire osteosynthesis of distal radial fractures. *J Bone Joint Surg Am* 2004; 86: 2621-8.

21. Singh S, Trikha P, Twyman R. Superficial radial nerve damage due to Kirschner wiring of the radius. *Injury* 2005; 36: 330-2.

22. Hochwald NL, Levine R, Tornetta P, 3rd. The risks of Kirschner wire placement in the distal radius: a comparison of techniques. *J Hand Surg Am* 1997; 22A: 580-4.

23. Habernek H, Weinstabl R, Fialka C, Scmhid L. Unstable distal radius fractures treated by modified Kirschner wire pinning; anatomic considerations, technique, and results. *J Trauma* 1994; 36: 83-8.

24. Harrison MR, Hamilton S, Johnstone AJ. Pseudo-rupture of extensor pollicis longus following Kirschner wire fixation of distal radius fractures. *Acta Orthop Belg* 2004; 70(5): 492-4.

25. Dicpinigaitis P, Wolinsky P, Hiebert R, Egol K, Koval K, Tejwani N. Can external fixation maintain reduction after distal radius fractures? *J Trauma* 2004; 57(4): 845-50.

26. Kapoor H, Agarwal A, Dhaon BK. Displaced intra-articular fractures of distal radius: a comparative evaluation of results following closed reduction, external fixation and open reduction with internal fixation. *Injury* 2000; 31(2): 75-9.

27. Lin C, Sun JS, Hou SM. External fixation with or without supplementary intramedullary Kirschner wires in the treatment of distal radial fractures. *Can J Surg* 2004; 47(6): 431-7.

28. Werber KD, Raeder F, Brauer RB, Weiss S. External fixation of distal radial fractures: four compared with five pins: a randomized prospective study. *J Bone Joint Surg Am* 2003; 85-A(4): 660-6.

29. Krishnan J, Wigg AE, Walker RW, Slavotinek J. Intra-articular fractures of the distal radius: a prospective randomised controlled trial comparing static bridging and dynamic non-bridging external fixation. *J Hand Surg Br* 2003; 28(5): 417-21.

30. Atroshi I, Brogren E, Larsson GU, Kloow J, Hofer M, Berggren AM. Wrist-bridging versus non-bridging external fixation for displaced distal radius fractures: a randomized assessor-blind clinical trial of 38 patients followed for 1 year. *Acta Orthop* 2006; 77(3): 445-53.

31. McQueen MM. Redisplaced unstable fractures of the distal radius. A randomised, prospective study of bridging versus non-bridging external fixation. *J Bone Joint Surg Br* 1998; 80(4): 665-9.

32. Carter PR, Frederick HA, Laseter GF. Open reduction and internal fixation of unstable distal radius fractures with a low-profile plate: a multicenter study of 73 fractures. *J Hand Surg Am* 1998; 23(2): 300-7.

33. Ring D, Jupiter JB, Brennwald J, Buchler U, Hastings H 2nd. Prospective multicenter trial of a plate for dorsal fixation of distal radius fractures. *J Hand Surg Am* 1997; 22(5): 777-84.

34. Kambouroglou GK, Axelrod TS. Complications of the AO/ASIF titanium distal radius plate system (Pi plate) in internal fixation of the distal radius: a brief report. *J Hand Surg Am* 1998; 23(4): 737-41.

35. Simic PM, Robison J, Gardner MJ, Gelberman RH, Weiland AJ, Boyer MI. Treatment of distal radius fractures with a low-profile dorsal plating system: an outcomes assessment. *J Hand Surg Am* 2006; 31(3): 382-6.

36. Rozental TD, Beredjiklian PK, Bozentka DJ. Functional outcome and complications following two types of dorsal plating for unstable fractures of the distal part of the radius. *J Bone Joint Surg Am* 2003; 85-A(10): 1956-60.

37. Kamano M, Honda Y, Kazuki K, Yasuda M. Palmar plating for dorsally displaced fractures of the distal radius. *Clin Orthop Relat Res* 2002; 397: 403-8.

38. Kamano M, Koshimune M, Toyama M, Kazuki K. Palmar plating system for Colles' fractures - a preliminary report. *J Hand Surg Am* 2005; 30(4): 750-5.

39. Rozental TD, Blazar PE. Functional outcome and complications after volar plating for dorsally displaced, unstable fractures of the distal radius. *J Hand Surg Am* 2006; 31(3): 359-65.

40. Orbay JL, Fernandez DL. Volar fixation for dorsally displaced fractures of the distal radius: a preliminary report. *J Hand Surg Am* 2002; 27(2): 205-15.

41. Orbay JL, Fernandez DL. Volar fixed-angle plate fixation for unstable distal radius fractures in the elderly patient. *J Hand Surg Am* 2004; 29(1): 96-102.

42. Wong KK, Chan KW, Kwok TK, Mak KH. Volar fixation of dorsally displaced distal radial fracture using locking compression plate. *J Orthop Surg* (Hong Kong) 2005; 13(2): 153-7.

43. Musgrave DS, Idler RS. Volar fixation of dorsally displaced distal radius fractures using the 2.4-mm locking compression plates. *J Hand Surg Am* 2005; 30(4): 743-9.

44. Ruch DS, Papadonikolakis A. Volar versus dorsal plating in the management of intra-articular distal radius fractures. *J Hand Surg Am* 2006; 31(1): 9-16.

45. Letsch R, Infanger M, Schmidt J, Kock HJ. Surgical treatment of fractures of the distal radius with plates: a comparison of palmar and dorsal plate position. *Arch Orthop Trauma Surg* 2003; 123(7): 333-9.

46. Edwards CC 2nd, Haraszti CJ, McGillivary GR, Gutow AP. Intra-articular distal radius fractures: arthroscopic assessment of radiographically-assisted reduction. *J Hand Surg Am* 2001; 26(6): 1036-41.

47. Kamano M, Koshimune M, Kazuki K, Honda Y. Palmar plating for AO/ASIF C3.2 fractures of the distal radius with arthroscopically-assisted reduction. *Hand Surg* 2005; 10(1): 71-6.

48. Ruch DS, Vallee J, Poehling GG, Smith BP, Kuzma GR. Arthroscopic reduction versus fluoroscopic reduction in the management of intra-articular distal radius fractures. *Arthroscopy* 2004; 20(3): 225-30.

49. Kreder HJ, Agel J, McKee MD, Schemitsch EH, Stephen D, Hanel DP. A randomized, controlled trial of distal radius fractures with metaphyseal displacement but without joint incongruity: closed reduction and casting versus closed reduction, spanning external fixation, and optional percutaneous K-wires. *J Orthop Trauma* 2006; 20(2): 115-21.

50. Harley BJ, Scharfenberger A, Beaupre LA, Jomha N, Weber DW. Augmented external fixation versus percutaneous pinning and casting for unstable fractures of the distal radius - a prospective randomized trial. *J Hand Surg Am* 2004; 29(5): 815-24.

51. Grewal R, Perey B, Wilmink M, Stothers K. A randomized prospective study on the treatment of intra-articular distal radius fractures: open reduction and internal fixation with dorsal plating versus mini open reduction, percutaneous fixation, and external fixation. *J Hand Surg Am* 2005; 30(4): 764-72.

52. Wright TW, Horodyski M, Smith DW. Functional outcome of unstable distal radius fractures: ORIF with a volar fixed-angle Tine plate versus external fixation. *J Hand Surg Am* 2005; 30(2): 289-99.

53. Andersen DJ, Blair WF, Steyers CM Jr, Adams BD, el-Khouri GY, Brandser EA. Classification of distal radius fractures: an analysis of interobserver reliability and intraobserver reproducibility. *J Hand Surg Am* 1996; 21(4): 574-82.

54. Kreder HJ, Hanel DP, McKee M, Jupiter J, McGillivary G, Swiontkowski MF. Consistency of AO fracture classification for the distal radius. *J Bone Joint Surg Br* 1996; 78(5): 726-31.

55. Geissler WB, Freeland AE, Savoie FH, McIntyre LW, Whipple TL. Intracarpal soft-tissue lesions associated with an intra-articular fracture of the distal end of the radius. *J Bone Joint Surg Am* 1996; 78(3): 357-65.

56. Mudgal C, Hastings H. Scapho-lunate diastasis in fractures of the distal radius. Pathomechanics and treatment options. *J Hand Surg Br* 1993; 18(6): 725-9.

Chapter 15

What's new in pelvic and acetabular surgery?

Peter V Giannoudis MD EEC (Orth)

Professor, Trauma & Orthopaedics

Christopher Tzioupis MD

Trauma Fellow, Trauma & Orthopaedics

ACADEMIC DEPARTMENT OF TRAUMA & ORTHOPAEDICS, SCHOOL OF MEDICINE
ST. JAMES'S UNIVERSITY HOSPITAL, LEEDS, UK

Introduction

Since the early 1960s, following the pioneer work of Judet and Letournel, there has been an ongoing evolution in the field of pelvic and acetabular surgery. It is now recognised as a well-developed sub-specialty in the field of trauma & orthopaedic surgery. Over a thousand manuscripts have been published on pelvic and acetabular surgery in peer review journals, reflecting the advances made in this surgical field. It is envisaged that more progress will follow in the years to come.

These advances affect every step in the management of patients with pelvic and acetabular fractures, including fracture classification, imaging, surgical approaches, reconstruction techniques, outcome evaluation and the treatment of complications. In this chapter a critical assessment of the relevant studies is made, addressing all the developments mentioned above, in order to present the reader with the best of the available evidence in this field.

Methodology

A broad search of the literature identified the trends and evolving concepts in pelvic and acetabular surgery and these are presented. Additionally a systematic review of the current literature on the aforementioned topics was conducted using the Cochrane library, Medline and Embase from 1999 until 2005. Studies identified in this way were appraised for their methodology. In total, 37 publications concerning the classification of acetabular fractures [1, 2], imaging techniques [3-7], surgical approaches to the acetabulum [8, 9], percutaneous techniques [10-16], Computer-Assisted Orthopaedic Surgery (CAOS) [17-19], Minimally Invasive Surgery (MIS) [20, 21], enhanced fixation of vertically unstable pelvic injuries [22, 23], urologic injuries [24], haemorrhage treatment in pelvic fractures [25-28], open pelvic fractures [29], the outcome of treatment in displaced acetabular fractures [30-33] and complications [34-37] were acknowledged. This chapter focuses on the current trends in the evolution of pelvic and acetabular surgery reported in these publications.

Classification of acetabular fractures

To be useful a fracture classification must have clinical relevance, be inclusive, provide fracture-type specificity and be easily understood by all physicians involved in the diagnosis and treatment of the fracture being classified.

Letournel's first description of the anterior column extending to the iliac crest remains the most widely recognised and accepted definition today. It represents a major advance in the recognition and treatment of acetabular fractures that has stood the test of time [38].

However, the Letournel definition of the anterior column can lead to uncertainty in diagnosis. For example, the Letournel 'elementary' anterior column fracture could be confined to the anatomic anterior column of the acetabulum, whereas the same Letournel fracture type would also apply to an anterior column fracture with extension into the iliac wing. Similar lack of clarity can apply to the Letournel associated fracture, that is anterior column or wall with hemitransverse, which could either be confined to the anatomic acetabulum or have superior extension into the iliac wing [39].

The Letournel classification consists of only ten specific fracture categories requiring the 'infinite' number of acetabular fracture patterns to fit in one of these fracture types. However, these characteristics result in remarkable variation in the designation and therefore diagnosis of acetabular fractures that have similar axial CT appearances [40].

In order to address such problems Harris et al [2] proposed a new fracture classification. The categories of this proposed classification [1, 2], which are based on the axial CT illustration of wall or column fracture location and fracture extension, are sufficiently broad to include the 'infinite' number of fracture patterns **(Ib/A)**. At the same time, the category and subcategory definitions retain fracture-type specificity. By using the anatomical display of the anterior and posterior columns, as shown on axial CT scans, this classification identifies which columns are fractured, whether anterior, posterior, or combined anterior and posterior, thereby guiding the surgeon in the selection of surgical approach **(Ib/A)**. Redefining the superior extent of the anterior column to coincide with that of Letournel's posterior column, provides a rationale for two-column fractures with inferior extension (Letournel T-shaped and its variants), superior extension (into the iliac wing), or simultaneous superior and inferior extension. Although based on the axial CT appearance of acetabular fractures, this classification has direct application to 3D reformatted images as well.

In Figure 1 the proposed classification is presented along with its correlation with the Letournel classification [2].

Imaging of pelvic and acetabular fractures

Over the past two decades there have been numerous technological advances in the field of imaging of the hips and bony pelvis. Conventional radiography remains the initial choice in virtually all cases, but options for more sophisticated imaging have increased considerably. Tomography has been virtually replaced by computed tomography (CT) and magnetic resonance imaging (MRI), whilst nuclear medicine techniques have been refined. In some instances, technological advances have occurred so quickly that they have outpaced the ability to adequately evaluate their accuracy and effectiveness.

The radiographic assessment of patients with pelvic trauma begins with the AP radiograph [41]. The AP radiograph, in conjunction with the pelvic inlet and outlet views, gives much information on the probable mechanism of injury, pelvic stability and any associated injuries. A thorough knowledge of the radiographic landmarks on the three standard pelvic films and their anatomic significance is essential when treating patients with pelvic fractures [42].

CT allows for better demonstration of the location, size, and displacement of fractures, particularly those arising from the posterior acetabular column [43] **(III/B)**. Spiral CT is a powerful modality for the evaluation of the musculoskeletal system, particularly when coupled with real-time, volume-rendering techniques. 3D spiral CT images have become a valuable part of the assessment (Figure 2); indeed, CT findings provide the basis for treatment of the injured patient. The hypothesis that

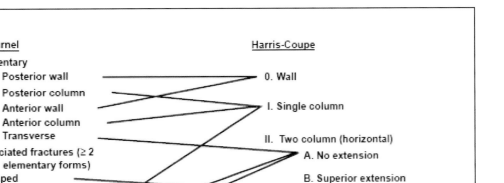

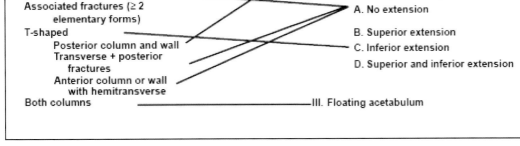

Figure 1. The Letournel's classification [2] and its relationship to the Harris-Coupe classification.

measurement of pelvic haemorrhage on CT scans can estimate the pelvic fracture component of total patient blood loss and predict the need for angiography has been addressed in many studies. CT has also been used to evaluate the results after operative treatment of posterior wall acetabular fractures in relationship to the quality of the fracture reduction, as assessed by postoperative two-dimensional CT [44].

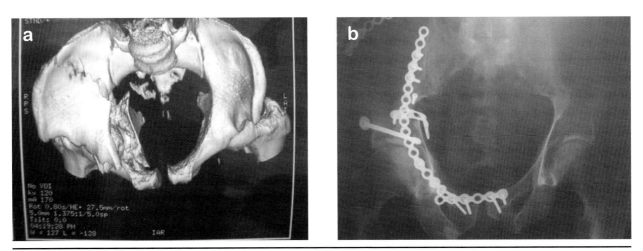

Figure 2. a) 3-D CT illustrating a complex pelvic/acetabular fracture (two column with disruption of the pubis symphysis). b) Fracture at 12 months follow-up reconstructed with plates and an AP column screw.

Despite the valuable contribution of plain radiographs to the initial evaluation of pelvic injuries, there are limitations in determining acetabular fracture displacement, which have been identified by studies comparing variations between the findings of conventional X-rays and CT **(IIb/B)**.

Surgical approaches to the pelvis and acetabulum

The goal of acetabular fracture surgery is to achieve anatomic reduction and stable fracture fixation. Achieving this goal requires adequate visualisation of fracture reduction and placement of hardware. No surgical approach is ideal for all fractures of the acetabulum. Choosing the appropriate approach begins with a careful analysis of the fracture pattern.

Of all the available approaches the classic ilio-inguinal approach has become established in the treatment of acetabular fractures [45] **(III/B)**. It allows exposure of the entire anterior column, from the symphysis to the sacroiliac joint, and is currently the standard approach for most anterior wall, anterior column, transverse, and both column fractures. However, in certain cases with extensive low anterior column or anterior wall fractures, less than optimal exposure may be obtained.

Karunakar et al [8, 9], in order to solve the above problem, have proposed a modification of the classic ilio-inguinal approach. The reasons for the proposed modification of this approach are:

- in cases with comminution of the anterior wall and/or low anterior column there is a need for better visualisation to allow exact anatomic reduction and internal fixation;
- when using the ilio-inguinal approach there is no option for intra-articular inspection; it relies on the perfect apposition of the visible extra-articular surfaces for joint congruence;
- mobilisation of the iliopsoas muscle during the classic ilio-inguinal approach requires separation of the iliocapsularis muscle;
- the frequent postoperative complication of injury to the lateral femoral cutaneous nerve (LFCN), as seen after the ilio-inguinal approach, can be a worrisome problem for the patient and surgeon [8, 9].

The proposed approach [8] represents a combination of the classic ilio-inguinal and a modified Smith-Petersen approach [46], with a modified skin incision addressing the aforementioned issues. This modification of the ilio-inguinal approach is a useful addition to the armamentarium of the acetabular and hip surgeon in selected fracture types **(III/B)**. It is clearly not proposed to replace the classic ilio-inguinal approach, but rather to expand its versatility in specific cases.

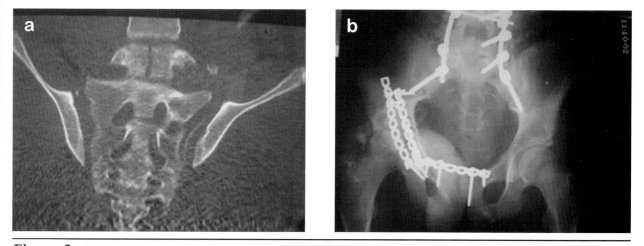

Figure 3. a) Sacral fracture associated with bilateral sacroiliac dislocations. **b)** Fracture was part of the pelvic ring injury that was stabilised via a Pfannenstiel and a Kocher-Langenbeck approach as shown.

In 1994, Cole and Bolhofner [47] described the modified Stoppa intrapelvic approach for the treatment of acetabular fractures. The primary feature of this approach is dissection along the pelvic brim with elevation of the iliopectineal and obturator fascias. Reported advantages of this approach include an improved mechanical advantage in the reduction and fixation of medially displaced fractures.

Another proposed modification [9] of the classic ilio-inguinal approach is based on the development of a larger medial window based on the Pfannenstiel (Figure 3) and modified Stoppa approaches. This eliminates the need for dissection around the lymphatics, limits the release of the inguinal ligament, allows for easier plate passage, and provides access to the entire pubis symphysis [9]. This approach is ideal for fractures with medial protrusio of the femoral head (medial displacement of the quadrilateral surface). Anterior pelvic ring injuries (symphyseal disruption) and the contralateral pubic rami fractures are also readily accessible through this approach.

Percutaneous stabilisation

The surgical treatment of pelvic and acetabular fractures is technically demanding. Percutaneous pelvic fixation has been receiving increasing attention as it attempts to overcome the need for extensile surgical approaches. These procedures may save surgical time and reduce exposure-related hazards, but they can jeopardize intrapelvic organs due to narrow 'safe zones'.

During the past few years the technique of percutaneous posterior sacroiliac screw fixation has gained increasing popularity among orthopaedic trauma surgeons [48] **(III/B)**. Its many advantages include the limited dissection necessary, minimal blood loss and a decreased risk of infection. Alternatively, many surgeons prefer sacroiliac screw fixation after open reduction of the posterior pelvic ring. Iliosacral screw placement has become the standard means of internal fixation for fractures and fracture-dislocations of the sacrum and sacroiliac joints. Nevertheless, the complexity and variations in sacral anatomy make the optimum placement of iliosacral screws technically difficult to achieve. Complications of the misplacement

of iliosacral screws can be devastating and include damage to the iliac and the superior gluteal vessels, damage to the fourth or fifth lumbar or first sacral nerve roots and to the sympathetic chain [49] **(III/B)**.

Recently, the technique of percutaneous fixation has expanded to other fracture patterns of the pelvic ring, such as anterior column fractures and iliac wing fractures.

Computer-assisted orthopaedic surgery (CAOS)

Percutaneous internal fixation of pelvic fractures has gained popularity allowing rapid patient mobilisation with reduced surgery-related morbidity. However, this method depends on conventional fluoroscopy, which exposes the patient and the surgeon to a significant amount of radiation.

Navigation procedures based on CT data were introduced into spinal surgery in 1994. Since then, the method has been used in other areas such as joint replacement, reconstructive surgery and tumour surgery, because of its high precision and reduced radiation exposure [50] **(IIa/B)**. The original CT-based spine module can be adjusted for pelvic surgery with the prerequisite that the positioning of the fragments is identical in CT and in the OR; otherwise a new dataset has to be acquired.

We should not forget that we are dealing with 'improved fluoroscopy', which is still limited and cannot be of assistance in the treatment of displaced fractures. However, the next generation of equipment will be able to provide the ability and means necessary for fracture reduction, prior to percutaneous fixation. Thus, more extensive use of the navigation system in more complex pelvic fractures will be possible.

Minimally invasive surgery (MIS)

Anterior pelvic stabilisation is usually achieved by internal fixation through the ilio-inguinal or Pfannenstiel exposures [51]. Frequent problems with these approaches arise from detachment and reattachment of the rectus abdominus muscle, dissection across complex anatomic structures (such as the inguinal canal) and potential damage to inguinal and pubic vessels [52]. High blood loss, infection, retractile scars, nerve entrapment, and incisional hernias, as well as weakening of the abdominal wall, are also factors to consider when performing surgery in this region [53]. Some reports have supported the convenience of minimally invasive fixation techniques, including retrograde medullary superior ramus screws, to avoid extensile dissections [54] **(IIb/B)**. Until now, by using these percutaneous techniques, reduction of displaced fragments remained an unsolved problem often requiring a limited blind approach across the inguinal canal.

Compared with the conventional ilio-inguinal approach, the use of an endoscopic technique for anterior pelvic fracture stabilisation minimises the soft tissue damage caused by the surgical approach. The avoidance of skeletalisation might decrease the development of heterotopic ossification and the occurrence of postoperative hernias and thrombosis. Additionally, the soft tissue envelope is maintained as a barrier to infection and wound breakdown. Another advantage is that with less soft tissue damage, patients have less pain allowing functional rehabilitation to begin more rapidly [21]. In the area of minimally invasive surgery, Rubel et al [20] described a technique for endoscopic fixation of pubic symphysis disruptions. The recommendations for the use of this technique are summarised at the end of this chapter.

Enhanced fixation of vertically unstable pelvic injuries

The goals of treatment for vertically unstable pelvic injuries are anatomical reduction and stabilisation. The method of fixation used is dependent on the fracture patho-anatomy. However, when the posterior injury consists of a sacral alar fracture (Denis Zone I) [55], the treatment options are fairly limited. Direct anterior fixation of sacral fractures is precluded due to the risk to the neurovascular structures [56].

Percutaneous iliosacral screw fixation is a useful technique in the management of vertically unstable pelvic fractures, but a vertical sacral fracture should

make the surgeon more wary of fixation failure and loss of reduction [57] **(IIb/B)**.

This ongoing surgical challenge has been addressed in different studies comparing lumbopelvic triangular SI screw osteosynthesis with standard iliosacral screw fixation in a transforaminal fracture model using 12 human cadavers. In another biomechanical study, S1 pediculo-iliac (as opposed to lumbopelvic) screw fixation was compared with iliosacral screw fixation and with anterior symphyseal double plating in polyurethane pelvic bone analogues.

Urologic injuries in pelvic ring disruptions

Pelvic ring disruptions are the result of high energy blunt trauma and are associated with other significant injuries in more than 50% of the cases. These injuries may involve neurovascular structures and other organ systems. Lower urinary tract injuries may occur in as many as 25% of patients with pelvic ring disruptions. Co-ordinated care between the orthopaedist and urologist is required for successful treatment of concurrent urologic and pelvic injury. Of primary importance to the orthopaedist is the potential for infection after open stabilisation of the anterior arch. When contaminated urine communicates with the anterior arch, the possibility of infection exists. Early repair of bladder disruptions with simultaneous anterior arch plating minimises this risk [58] **(IIb/B)**.

Haemorrhage control and treatment strategies in pelvic fractures

Pelvic ring disruptions are frequently severe, life-threatening injuries. Primary steps in resuscitation include control of airway, breathing and circulation. It is important to assess the haemodynamic status of the patient and to do a brief neurologic evaluation. Life-threatening problems recognised during initial assessment should be addressed. Patients who are haemodynamically unstable may require abdominal ultrasound or diagnostic peritoneal lavage (DPL). Pelvic instability, neurologic injury, or evidence of urethral injury may alert the physician that the retroperitoneum has been disrupted. In these instances, closure of the pelvic cavity decreases the retroperitoneal volume and may decrease blood loss.

Rapid control of retroperitoneal haemorrhage in patients with unstable pelvic fractures is essential to prevent early death, reduce the complications associated with massive transfusions, and to improve overall outcome. Previous attempts to control retroperitoneal bleeding by surgical ligation of the internal iliac artery have proven futile because of the extensive collateral circulation within the pelvis [59].

Pelvic bleeding is multifactorial and potential bleeding sites include fracture edges, veins, and arteries [60]. Delay in diagnosis can dramatically reduce survival. Treatment alternatives include pneumatic anti-shock garments, pelvic binders, external fixation, specially designed pelvic clamps, angiography with embolisation and laparotomy with pelvic packing [61] **(IIb/B)**.

In most patients with stable pelvic ring injuries and stable vital signs, bleeding into the closed pelvic space will be self-limiting. By contrast, unstable pelvic fractures will frequently be associated with disruption of retroperitoneal muscle compartments. This can lead to uncontrolled haemorrhage creeping cranially above the psoas muscle or along the gluteal muscles, with the risk of exsanguination or pelvic and abdominal compartment syndromes - the chimney effect [62].

During the past decade, direct pelvic compression using a pelvic sling has been introduced for emergency stabilisation of pelvic fractures. It achieves satisfactory pelvic compression without seriously limiting access to the patient. Prophylactic application at the accident scene or in the emergency department appears to be warranted [63].

Several investigators have shown that the application of anterior pelvic frames has reduced acute haemodynamic mortality and should be applied immediately in patients with pelvic ring disruption and haemodynamic instability **(IIb/B)**. The physician must have a high index of suspicion for associated injuries and the possibility of retroperitoneal haemorrhage with the recognition of pelvic ring disruption. It is in

this situation that the orthopaedic surgeon must play a major role by applying a provisional anterior pelvic external fixation device, which can be lifesaving in the haemodynamically unstable patient. The pelvic external fixator can be applied in the emergency room setting or in the operating room. If the fixator is placed prior to laparotomy, a frame must be constructed that will not impede access to the abdomen. If, at the time of laparotomy, an expanding haematoma is noted, external fixation can be applied in the operating room. In a haemodynamically stable patient with an unstable fracture, pelvic external fixation, with or without posterior stabilisation, may provide the stability and pain control to allow mobilisation of the patient. In haemodynamically unstable patients with unstable pelvic fractures, anterior stabilisation should be performed immediately. Patients with stable pelvic fractures or patients who remain haemodynamically unstable after pelvic external fixation may need emergency pelvic angiography and selective embolisation [64] **(IIb/B)**.

The application of the pelvic C-clamp provides compression and stability at the posterior aspect of the ring at the point where the greatest bleeding usually occurs and thus offers effective pelvic tamponade. However, its use may be compromised in the presence of fractures of the ilium and trans-iliac fracture dislocations. Potential complications include iatrogenic injury to the gluteal neurovascular structures and secondary injury as a result of over-compression in sacral fractures [65].

It is not uncommon for the patient with a pelvic fracture to have one or more arterial sources contributing to their total blood loss. If outcome is to be improved it is essential that all bleeding sources be identified and controlled in an expedient manner.

Controversy exists about the indications and optimal timing of angiography in haemodynamically unstable patients with severe pelvic fractures. Its efficacy has been questioned, as mortality figures of up to 50% have been reported despite effective bleeding control. Furthermore, as the procedure can be time-consuming, the management of other associated injuries can be compromised [66]. The indication for angiography with the added option of therapeutic embolisation exists if pelvic bleeding persists even after reposition and operative fixation of the injury. The use of intravenous contrast material in the evaluation of trauma cases allows simultaneous evaluation of osseous and vascular structures within the affected area. It is thought that for selected patients angiography is both diagnostic and therapeutic. This technique offers the advantage of localising multiple bleeding sites and occluding them at the level of injury. It also has the advantage of leaving the retroperitoneum undisturbed, thereby preserving the tamponade effect and reducing the risk of infecting a pelvic haematoma. Early control of haemorrhage reduces transfusion requirements and its associated complications and in addition, allows expeditious treatment of the patient's other injuries. It is thought that angiography and transcatheter embolisation continues to play an important role in specific cases in the multidisciplinary approach to the patient who is unstable and has a pelvic fracture.

The technique of retroperitoneal packing has been successfully used in some institutions where tamponades are applied in the paravesical and presacral spaces in an attempt to tamponade bleeding. Immediate posterior ring stabilisation with the pelvic C-clamp or an external fixator provides mechanical stability for pelvic tamponade and fracture reduction leads to a reduction in fracture haemorrhage. The presacral and paravesical regions are then packed from posterior to anterior using standard surgical techniques. The packing is changed or removed 48 hours after injury.

Mortality from pelvic fractures could be classified as:

- early, secondary to uncontrolled haemorrhage; and
- late, due to post-traumatic complications such as acute respiratory distress syndrome (ARDS)/multiple organ dysfunction syndrome (MODS).

It is clear today that the development of ARDS and MODS is due to multiple alterations in inflammatory and immunological function, which occurs shortly after trauma and haemorrhage (first-hit phenomenon). The effect of surgery on the immune response of the polytraumatised patient (the second-hit phenomenon), is nowadays considered to be a critical factor directly affecting the clinical outcome of the patient [67].

'Damage control orthopaedics' is the current treatment of choice for the severely injured patient, especially those with an unstable pelvic ring injury associated with haemodynamic instability. Management of the pelvic fracture should be conceived as part of the resuscitative effort. By maintaining circulating blood volume and tissue oxygenation whilst performing a rapid and limited surgical intervention where indicated, the damage induced by any procedure is minimised. Immediate external fixation of the unstable pelvis with pelvic packing to control pelvic haemorrhage is a practical approach to those borderline unstable patients, or those *in extremis*. Angiographic embolisation can only be recommended in the more stable patient [68] **(IIb/B)**.

Open pelvic fractures

Open pelvic fractures constitute one of the most devastating injuries in musculoskeletal trauma and must be treated aggressively, incorporating a multidisciplinary approach. Early treatment, focusing on prevention of haemorrhage and sepsis, is essential **(IIb/B)**.

The management of associated soft tissue injuries must be aggressive, including early administration of broad-spectrum antibiotics and repeated, meticulous wound debridement and irrigation. Selective faecal diversion, dictated by wound location may be essential to minimise the risk of sepsis and to reduce mortality **(IIb/B)**. Recommendations are summarised at the end of the chapter.

Outcome after treatment of displaced acetabular fractures

Functional outcome is important and can be assessed and quantified in several ways. Health surveys, employment status, activity level, clinical examination, radiographs and CT scans are useful tools in evaluating patient outcome. The most vital issue in determining the success of treatment is the patient's ability to return to their previous activities. Unfortunately, evaluating this goal is sometimes difficult because it is hard to quantify the ability to work, to perform household activities and to engage in recreational activities.

The functional outcome of acetabular fracture treatment, as determined on the basis of limb-specific or joint-specific outcome measures and the physical function components of general-health status, have become a major focus of interest. Open reduction and internal fixation is thought to offer the highest likelihood of a favourable outcome for patients with displaced acetabular fractures. However, acetabular fractures associated with extensive impaction or erosion of the acetabulum or femoral articular cartilage or with marked comminution and osteopenia have an intrinsically poor prognosis.

Complications of pelvic fracture

Deep venous thrombosis

Thrombo-embolic complications are the most common preventable cause of morbidity and mortality in the patient with trauma. Their management is controversial, and much remains to be determined regarding the prevention, detection, and treatment of deep venous thrombosis and pulmonary embolism in injured patients. Pulmonary embolism is a particularly devastating complication because of its sudden onset, unpredictable nature, and often fatal outcome, typically striking the patient who has recently stabilised from other more apparent injuries [69].

In the multiply injured patient, classic anticoagulation is often contraindicated because of the risk of bleeding. Mechanical lower limb compression has been recommended as an alternative to pharmacological prophylaxis in this high-risk group of patients. Mechanical prophylaxis provides protection without increasing the risk of blood loss and such devices work by improving venous blood flow as well as by stimulating endogenous fibrinolytic activity [70] **(Ia/A)**.

Ultrasound is notoriously poor at detecting pelvic clots. This problem is exacerbated in the setting of trauma by the presence of a pelvic haematoma. Ascending venography is invasive and also lacks sensitivity for detecting pelvic deep vein thromboses.

The accuracy of magnetic resonance venography depends upon experienced interpretation by radiologists familiar with the technique in patients with traumatic injury. It has a high sensitivity and may detect clots that are small and not at risk for embolisation. Magnetic resonance venography has the major advantage of being able to detect thromboses in the pelvic veins as well as in the thigh [71] **(III/B)**.

Heterotopic ossification

Heterotopic ossification is a well-known complication of surgical approaches to the hip that involve dissection of the gluteal muscles. The exact mechanism for heterotopic bone formation has not been thoroughly elucidated; however, it appears to involve pluripotent mesenchymal cell differentiation into osteoprogenitor cells after tissue injury or dissection.

Reported risk factors for heterotopic ossification following acetabular surgery include thoracic and abdominal trauma, male gender, closed head injury, high 'Injury Severity Score', delay in fracture fixation, T-type fracture, and extensile approaches. The extended iliofemoral, combined anterior and posterior, and Kocher-Langenbeck approaches are associated with the highest prevalences of heterotopic ossification (57%, 45.4%, and 26.3%, respectively), whereas non-operative treatment and anterior approaches that do not violate the gluteal muscles are believed to be associated with a lower rate of heterotopic ossification [8].

Both radiation therapy and indomethacin provide effective prophylaxis against heterotopic bone formation **(Ia/A)**. Radiation prevents heterotopic ossification when administered 24 hours before surgery or within 72 hours afterwards. Indomethacin reduces the rate of heterotopic ossification after surgical treatment of acetabular fractures by 30% to 45%.

There is controversy surrounding the relative effectiveness of local irradiation and oral indomethacin for prophylaxis against heterotopic ossification following surgical treatment of acetabular fractures. Heterotopic ossification after an extensile approach to the hip is not uncommon, and often leads to a decreased range of hip motion and to pain.

Nerve injuries

The rising number of high-speed vehicular accidents has resulted in an increasing incidence of polytrauma, often including severe pelvic injuries. Improved initial resuscitation has lowered overall mortality rates and newer techniques of fixation have improved late morbidity. Neurologic injury, however, continues to be a major cause of long-term morbidity after pelvic disruption. The true incidence of neurologic injuries associated with fractures of the pelvis remains a subject of much debate. Early series of large numbers of pelvic fractures reported a very low incidence of associated neurologic injury. Clinically, most neurologic injuries associated with pelvic ring fractures involve the L5 or S1 nerve roots. The incidence of neurologic injuries associated with fractures of the pelvic ring is undoubtedly multifactorial. Common sense dictates that the proximity of the posterior ring injury to the neurologic structures and the initial displacement should play a role [72].

Injury to the sciatic nerve is one of the more serious complications of acetabular fracture and traumatic dislocation of the hip, both in the short and long term. Injury to the femoral nerve can occur as well. Patient satisfaction and functional outcome will be compromised when these complications develop.

Conclusions

Pelvic and acetabular surgery has evolved into an acknowledged area of clinical expertise within the scope of orthopaedic surgery. Despite the introduction of organised trauma systems, pelvic ring disruptions continue to be a significant source of morbidity and mortality. Their management is challenging to the most experienced trauma surgeons and often requires a multidisciplinary approach involving a variety of specialties. The goal of acetabular fracture surgery is to achieve an anatomic reduction and stable fixation of the fracture. Achieving this goal requires adequate visualisation for fracture reduction and placement of hardware. Careful interpretation and new innovative redefinitions of fracture classifications can eliminate diagnostic ambiguity and contribute to the appropriate surgical approach. Advances in the existent surgical approaches allow reconstruction without the need for extensile dissections. CT scans are essential and should continue to be used in conjunction with plain radiographs in the pre-operative evaluation of displaced acetabular fractures and perhaps should be considered in the postoperative assessment of fracture reduction. New percutaneous and minimally invasive surgical techniques, in conjunction with innovative computer-based imaging modalities, provide promising treatment alternatives. Pelvic and acetabular fractures are usually associated with other injuries and play an important role in the prognosis of multiply injured patients. Damage control orthopaedics is the current treatment of choice for the severely injured patient, especially those with an unstable pelvic ring injury associated with haemodynamic instability. The care of the patient with pelvic and acetabular fractures is challenging, but rewarding. Becoming accustomed with these areas should help to improve care for patients with musculoskeletal injuries.

Recommendations	Evidence level

Classification of acetabular fractures

- The axial CT display of acetabular fracture patterns provides a basis for a classification of acetabular fractures that is simple, unambiguous, readily understood by both radiologists and orthopaedic surgeons.   Ib/A
- It provides clear direction for both diagnosis and surgical treatment planning.   Ib/A
- Category and subcategory fracture specificity creates a mechanism for intra- and interdepartmental postoperative assessment of any of the individual acetabular fracture types.   Ib/A

Imaging of pelvic and acetabular fractures

- Plain radiographs show poor sensitivity for the detection of step and gap deformities in patients with acetabular fractures relative to CT scans.   IIb/B
- Differences between CT and plain radiographs are greatest with the most clinically relevant deformity, i.e. step.   IIb/B
- Computed tomography determines the exact nature of the posterior pelvic ring injury, discriminates between the type and location of injury, and is also useful as an adjunct in defining associated acetabular injuries.   III/B

CT scanning is recommended for the following situations:

- Single breaks in the pelvic ring in which a significant posterior ring injury is suspected but cannot be confirmed by radiography.   III/B
- Double vertical fractures of the pelvis in which radiography cannot conclusively demonstrate the stability of the pelvis.   III/B
- Evaluation of fracture extension into the articular portion of the acetabulum.   III/B
- Injuries to the pelvis under consideration for open reduction and internal fixation.   III/B
- Evaluation of intrapelvic soft tissue injuries.   III/B
- The degree of residual fracture displacement is detected more accurately on postoperative computed tomography scans than on plain radiographs. The accuracy of surgical reduction as assessed on postoperative computed tomography is highly predictive of the clinical outcome.   III/B
- Pelvic haemorrhage volumes derived from pelvic CT scans are predictors of the need for pelvic arteriography and transfusions.   III/B
- CT scans are essential and should continue to be used in conjunction with plain radiographs in the pre-operative evaluation of displaced acetabular fractures and should be considered in the postoperative assessment of fracture reduction.   IIb/B

Recommendations	Evidence level

Surgical approaches to the pelvis and acetabulum

- Advantages of the modified ilio-inguinal approach are intra-articular visualisation, better access to the quadrilateral surface and a lower risk of iatrogenic injury to the lateral femoral cutaneous nerve.   III/B
- It can be used when there is comminution of the anterior wall and/or low anterior column where there is a need for articular inspection.   III/B
- The modified ilio-inguinal approach provides exposure to the anterior pelvis and quadrilateral plate.   III/B
- It avoids some of the potential complications associated with the classic ilio-inguinal approach.   III/B
- It allows surgeons to extend the utility of the ilio-inguinal approach by providing direct access to the quadrilateral surface and anterior pelvic ring for fracture fixation.   III/B

Percutaneous stabilisation

- Exhaustive attempts at reduction must be made because screw placement with residual displacement of 10mm can endanger the adjacent neurovascular structures and is associated with compromised outcome and function.   IIb/B
- To ensure safe insertion, iliac screws must be positioned in the geometric centre of the sacral ala. Anything except this could represent unintentional extra-osseous placement.   III/B
- Electromyographic monitoring can enhance the safety of percutaneous placement of iliosacral screws.   III/B
- Percutaneous stabilisation should be limited to elementary fracture patterns in young patients. Comminuted or complex fractures still require open procedures.   III/B
- For elderly patients whose physical demands are lower, the technique may have broader indications for use because imperfect reductions may be more acceptable.   III/B
- The use of the percutaneous acetabular fixation technique is associated with an extremely low complication rate in the treatment of anterior column acetabular fractures.   III/B
- Percutaneous iliosacral screw fixation is a useful technique in the management of vertically unstable pelvic fractures, but a vertical sacral fracture should make the surgeon more wary of fixation failure and loss of reduction.   IIb/B
- Percutaneous fixation diminishes potential blood loss and operative times in U-shaped sacral fractures and allows subsequent sacral decompression of the local neural elements using open techniques when necessary.   III/B

Recommendations	Evidence level

Percutaneous stabilisation *continued:*

- Patients with significant soft tissue injuries that would complicate or prevent open techniques can be treated. These patients include those with severe open fractures, faecal or environmental contamination, extensive closed degloving injuries and abrasions or lacerations. III/B
- Contraindications to percutaneous pelvic fixation include sacral dysmorphism and other unusual pelvic anatomic variations. III/B
- Percutaneous sacroiliac screws can be positioned safely, in experienced hands, using peri-operative fluoroscopic techniques. A position in the first sacral vertebral body has a significantly lower incidence of neurologic injury compared with a position in the second. In the case of postoperative neurologic deficit, only a CT scan can predict the clinical outcome. III/B

Computer-assisted orthopaedic surgery (CAOS)

- Current results indicate that computer-aided frameless navigation of iliosacral screw stabilisation is a safe technique with the outlined conditions. It provides an excellent intra-operative detailed view of the anatomy during implantation and may reduce access-related peri-operative complications associated with the traditional method. IIa/B

At this stage, a selective population with traumatic pelvic fractures can be treated percutaneously with the use of the computerised navigation system:

- Displaced fractures with a feasible closed reduction. III/B
- Complex fractures in which a combination of closed and open reduction is necessary. III/B
- Cases of minimally displaced pelvic or acetabular fractures. III/B

Minimally invasive surgery (MIS)

- MIS is indicated in complex anterior pelvic ring fractures, especially anterior pelvic ring fractures with extension close to the acetabulum where the anterior stabilisation has to be achieved with a plate from the symphyseal region to the iliac wing. IIb/B
- Endoscopy permits placement of plates and screws on top of the symphysis pubis, reduction of internally displaced fragments, and performance of percutaneous procedures that do not harm anatomic structures. III/B
- It can also be applied to the treatment of the Morel-Lavallee lesion (the collection of fluid and devitalised fat resulting from the shearing and separation of subcutaneous tissue from the underlying fascia) through a small proximal and distal incision with a long plastic brush and copious pulse lavage. III/B

Chapter 15

Recommendations	Evidence level

Enhanced fixation of vertically unstable pelvic injuries

- Triangular osteosynthesis demonstrates smaller displacement under initial peak loads, as well as fewer failures after 10,000 cycles of loading. — IIb/B
- Iliosacral screw fixation was found to be more stable in terms of early and ultimate failure loads when used for the treatment of zone-I sacral fractures and sacroiliac joint disruption. — IIb/B

Urologic injuries in pelvic ring disruptions

- With regard to the issue of urethra early versus late rupture repair following pelvic fractures, current evidence supports the view that early realignment followed by delayed repair is associated with more favourable results in terms of sexual function. — IIb/B
- The development of long-term strictures appears not to be significant, irrespective of the time of definitive reconstruction. — IIb/B

Haemorrhage control and treatment strategies in pelvic fractures

Application of pelvic frame

- Patients with evidence of unstable fractures of the pelvis not associated with hypotension but who do require a steady and ongoing resuscitation should be considered for some form of external pelvic stabilisation. — III/B
- Patients with evidence of unstable fractures of the pelvis associated with hypotension should be considered for some form of external pelvic stabilisation. — IIb/B
- Patients with evidence of unstable pelvic fractures who warrant laparotomy should receive external pelvic stabilisation prior to laparotomy incision. — IIb/B

Indications for angiography and embolisation

- The morphology of the fracture is not a reliable guide to an associated vascular injury. — IIb/B
- CT can help predict the specific bleeding artery and therefore potentially guide angiographic intervention. — III/B
- Patients with a major pelvic fracture who have signs of ongoing bleeding after non-pelvic sources of blood loss have been ruled out should be considered for pelvic angiography and possible embolisation. — IIb/B
- Laparotomy and packing of the pelvic retroperitoneum has been suggested as a therapeutic alternative for the treatment of catastrophically injured patients. — IIb/B
- Patients with major pelvic fracture who are found to have bleeding in the pelvis, which cannot be adequately controlled at laparotomy, should be considered for pelvic angiography and possible embolisation. — IIb/B

Recommendations	Evidence level

Haemorrhage control and treatment strategies in pelvic fractures *continued:*

Treatment strategies

- The physical examination of the patient with a pelvic ring injury is extremely important. — III/B
- Initial evaluation of the patient with a suspected pelvic ring injury should be directed towards identifying potential instability and deformity. — III/B
- Careful examination of the soft tissues about the pelvis is required to ensure that an open pelvic fracture is not overlooked. — III/B
- The initial assessment of the patient must include assessment of the immediate life-threatening problems that are often associated with pelvic fractures. — III/B
- The initial treatment of patients who have a major pelvic ring injury involving disruption of the posterior pelvic ring, and who are haemodynamically unstable, involves aggressive fluid resuscitation, evaluation to rule out ongoing intra-abdominal and/or intrathoracic haemorrhage and early stabilisation of the pelvic ring. — III/B
- If haemodynamic instability persists after pelvic stabilisation, without evidence of abdominal or thoracic haemorrhage, the patient should have urgent angiography to exclude a pelvic arterial bleed which may be suitable for embolisation. — III/B
- Laparotomy and packing of the pelvic retroperitoneum has been suggested as a therapeutic alternative for the treatment of catastrophically injured patients. — IIb/B

Open pelvic fractures

- Haemorrhage control has the highest priority and can be achieved by aggressive resuscitation with intravenous fluids and blood products, with the early application of antiseptic pressure dressings to obvious bleeding sites. — IIb/B
- Emergency stabilisation of pelvic ring fractures using circumferential sheets or external fixation devices is mandatory. — IIb/B
- A thorough clinical examination of the patient, including meticulous inspection of perineal tissues, examination of the vaginal vault and rectal digital examination, is essential in order to discover occult open fractures. — IIb/B
- Treatment of soft tissue injuries must be aggressive, including early administration of broad-spectrum antibiotics and repeated, meticulous wound debridement and irrigation. Open wound care is imperative in these injuries and is initiated in the trauma room. — IIb/B
- Selective faecal diversion based on wound location (zone I or pelvi-perineal wounds) is compulsory and safe. Faecal diversion must include a meticulous distal rectal evacuation, possible sphincter repair and local open wound management. — IIb/B

Chapter 15

Recommendations	Evidence level

Open pelvic fractures *continued:*

- Vaginal lacerations and intraperitoneal bladder disruptions require prompt repair. Urethral injuries are best treated by early realignment, if possible, and delayed end-to-end repair. — IIb/B
- Definitive stabilisation of pelvic fractures should be performed according to the principles of 'damage control orthopaedics'. — IIb/B
- Fixation techniques, including external fixation with minimally invasive, or open internal fixation, need to be adjusted according to the site, condition and contamination of open wounds. — IIb/B
- Long-term sequelae of open pelvic fractures include chronic pain, residual disability, incontinence, impotence and dyspareunia. — IIb/B

Outcome after treatment of displaced acetabular fractures

- Residual displacement of 1-2mm may lead to an increased incidence of post-traumatic arthritis and a poor clinical outcome. — IIa/B
- The percentage of good and excellent results correlated closely with the percentage of anatomic reductions. — IIa/B
- Only surgeons who have the appropriate training and experience should perform these complex procedures. — III/B
- Poor outcome after open reduction and internal fixation is associated with fracture comminution, marginal impaction, and the inability to achieve an anatomic reduction. — IIa/B
- Risk factors for an unsatisfactory result include an age of more than 55 years, a delay of more than 24 hours from the time of injury to the time of reduction of a hip dislocation, intra-articular fracture comminution, and a residual fracture gap of >1 cm. — IIa/B
- Hip flexion and extension strength are negatively affected following the open reduction and internal fixation of an acetabular fracture. — IIb/B
- The functional outcome of operative treatment of acetabular fractures in geriatric patients were comparable with those in an age-matched cohort without a history of acetabular fracture, with good to excellent results in two-thirds of the patients studied. — IIb/B
- Patients who have undergone total hip arthroplasty for the treatment of post-traumatic arthritis after an acetabular fracture have shown inferior results compared with the results for patients who have undergone the procedure for the treatment of non-traumatic arthritis. — III/B
- Patients who had a total hip replacement after a previous acetabular fracture had worse function than those who had had a total hip replacement for the treatment of osteoarthritis. — III/B
- Total hip arthroplasty performed after an acetabular fracture was a more extensive procedure and was associated with greater blood loss, especially in patients with previous internal fixation. — III/B

Chapter 16

Hip fracture management trends

Martyn J Parker MD FRCS (Ed)

Orthopaedic Research Fellow

PETERBOROUGH AND STAMFORD HOSPITAL NHS FOUNDATION TRUST,
PETERBOROUGH DISTRICT HOSPITAL, PETERBOROUGH, UK

Introduction

A hip fracture is the commonest reason for an elderly person to be admitted to an acute orthopaedic ward. The average age of patients sustaining a hip fracture is about 80 years and 80% are female. Most fractures are due to a fall from standing height. Aetiological factors include loss of protective mechanisms in falling and reduced bone strength. Globally, numbers of hip fractures were estimated at 1.26 million in 1990 and this number is expected to increase to between 7.3 to 21.3 million by 2025 [1]. The age-specific incidence of this condition, which has been increasing in industrialised countries, may now be levelling out, although the total number of hip fractures occurring each year continues to increase as more of the population live to their eighties. Much of this increase in hip fracture incidence in the next 20 years will occur in developing countries.

Radiographically, hip fractures can be subdivided into intracapsular and extracapsular fractures. Intracapsular fractures are further subdivided into displaced and undisplaced fractures [2]. Extracapsular fractures may be subdivided into trochanteric and subtrochanteric fractures. Trochanteric fractures may be further subdivided into stable (two-part fractures) and unstable fractures (more than two parts) [3].

Methodology

The search strategy involved Medline and Cochrane databases (March 2005) using the term 'hip fracture'. Abstracts of all these articles from the last 50 years have been reviewed by the author, with further study of those articles considered relevant. Extensive search strategies for randomised trials on the topic of hip (proximal femur) fracture have been undertaken by the Musculoskeletal Group of the Cochrane Collaboration. This group has completed reviews on all aspects of hip fracture management.

Peri-operative care

Resuscitation

Pre-operative preparation for theatre, the timing of surgery and use of intravenous fluids for resuscitation has not been adequately evaluated within randomised trials. One systematic review identified two randomised trials on pre and peri-operative fluids [4]. The use of more invasive monitoring demonstrated that many patients were hypovolaemic prior to surgery and appropriate infusion of intravenous fluids could correct this. Within the limited number of patients studied (130), no difference in mortality was demonstrated, but there was a trend towards a reduced hospital stay in those managed by more invasive monitoring (IIa/B).

Traction

Prior to the surgical treatment of a hip fracture the injured limb may be immobilised with traction. One systematic review of eight RCTs with 1349 participants in total found no evidence of any benefit of traction, whether this be applied to the skin or as skeletal traction [5] (Ia/A).

Analgesia

Conventional analgesics for pain related to hip fractures are opiates (parenteral or oral), paracetamol (acetaminophen) and codeine. Non-steroidal anti-inflammatory drugs can be used, but many physicians prefer to avoid these during the peri-operative period because of the potential risk of gastrointestinal irritation and renal impairment. Nerve blocks may be used as an adjunct to analgesic drugs. A systematic review of eight RCTs of 328 participants found that nerve blocks reduced reported pain levels and the need for oral or parenteral analgesic [6]. No clear-cut reduction in the occurrence of peri-operative complications was demonstrated (Ib/A).

Thrombo-embolic prophylaxis

Despite the abundant research material on this topic, thrombo-embolic prophylaxis remains a controversial subject. Supporting arguments can be made for extended prophylaxis, but at the other end of the spectrum there is a case for not using any pharmacological prophylaxis. Standard measures that may be used to reduce the incidence of thrombo-embolic complications include the avoidance of delays

to surgery, early mobilisation, spinal anaesthesia and avoidance of over-transfusion. These measures can then be supplemented by pharmacological and/or mechanical methods.

A systematic review of heparin use found that this agent reduced the incidence of deep vein thrombosis, as measured by routine venography (13 RCTs, 124/474 [26.2%] versus 219/519 [42.2%], RR 0.60, 95% CI 0.50 to 0.71) [7]. No difference for pulmonary embolism was noted (ten RCTs, 13/404 [3.2%] versus 14/454 [3.1%], RR 1.00, 95% CI 0.49 to 2.02). Mortality was slightly higher with heparin (eight RCTs, 42/356 [11.8%] versus 38/374 [10.2%], RR 1.16, 95% CI 0.77 to 1.74). There were limited data on the incidence of wound haematomas, wound infection, blood loss and the need for blood transfusion, which showed no difference between heparin and placebo groups.

Antiplatelet drugs, notably low-dose aspirin, have been advocated for thrombo-embolic prophylaxis [8]. One systematic review [9] and a large multicentre randomised trial [10], found that antiplatelet drugs significantly reduced the incidence of 'venographic' venous thrombosis (35.9% versus 41.9%), clinical venous thrombosis (1.0% versus 1.5%), pulmonary embolism (2.8% versus 6.9%), and fatal pulmonary embolism (0.3% versus 0.6%). There was no significant effect on mortality in either of the studies. Antiplatelet drugs did, however, increase the risk of postoperative bleeding complications requiring transfusion in the multicentre study (197/6679 [2.9%] versus 157/6677 [2.3%], RR 1.25, 95% CI 1.02 to 1.54) [10].

Graduated elastic compression stockings have been evaluated for elective surgical operations, where they have been shown to be effective in reducing the occurrence of deep vein thrombosis. They have not been evaluated on hip fracture patients within randomised trials. Cyclical compression devices (foot or calf pumps) have been evaluated within five randomised trials and the results have been summarised in a systematic review [7]. The incidence of deep venous thrombosis was reduced from 52/229 (22.7%) to 16/221 (7.2%) with the use of compression devices (RR 0.31, 95% CI 0.19 to

0.51). No significant difference in the incidence of pulmonary embolism or mortality was noted.

In summary, both pharmacological methods and compression devices are effective in reducing the occurrence of venous thrombosis, but neither method has been shown to have a demonstrable effect on mortality. The pharmacological methods may be associated with an increased risk of bleeding complications **(Ia/A)**.

Nutrition

One systematic review of 17 RCTs involving 1266 participants found some evidence that oral protein and energy supplementary feeds reduce the occurrence of postoperative complications. No definite effect on mortality could be demonstrated [11] **(Ia/A)**.

Surgery

Type of anaesthesia

Anaesthesia for hip fracture surgery can be broadly divided into those techniques that render the patient unconscious (general anaesthesia) and regional anaesthesia techniques (spinal or epidural). One systematic review of 22 RCTs with 2567 participants, which compared general with regional anaesthesia, found a tendency to less postoperative confusion (five RCTs, 11/117 [9.4%] versus 23/120 [19.2%], RR 0.50, 95% CI 0.26 to 0.95) and less deep vein thrombosis (four RCTs, 39/129 [30.2%] versus 61/130 [46.9%], RR 0.64, 95% CI 0.48 to 0.86) with regional anaesthesia [12]. No conclusive differences were demonstrated for any other outcomes including mortality between anaesthetic techniques **(Ia/A)**.

Peri-operative antibiotics

Two systematic reviews of 15 RCTs [13] and 22 RCTs [14] studied the use of one to three doses of antibiotic prophylaxis, starting at the time of surgery. Deep wound infections were reported in 11 RCTs and reduced from 40/935 (4.3%) without antibiotics to 12/961 (1.2%) with antibiotics (RR 0.29, 95% CI

0.15 to 0.65). Seven RCTs reported on superficial wound infection rates, which were also reduced from 38/661 (5.7%) to 22/705 (3.2%) (RR 0.48, 95% CI 0.28 to 0.81). Some benefit was also seen for a reduction in urinary tract infections **(Ia/A)**.

Operative versus conservative

The first question about the specific management of the hip fracture which the orthopaedic surgeon has to ask is, should the fracture be managed operatively or by conservative methods? This decision is strongly influenced by the radiographic classification of the fracture. Undisplaced intracapsular fractures may be managed by either method; operative treatment by internal fixation reduces the risk of displacement of the fracture. The one small randomised trial of only 23 patients on this topic was abandoned in favour of operative treatment [15] **(IIa/B)**. No randomised trials have been reported comparing operative versus conservative treatment for displaced intracapsular fractures. Clinical experience from historical case series indicates markedly improved outcomes for operative treatment **(III/B)**. For trochanteric (extracapsular) fractures, a systematic review of four studies including 405 participants found no difference in mortality between treatment methods, but operative treatment reduced the length of hospital stay, limb deformity and increased the number of patients who returned home [15] **(Ia/A)**.

Intracapsular fractures

Internal fixation versus arthroplasty

For patients with undisplaced fractures and younger patients (aged less than 60 to 70 years), internal fixation is recommended in order to preserve the femoral head. For older patients controversy exists about internal fixation or arthroplasty for displaced intracapsular fractures. The recent systematic review [16] and Cochrane review on this topic [17], identified 13 RCTs with 2091 participants and came to the same conclusions. There was a trend to a lower early mortality after internal fixation, but this was no longer apparent at one year from surgery. Internal fixation had shorter operative times, lower operative blood loss, less transfusion requirements and wound infections, but had a markedly increased re-operation rate (13 RCTs, 331/990 [33.4%] for internal fixation versus 123/1102 [11.1%] for arthroplasty, RR 3.09, 95% CI 2.55 to 3.75). No difference was found between treatment methods for length of hospital stay, occurrence of general medical complications, regain of mobility and residential status, and degree of residual pain **(Ia/A)**.

Internal fixation for intracapsular fractures - choice of implant

Numerous designs of implant are available for the internal fixation of intracapsular fractures. Many case series reports and randomised trials exist but because of differences in the selection of patients for internal fixation, case series are of very limited value in determining the choice of implant. The Cochrane review on this subject identified 28 RCTs involving 5547 participants, which compared different implants [18]. No notable differences in the incidence of fracture healing complications were noted between implants **(Ia/A)**.

Internal fixation for intracapsular fractures - surgical techniques

The limited randomised trials available on this topic indicate no benefit from compression or impaction of the fracture at the time of surgery (two RCTs, 323 participants) or open versus closed reduction (two RCTs, 151 participants) [19] **(Ib/B)**. Fracture reduction to an anatomical or slight valgus position is associated with a reduced incidence of fracture healing complications **(III/B)**. Implant positioning is more the subject of dogma than good clinical studies, with an inferior/central position of the implant on the anteroposterior X-ray and a central position on the lateral X-ray being generally favoured **(III/B)**.

Choice of arthroplasty

Key decisions related to the choice of arthroplasty are: should the implant be cemented in place?; whether the implant should be a hemiarthroplasty or total hip replacement (THR)?; and, if a hemiarthroplasty is chosen, what design should it be? Five RCTs of 482

participants have compared cemented versus uncemented hemiarthroplasties. Those with a cemented prosthesis had less residual pain at one year (two RCTs, 16/52 [30.8%] versus 28/45 [62.2%], RR 0.51, 95% CI 0.31 to 0.81) and were more likely to regain pre-fracture mobility (three RCTs, 40/58 [69.0%] versus 33/89 [37.1%], RR 0.60, 95% CI 0.44 to 0.82). No difference in mortality or other peri-operative outcomes were noted [20] **(Ia/A)**.

Seven RCTs of 857 participants have compared unipolar with bipolar hemiarthroplasty and have not found any notable difference between these types of prosthesis [20] **(Ia/A)**. A systematic review of case series reports found no difference in the incidence of dislocation between unipolar and bipolar hemiarthroplasties after adjustment for surgical approach and the use of cement (adjusted odds ratio bipolars versus unipolars 0.93, 95% CI 0.58 to 1.50) [21]. Only two RCTs of 269 participants have been identified comparing a hemiarthroplasty with a total hip replacement (THR). No notable differences were reported for mortality, wound infection or failure to regain mobility [20] **(Ib/A)**.

Surgical techniques - arthroplasty

Only one randomised trial of 114 patients has addressed the choice of surgical approach for an arthroplasty [22]. Results favoured an anterior-lateral approach. A systematic review of case series reports, found the anterior-lateral approach was favoured because of its lower risk of dislocation (397/7912 [5.1%] versus 128/6026 [2.4%]) [21] **(IIa/B)**.

Extracapsular fractures

Choice of implant - extramedullary versus intramedullary

Numerous randomised trials have compared various intramedullary nails with plate and sliding screw devices for the internal fixation of trochanteric fractures. The Cochrane review for nails that are inserted in a proximal to distal direction was able to utilise data from 24 RCTs involving 3403 participants [23]. No significant differences were found for the final outcome measures of mortality, pain and regain of hip function. Neither was there any difference in the incidence of the surgical complications of wound infection, blood transfusion requirements and cut-out of the implant. An increased risk of later fracture below the implant for the nails compared to sliding hip screws was clearly demonstrated (36/1325 [2.7%] versus 2/1337 [0.2%], RR 5.38, 95% CI 2.53 to 11.45). This specific complication of these nails results in an increased re-operation rate for them in comparison to the sliding hip screw (76/1318 [5.8%] versus 47/1357 [3.5%], RR 1.64, 95% CI 1.16 to 2.32)**(Ia/A)**. These findings only apply to trochanteric fractures. For other fracture patterns such as reversed fracture lines and subtrochanteric fractures, then intramedullary fixation may be superior **(III/B)**.

Nails that are inserted from the knee and passed up across the fracture site towards the femoral head have also been evaluated against both fixed extramedullary fixation implants and the sliding hip screw. Eleven RCTs of 1667 participants were identified for a systematic review, which found these nails, mainly of the Enders type, had an increased risk of fixation failure, re-operation, limb shortening, limb deformity and residual pain in comparison to extramedullary fixation [24] **(Ia/A)**.

Choice of implant - extramedullary implants

Extramedullary implants for the fixation of an extracapsular hip fracture, can be divided into those without sliding capacity (static), or those that have the capacity to slide as the fracture collapses (dynamic). Three RCTs of 355 participants and a systematic review of non-randomised comparative studies (13 studies, 2855 participants), demonstrated an increased risk of fixation failure, re-operation, impaired mobility and mortality for the fixed nail plates [25, 26] **(Ia/A)**.

A number of modifications to the sliding hip screw have recently been introduced, such as a supplementary trochanteric stabilising plate, variable angle plate, Medoff slide plate and a percutaneously inserted plate. Two RCTs of 292 participants have compared the Medoff sliding plate with the sliding hip screw and found a lower risk of fixation failure for the

Medoff plate (2/123 [1.6%] versus 14/151 [9.3%], RR 0.20, 95% CI 0.05 to 0.74), although operative time and blood loss were increased for the Medoff [25]. Two RCTs of 226 participants have compared the Gotfried percutaneous compression plate with a sliding hip screw and found a reduced blood transfusion requirement for the percutaneous plate but a higher fixation failure rate with the percutaneous plate (11/108 [10.2%] versus 4/118 [3.4%], RR 3.03, 95% CI 1.00 to 9.17) [25]. Until further evidence is obtained the use of these modifications to the sliding hip screw cannot be advocated **(Ib/A)**.

Choice of implant - arthroplasty

An alternative treatment for an extracapsular femoral fracture is arthroplasty. Generally a cemented long-stem hemiarthroplasty has been described in a number of case series reports and one randomised trial of 90 patients with an unstable trochanteric fracture [27]. Although the reports to date seem to give comparable results to internal fixation, because of the limited reported results of this method of treatment, arthroplasty cannot be recommended as a method of treatment **(III/B)**.

Choice of implant - external fixation

An alternative method of fixation for an extracapsular proximal femoral fracture is using an external fixation device. A number of case series reports have described the use of the external fixator and one RCT of 100 participants have compared an external fixator with the sliding hip screw. The RCT demonstrated a reduced need for blood transfusion with the external fixator and a reduced length of hospital stay, but no difference in mortality and regain of walking ability [25]. Further reports are required before definite conclusion can be made on this method of treatment **(III/B)**.

Surgical techniques - extracapsular fracture fixation

Few randomised trials have examined different aspects of surgical technique for the internal fixation of extracapsular fractures [28]. Four trials involving 465 participants compared osteotomy with anatomical fracture reduction in conjunction with a sliding hip screw fixation. Osteotomy was associated with an increased operative blood loss, length of surgery and a tendency to an increased risk of fracture healing complications **(Ib/A)**. Other aspects of surgical technique related to fracture reduction and implant positioning have only been studied in case series reports. They generally favour an anatomical or valgus reduction with central positioning of the implant **(III/B)**.

Postoperative care and rehabilitation

Mobilisation and physiotherapy

After surgery various mobilisation strategies and different exercise regimes have been used to aid the patient's regain of mobility. One systematic review of six RCTs of these different regimes found no major differences between 'normal' and more intensive physiotherapy regimes and different exercise programmes [29] **(Ib/B)**.

Weight-bearing

The one identified systematic review on this topic found insufficient evidence to draw any conclusions on this topic [29]. The single randomised trial on weight-bearing after internal fixation of intracapsular fractures found no benefit from delayed weight-bearing [29] **(IIa/B)**.

Inpatient rehabilitation

One systematic review identified nine RCTs involving 1887 participants, which compared 'usual care', generally on the orthopaedic ward, to co-ordinated multidisciplinary rehabilitation [30]. No significant difference in mortality (eight RCTs, 163/909 [17.9%] for multidisciplinary care versus 188/951 [19.8%] for usual care, RR 0.91, 95% CI 0.75 to 1.10), need for institutional care, length of hospital stay or change in functional status was seen between groups. There was a tendency within some

of the studies identified to slightly better outcomes and reduced complications for those allocated to multidisciplinary care, but no firm conclusions could be made **(Ib/A)**.

Care home rehabilitation

No RCTs were identified by the systematic review for hip fractures to compare conventional inpatient rehabilitation and care home or skilled nursing home rehabilitation [31] **(IV/C)**.

Community rehabilitation

Three RCTs have compared early discharge schemes using supported community services with conventional inpatient rehabilitation [32-34]. These studies found early supported discharge reduced hospital inpatient stay, but increased the overall time in rehabilitation care. No significant difference in mortality, falls, readmissions or quality of life was noted. There was some support for those allocated to community rehabilitation to have improved mobility at one year, increased confidence in avoiding falls and a reduce dependency on community support **(Ib/B)**.

Conclusions

The common occurrence of fractures of the proximal femur has enabled a good evidence base for the treatment of this condition to be established. Case series reports are too numerous to mention. Of more importance in determining the best treatment method are randomised trials, for which there are in excess of 250 reported studies on various aspects of hip fracture care. Most of these studies have been summarised within Cochrane reviews. In addition, an excellent evidence-based guideline for the management of hip fractures has been produced [8]. Despite this, areas of uncertainty remain about many aspects of peri-operative care, optimum choice of implant and different aspects of surgical treatment and rehabilitation. Furthermore, new developments in surgical technique and implant require evaluation, preferably within the context of randomised trials.

Recommendations	Evidence level
◆ Pre-operative traction is not appropriate.	Ia/A
◆ Nerve blocks are effective in reducing pain.	Ib/A
◆ Thrombo-embolic prophylaxis is effective at reducing the risk of deep vein thrombosis but has no demonstrable effect on mortality and may increase the risk of bleeding complications.	Ia/A
◆ Nutritional supplements may reduce the occurrence of postoperative complications.	Ia/A
◆ Little difference in outcome exists between regional and general anaesthesia.	Ia/A
◆ Peri-operative antibiotic prophylaxis against infection is effective.	Ia/A
◆ Most hip fractures require operative treatment.	Ib/A
◆ Undisplaced intracapsular fractures and displaced intracapsular fractures in younger patients should be managed by internal fixation of the fracture.	IIa/B
◆ Displaced intracapsular fracture in the elderly can be managed by either internal fixation or arthroplasty.	Ia/A
◆ No notable difference in fracture healing complications has been demonstrated between different types of implant for the internal fixation of intracapsular fractures.	Ia/A
◆ No notable difference has yet been demonstrated between unipolar and bipolar hemiarthroplasties or THRs.	Ia/A, Ib/A
◆ Cementing a prosthesis in place results in less pain and better regain of mobility.	Ia/A
◆ An anterior surgical approach is preferred to a posterior approach for insertion of a hemiarthroplasty.	IIa/B
◆ The sliding hip screw is the implant of choice for trochanteric fractures.	Ia/A
◆ Replacement arthroplasty and external fixation for extracapsular fractures are of unproven effectiveness.	III/B
◆ Osteotomy of the femur for reducing a trochanteric hip fracture prior to fixation is not appropriate.	Ib/A
◆ Insufficient evidence exists between different aspects of different inpatient or community-based rehabilitation programmes to determine which is the best method.	Ib/A

Chapter 16

References

1. Gullberg B, Johnell O, Kanis JA. World-wide projections for hip fracture. *Osteoporosis Int* 1997; 7: 407-13.

2. Thorngren K-G. Femoral neck fractures. In: *Oxford Textbook of Orthopaedics and Trauma.* Bulstrode C, Buckwalter J, Carr A, *et al*, Eds. Oxford: Oxford University Press, 2002: 2216-27.

3. Parker MJ. Trochanteric and subtrochanteric fractures. In: *Oxford Textbook of Orthopaedics and Trauma.* Bulstrode C, Buckwalter J, Carr A, *et al*, Eds. Oxford: Oxford University Press, 2002: 2228-39.

4. Price JD, Sear JW, Venn RM. Perioperative fluid volume optimization following proximal femoral fracture. In: *The Cochrane Library*, Issue 1, 2004. Chichester, UK: John Wiley & Sons, Ltd.

5. Parker MJ, Handoll HHG. Pre-operative traction for fractures of the proximal femur. In: *The Cochrane Library*, Issue 3, 2004. Chichester, UK: John Wiley & Sons, Ltd.

6. Parker MJ, Griffiths R, Appadu BN. Nerve blocks (subcostal, lateral cutaneous, femoral, triple, psoas) for hip fractures. In: *The Cochrane Library*, Issue 3, 2004. Chichester, UK: John Wiley & Sons, Ltd.

Chapter 16

7. Handoll HHG, Farrar MJ, McBirnie J, *et al*. Heparin, low molecular weight heparin and physical methods for preventing deep vein thrombosis and pulmonary embolism following surgery for hip fractures. In: *The Cochrane Library*, Issue 3, 2004. Chichester, UK: John Wiley & Sons, Ltd.

8. Scottish Intercollegiate Guidelines Network (SIGN). Prevention and management of hip fracture in older people; a national clinical guideline. Royal College of Physicians, Edinburgh, 2002: 56. (www.sign.ac.uk).

9. Antiplatelet Trialists' Collaboration. Collaborative review of randomized trials of antiplatelet therapy. III: reduction in venous thrombosis and pulmonary embolism by antiplatelet prophylaxis among surgical and medical patients. *Br Med J* 1994; 308: 235-46.

10. Anonymous. Prevention of pulmonary embolism and deep vein thrombosis with low dose aspirin: Pulmonary Embolism Prevention (PEP) trial. *Lancet* 2000; 355: 1295-302.

11. Avenell A, Handoll HHG. Nutritional supplementation for hip fracture aftercare in the elderly. In: *The Cochrane Library*, Issue 3, 2004. Chichester, UK: John Wiley & Sons, Ltd.

12. Parker MJ, Handoll HHG, Griffiths R. Anaesthesia for hip fracture surgery in adults. In: *The Cochrane Library*, Issue 4, 2004. Chichester, UK: John Wiley & Sons, Ltd.

13. Southwell-Keely JP, Russo RR, March L, *et al*. Antibiotic prophylaxis in hip fracture surgery: a meta-analysis. *Clin Orthop* 2004; 419: 179-84.

14. Gillespie WJ, Walenkamp G. Antibiotic prophylaxis for surgery for proximal femoral and other closed long bone fractures. In: *The Cochrane Library*, Issue 3, 2004. Chichester, UK: John Wiley & Sons, Ltd.

15. Parker MJ, Handoll HHG. Conservative versus operative treatment for hip fractures. In: *The Cochrane Library*, Issue 3, 2004. Chichester, UK: John Wiley & Sons, Ltd.

16. Bhandari M, Devereaux PJ, Swiontkowski MF, *et al*. Internal fixation compared with arthroplasty for displaced fractures of the femoral neck. *J Bone Joint Surg Am* 2003; 85: 1673-81.

17. Masson M, Parker MJ, Fleischer S. Internal fixation versus arthroplasty for intracapsular proximal femoral fractures in adults. In: *The Cochrane Library*, Issue 3, 2004. Chichester, UK: John Wiley & Sons, Ltd.

18. Parker MJ, Stockton G, Gurusamy K. Internal fixation implants for intracapsular proximal femoral fractures in adults. In: *The Cochrane Library*, Issue 3, 2004. Chichester, UK: John Wiley & Sons, Ltd.

19. Parker MJ, Dynan Y. Surgical approaches and ancillary techniques for internal fixation of intracapsular proximal femoral fractures. In: *The Cochrane Library*, Issue 3, 2000. Oxford: Update Software.

20. Parker MJ, Gurusamy K. Arthroplasties (with and without bone cement) for proximal femoral fractures in adults. In: *The Cochrane Library*, Issue 3, 2004. Chichester, UK: John Wiley & Sons, Ltd.

21. Varley J, Parker MJ. Stability of hip hemiarthroplasties. *Int Orthop* 2004; 28: 274-7.

22. Sikorski JM, Barrington R. Internal fixation versus hemiarthroplasty for the displaced subcapital fracture of the femur: a prospective randomised study. *J Bone Joint Surg* 1981; 63-B: 357-61.

23. Parker MJ, Handoll HHG. Gamma and other cephalocondylic intramedullary nails versus extramedullary implants for extracapsular hip fractures. In: *The Cochrane Library*, Issue 3, 2004. Chichester, UK: John Wiley & Sons, Ltd.

24. Parker MJ, Handoll HHG, Bhonsle S, *et al*. Condylocephalic nails versus extramedullary implants for extracapsular hip fractures. In: *The Cochrane Library*, Issue 3, 2004. Chichester, UK: John Wiley & Sons, Ltd.

25. Parker MJ, Handoll HHG. Extramedullary fixation implants and external fixators for extracapsular hip fractures. In: *The Cochrane Library*, Issue 3, 2004. Chichester, UK: John Wiley & Sons, Ltd.

26. Chinoy MA, Parker MJ. Fixed nail plates versus sliding hip systems for the treatment of trochanteric femoral fractures: a meta-analysis of 14 comparative studies. *Injury* 1999; 30: 157-63. Erratum for table 6: *Injury* 1999; 30: 452.

27. Parker MJ, Handoll HHG. Replacement arthroplasty versus internal fixation for extracapsular hip fractures. In: *The Cochrane Library*, Issue 3, 2004. Chichester, UK: John Wiley & Sons, Ltd.

28. Parker MJ, Tripuraneni G, McGreggor-Riley J. Osteotomy, compression and reaming techniques during internal fixation of extracapsular hip fractures. In: *The Cochrane Library*, Issue 2, 1998. Oxford: Update Software.

29. Handoll HHG, Parker MJ, Sherrington C. Mobilisation strategies after hip fracture surgery in adults. In: *The Cochrane Library*, Issue 3, 2004. Chichester, UK: John Wiley & Sons, Ltd.

30. Cameron ID, Handoll HHG, Finnegan TP, *et al*. Co-ordinated multidisciplinary approaches for inpatient rehabilitation of older patients with proximal femoral fractures. In: *The Cochrane Library*, Issue 3, 2004. Chichester, UK: John Wiley & Sons, Ltd.

31. Ward D, Severs M, Dean T, *et al*. Care home versus hospital and own home environments for rehabilitation of older people. In: *The Cochrane Library*, Issue 3, 2004. Chichester, UK: John Wiley & Sons, Ltd.

32. Richards SH, Coast J, Gunnell DJ, *et al*. Randomised controlled trial comparing effectiveness and acceptability of an early discharge, hospital at home scheme with acute hospital care. *Br Med J* 1998; 16: 1796-1801.

33. Crotty M, Whitehead C, Miller M, *et al*. Patient and caregiver outcomes 12 months after home-based therapy for hip fracture: a randomized controlled trial. *Arch Phys Med Rehabil* 2003; 84: 1237-9.

34. Kuisma R. A randomized, controlled comparison of home versus institutional rehabilitation of patients with hip fracture. *Clin Rehabil* 2002; 16: 553-61.

Chapter 17

Resurfacing arthroplasty of the hip

Nikhil Shah FRCS (Tr & Orth)
Consultant Orthopaedic Surgeon [1]

Martyn Porter FRCS (Tr & Orth)
Consultant Orthopaedic Surgeon [2]

1 NORTH MANCHESTER GENERAL HOSPITAL, MANCHESTER, UK
2 CENTRE FOR HIP SURGERY, WRIGHTINGTON HOSPITAL, LANCASHIRE, UK

Introduction

Metal-on-metal (MoM) resurfacing hip arthroplasty (RHA) is currently enjoying popularity among surgeons and patients. However, opinions are still divided regarding its role in current practice. Wagner recommended it as an 'in-between' procedure in young individuals to gain time before conventional total hip arthroplasty (THA)(Table 1) [1-6].

History and evolution

Earlier resurfacing designs consisted of metal-on-polyethylene bearings [6-9, 10-11]. In spite of initial enthusiasm, high failure rates were reported [8, 12, 13]. These were initially attributed to femoral neck fractures, avascular necrosis (AVN), loosening and impingement, but later shown to be due to polyethylene wear, osteolysis and loosening from biologically active particulate debris [14]. Although femoral bone stock was preserved, excess removal of bone from the acetabulum and destruction by osteolysis made revision surgery difficult [15-16].

First-generation MoM prostheses, such as the McKee Farrar, Muller, Huggler, Sivash and Ring, had high failure rates due to poor manufacturing, equatorial contact, high frictional torque and loosening [17-19]. Metallosis occurred in association with high wear or impingement. This, combined with the early success of the Charnley hip, and concerns about metal sensitivity and carcinogenicity, led many surgeons to abandon resurfacing [20].

Retrieval studies of few long-surviving MoM prostheses revealed substantially less wear than metal-on-polyethylene (MoP) bearings, a survivorship comparable to the Charnley system, and few osteolytic problems [21-24, 25, 26]. Second-generation MoM bearings were subsequently developed with superior alloys, precise manufacturing and excellent wear characteristics [20, 27-30]. Thinner acetabular shells and larger diameter femoral components made resurfacing possible [31-36]. Several resurfacing systems using modern bearings [25, 26, 37-46], which attempted to remove design flaws of earlier implants, have shown encouraging short-term results. This chapter presents a brief overview of the available evidence for modern MoM hip resurfacing, and examines some of the issues of concern [47-55].

Table 1. Potential advantages and disadvantages of RHA [31-36, 92, 94, 103-105, 110, 111].

Advantages

- Restoration of normal anatomy and biomechanics
- Better proprioception and range of movement
- Low risk of dislocation
- Bone conserving
- Normal femoral loading and reduced stress shielding
- Reduced wear of MoM bearings, improved longevity
- Reduced thrombo-embolism
- Early return to physical activity
- Smaller field of contamination should infection occur

Disadvantages

- Technically demanding. Increased surgical time
- Potential for fracture of neck of femur
- Osteonecrosis of femoral remnant
- Long-term concerns of metal ions
- Increased bone loss on acetabular side

Methodology

A broad search of the literature was initially performed using Medline. Free search text terms such as 'hip resurfacing', 'surface replacement', 'metal on metal bearings', amongst others, were used to identify relevant papers. A systematic review of current literature was conducted using Medline, Embase and Proquest. A manual search of major orthopaedic journals was done to ensure inclusion of available studies. Identified publications were assessed for their methodology and quality and references reviewed. Guidelines issued by the National Institute for Clinical Excellence [56] were reviewed.

Summary of available evidence

Wear studies

Wear of MoM bearings is difficult to measure on radiographs. Hip simulator and retrieval studies [57-62] have shown lower linear and volumetric wear rates (1-5mm^3) than MoP implants (50-100mm^3), both *in vitro*

and *in vivo*. First-generation MoM inplants were shown to have wear rates of 1-6mm^3/year, while second-generation implants showed wear rates of 0.3mm^3/year [63]. There is an initial run-in period of higher volumetric wear, followed by a lower, steady-state wear, possibly due to a shift in the lubrication regime to mixed film. Increased wear can occur from impingement, steep cup inclination and rim loading, subluxation, cup deformation during implantation, or too large or excessively small diametral clearance **(III/B, IV/C)**. The most significant ion load to the body is associated with the run-in phase, and could be reduced by optimising the diametral clearance [63].

Metal scratches have a 'self-polishing' capacity [57-62, 64, 65] **(IIa/B, III/B)**. The running-in process has been correlated with improvement in lubrication. Testing in a friction simulator has shown that as the wear test continued, the Stribeck curve analysis indicated a shift towards a more favourable lubrication regime along with lower wear in the later stages of testing. Measurement of surface roughness has revealed a progessive smoothening of protruding carbide features and improvement in surface topography [66] **(IIb/B)**.

Revision of a failed femoral component in RHA or MoM THA with a new unworn pristine femoral head running against a well-run-in retained original cup does involve an additional running-in period, but the volumetric wear was found to be less than the initial running-in wear. A similar effect was seen with head rotation and scratches **(IIb/B)** [67].

Metal wear particles are smaller (typically 20-90nm) and more numerous than submicron polyethylene particles, and have larger effective surface area. The majority of particles in histological studies were oval or round in shape but few were needle or shard-like in morphology [68]. Metal wear particles isolated from periprosthetic tissues of MoM THA with short implantation times have been found to be round to oval chromium oxide particles, whereas those from long-term implants showed a greater proportion of cobalt-chromium-molybdenum (Co-Cr-Mo) particles, mainly needle-shaped **(III/B)** [69].

Osteolysis is relatively uncommon [28, 34]. Histological examination of periprosthetic tissue has revealed a much less intense inflammatory reaction [70-75] **(III/B)**. Inflammation around MoM prostheses is dominated by perivascular lymphocytic infiltrates, whereas around MoP prostheses, it is predominantly histiocytic [76]. Although evidence of necrosis and necrobiosis has been identified along with large numbers of metal particles in retrieved tissues, an absence of multinucleated giant cells may explain the lack of osteolysis [68]. Osteolysis in a well fixed implant with an MoM bearing with minimal wear has also been attributed to transmission of joint fluid pressure [77].

Metallurgy, engineering and tribology

Alloy composition, carbon content, head diameter, diametral clearance and lubricating regime are important and interrelated determinants of wear behaviour in MoM bearings [78-81]. Wrought forged cobalt chrome alloy and as-cast materials in current designs have both demonstrated good clinical performance **(III/B)**. High carbon alloys (0.20% to 0.25%) have a lower wear rate than low carbon alloys (<0.10%), whether wrought or cast [82-89] **(IIa/B, IIb/B)** and have shown superior resistance to wear

corrosion. Carbon helps to stabilise a face-centred cubic crystal structure [90, 91].

Heat treatment was blamed for the high early failure rate of a particular batch of prostheses in one study, due to depletion of surface carbides [92]. However, other successful designs are manufactured using hot isostatic pressing and solution annealing [93-95]. Changes in alloy microstructure due to double heat treatment (hot isostatic pressing and solution annealing) did not appear to influence wear behaviour of high carbon cast alloys with similar chemical compositions **(IIa/B)** [96]. Surface engineering of alloy using thick chromium nitride coatings, may have a beneficial effect on wear, but nitrogen ion implantation does not [97-99] **(IIa/B)**. *In vitro* tests using 'severe wear' conditions to simulate severe gait, have shown increased volumetric wear.

Current resurfacing implants are manufactured to strict tolerances of sphericity, smooth surface finish and diametral clearance to facilitate polar contact. Large diameter MoM articulations with smaller clearances may support the development of fluid films (lambda coefficient >3) and reduce wear, with the additional advantage of increased stability [84-86, 100, 101].

Diametral clearance should be as low as practicable to ensure polar contact, mixed film lubrication and reduced wear. However, a very small diametral clearance leads to equatorial contact and clamping of the articulation. Clearance in the range of 120-200μm shows a linear wear rate below 5μm per year **(IIb/B, III/B)**. There is potential for the production of full or partial lubricating films during part of the cycle of articulation [84-86].

MoM joints may exhibit 'stick phenomena' due to interruptions in motion or rest periods during physiological locomotion. *In vitro* testing has shown increased static friction of MoM joints with rest but wear was unaffected. This friction may be transferred to the bone-implant interface *in vivo* and may have implications in the design features of the cup-bone interface of large diameter MoM joints [102].

Table 2. Patient selection.

Indications for resurfacing hip arthroplasty

- Osteoarthritis
- Osteonecrosis
- Slipped upper femoral epiphysis
- Perthes' disease
- Post-traumatic arthritis
- Ankylosing spondylitis
- Rheumatoid arthritis and JRA
- Arthrokatadysis
- Others - melorheostosis, neurometabolic

Absolute contraindications

- Elderly people with osteoporotic bone
- Known metal hypersensitivity
- Compromised renal function

Relative contraindications

- Inflammatory arthropathy
- Large areas of avascular necrosis
- Severe acetabular dysplasia
- Grossly abnormal proximal femoral morphology

Design considerations

Current systems offer hybrid fixation with a cemented femoral component, or totally uncemented femoral and acetabular components. Titanium plasma vacuum sprays and sintered cobalt chrome beads are both available for reliable socket fixation **(III/B)**. On the femoral side, controlled cement extrusion is important to permit complete seating of the component without undue force [92, 94, 95, 103] **(IV/C)**.

The stem aids in alignment and may transmit force if cemented or press-fit. Force transmission by the stem may result in stress shielding and bone loss, but on the other hand also protects osteopenic bone **(IV/C)**. No data are available on whether cementing the stem improves survivorship. Alignment guides are available to aid placement of the femoral guide pin. Some systems offer larger dysplasia cups with peripheral screw fixation capability [92, 94, 95, 103-105].

Cementation

An experimental study of cementing technique showed that a more consistent controlled cement mantle could be achieved with a high-viscosity cementing technique for that particular system **(IIb/B)** [106]. Excessive cement penetration of low-viscosity cement in the proximal femoral head could lead to possible thermal damage during exothermic polymerisation. It was also thought to be responsible for incomplete seating of the femoral component. However, other successful systems have shown good results with a low-viscosity cementing technique **(III/B)**. In a cadaveric study investigating cementing technique using two low-viscosity bone cements, cement penetration was found to be increased using pulse lavage and by increasing the cement standing time from 1.5 to three minutes. There was no difference between the different cement brands of comparable viscosity **(IIa/B)** [107]. A retrieval study of early failures due to fractures after RHA revealed deviations from the suggested cement mantle thickness and cement penetration and high trauma during implantation and attributed most failures to the 'learning curve' effect [108].

Patient selection and surgical technique

RHA is indicated in young, active patients who are likely to outlive the lifespan of a conventional THA, usually males under 65 and females under 60 years. Older, active patients with good bone stock may be candidates [92, 94, 95, 103-105, 109-111] **(III/B, IV/C)**. Common indications and contraindications mentioned in the literature are listed in Table 2.

Surgical aspects and blood supply

Since the head and neck are preserved, adequate surgical exposure is necessary to aid visualisation and accurate component placement [112]. Various surgical approaches have been used for RHA, but the posterior approach is most common [113]. Damage to the ascending branch of the medial femoral circumflex artery during surgery may compromise femoral blood supply, but can be avoided by leaving the tendon of obturator externus intact [113-116].

Freeman argued that the majority of blood supply to the arthritic femoral head was from intraosseous blood vessels [117]. This may explain the low rate of avascular necrosis reported in most series. However, this may not be true, and laser Doppler flowmetry has shown that damage to the extraosseous blood supply to the femoral head, induced by simulated notching of the femoral neck, can cause a significant decrease in intraosseous blood flow **(IIb/B)**. The authors suggested that femoral head vascularity in the osteoarthritic state is similar to the non-arthritic state and recommended a modified lateral approach which leaves the main branch of the medial femoral circumflex artery intact [118].

Variable damage to the blood supply of the femoral head has been demonstrated by intra-operative measurement of oxygen concentration during RHA through the posterior approach. A large necrotic fragment may compromise femoral fixation or lead to neck fracture [109, 119, 120]. On the other hand a nuclear imaging study of asymptomatic patients after Birmingham hip resurfacing (BHR) using a posterior approach, complete posterior capsulotomy, incision of obturator externus, and anterosuperior translocation of the hip, has revealed no long-term evidence of AVN of the femoral head in any of the patients **(III/B)**. The authors believe this to be due to increase in vascularity that occurs in osteoarthritis of the hip from intraosseous blood vessels [121].

A soft tissue-sparing approach has been described, based on the concept of surgical dislocation of the hip [109, 120], but there can be problems with trochanteric fixation. The choice of surgical approach has not been shown to have a significant effect on the outcome from currently available evidence. Careful attention to the blood vessels, avoidance of notching, and the use of alternative surgical approaches may avoid problems related to damage to the blood supply.

Component positioning and sizing

The acetabulum is placed in 25-30° anteversion and 45° of abduction. Less anteversion may result in groin pain [105]. The femoral component should be optimally placed in slight valgus orientation (140°), to avoid superolateral notching. Varus placement was associated with adverse clinical and radiological outcome in one biomechanical study [94, 122]. Hips with a lower mean stem shaft angle of <130° had an increased relative risk of an adverse outcome by a factor of 6.1, compared to the rest of the cohort. Excess valgus can also cause notching during cylindrical reaming **(III/B)**.

An undersized femoral component may conserve acetabular bone but risk notching of the neck. An oversized femoral component can result in more extensive bone removal from the acetabulum. Restoring the offset and careful removal of the anterior neck osteophyte is important to avoid impingement with the rim of the acetabulum or the component itself [94, 104, 105, 111]. Suction venting of the lesser trochanter may aid femoral cementation, reduce local thrombogenesis, and systemic embolisation [92, 103] **(IV/C)**.

Postoperative management varies between partial to early full weight-bearing. Most recommend a graded return to impact-loading activity, with avoidance of high impact activities during the first postoperative year [92, 94, 95, 103-105, 111] **(IV/C)**.

Risk factors

Patient height, large femoral head cysts, female gender, previous surgery, and small component size in male patients are risk factors for femoral component loosening. Beaulé *et al* developed a Surface Arthroplasty Risk Index (SARI) based on a six-point scoring system. A SARI score of >3 represented a 12-fold increased risk of early failure or adverse radiological changes [123] **(IIa/B)**.

Schmalzried *et al* have used a radiographic arthritic hip grading scale to assess four characteristics of the proximal femur: bone density, shape, biomechanics, and focal bone defects. Hips with a lesser degree of secondary arthritic changes have a higher arthritic hip grade and better outcomes with total hip resurfacing **(IIa/B)** [124].

Anatomical, biomechanical and imaging studies

Freeman recommended valgus placement of the femoral component in RHA in line with the load-bearing medial trabecular system. Varus positioning can create tensile stresses on the lateral surface of the neck and shear stresses at the prothesis-neck junction, increasing the chances of a femoral neck fracture [117, 122].

Bone conservation

A mean of 34% less bone was resected at resurfacing than at conventional THA, mainly on the femoral side. Another study concluded that it is a bone-conserving procedure on both sides in females, but not in males, compared to THA [125, 126] **(III/B)**. On the other hand, a study using dry pelvic and femoral Sawbones found that although 51.4% less Sawbone was removed from the femur, more bone (311.1%) was removed during acetabular preparation for RHA than for a hybrid THA, which may prove problematic should patients require future acetabular revision surgery **(IIa/B)** [127]. A recent retrospective series showed that more bone is removed from the acetabulum in hip resurfacing than during hybrid THA, a difference which is most marked in larger patients [128]. More robust and conclusive studies are needed to provide better evidence **(III/B)**.

Radiological measurement showed that patients undergoing THA had a more accurate restoration of femoral offset and overall leg length compared to RHA, leading to the conclusion that resurfacing does not restore hip biomechanics as accurately as THA. Arthritic hips with more than 1cm shortening or comparatively lower femoral offset may be better served with conventional THA [129, 130] **(III/B)**. However, another recent prospective randomised study comparing the biomechanical reconstruction of the hip in conventional THA versus RHA has shown better and more precise restoration of hip offset, leg length inequality and proximal femoral anatomy with RHA **(I/A)** [131]. Obviously more studies are needed to better evaluate this aspect of RHA.

Dual energy X-ray absorptiometry (DEXA) studies have shown preservation of proximal femoral bone mineral density, due to physiologic load transfer at two years using the hybrid BHR prosthesis. A similar beneficial effect on bone stock was noted with hemiresurfacing arthroplasty for osteonecrosis. Stress shielding was thought to be an unlikely cause of femoral neck fractures [132-135] **(III/B)**.

Two-dimensional finite element analysis (FEA) models demonstrated unnatural stress shielding and stress concentration in the proximal femur around RHA. FEA of the cemented McMinn component using three-dimensional models has shown cortical stress concentration around the postero-inferior cup-rim region, stress shielding in the anterior superior neck region, and stress concentration around the peg **(IIb/B)**. This may increase the risk of femoral neck fracture or loosening [136-138]. Others have suggested that elevated strain in the superior femoral neck was unlikely to cause femoral neck fracture. Increasing the stem diameter and increasing the percentage stem length in contact with bone both increased the degree of strain shielding in the superior femoral head. Bonding the metaphyseal stem produced the most dramatic strain shielding, but varying the cement mantle thickness had a negligible effect on the load transfer. After remodelling, bone resorption of 60%-90% was observed in the bone underlying the implant, which might be a concern for long-term fixation **(IIb/B)**. Regions of strain concentration at the head-neck junction, which may increase the initial risk of femoral neck fracture, are reduced with bone remodelling. Hence, the authors recommend avoidance of activities during the early rehabilitation period after surgery [139-140].

Roentgen stereophotogrammetric analysis has shown that the cemented femoral component and the hydroxyapatite-coated acetabular component of the BHR system, are stable at two years after implantation, with no evidence of excess early migration or loosening, suggesting that it is likely to perform well in the long term [141, 142]. The Einzel-Bild Roentgen Analyse-Femoral Component Analysis (EBRA-FCA) method was shown to be a valid and reliable tool for measuring migration of the femoral component, and can help predict early failure [143, 144] **(III/B)**. Other clinical studies have noted migration of the femoral component at medium-term follow-up in 3.9%-8% of the patients [94, 145].

In vivo fluoroscopy has shown that femoral head sliding and separation commonly occurs in MoP joints during the swing phase of gait, but not with MoM joints in clinically successful cases. This was

Table 3. Results and survivorship.

Authors	No. of hips	Prosthesis	Follow-up (years)	Femur survivorship & 95% CI, endpoint Survivorship acetabulum & 95% CI)
Howie 2005	-	Cemented McMinn	8.5(8-10)	Trial discontinued
McMinn 2004	446	McMinn 43 BHR 403 Hybrid	3.3 (1.1-8.2)	99.8% over 8 years
Treacy 2005	144	BHR hybrid	Min 5 years	5 years - 98% overall 99% for aseptic revisions
Amstutz et al 2004	400	Conserve plus hybrid	3.5 (2.2-6.2)	94.4% at 4 years (91-98%)
Beaulé et al 2004	42 1 died	McMinn cemented	8.7 (7.2-10)	7 years - 93% (82-100%) (aseptic loosening) 7 years - 80 % (67-93%)
Shimmin 2005	230	BHR hybrid	3 (2-4.4)	99.14% at 3 years
De Smet 2005	252	BHR hybrid	2.8 (2-5)	Not mentioned
Villar 2005	70	Cormet 2000 uncemented	2.4 (2-3.1)	Overall 97.1% at mean survival time 37.0 months. Femoral 98.6% at mean survival time 37.3 months
Grigoris 2005	200	Durom	2.2 (1-3.5)	Not reported

attributed to the formation of a thin fluid film, which may effectively connect and constrain the femoral head to the acetabular liner, and result in more favourable wear kinematics [146] **(III/B)**.

The cup deflection due to interference press-fit of a metallic one-piece resurfacing acetabular cup was shown by experimental and finite element methods to be mainly dependent on the cup wall thickness and the diametral interference between cup and prepared acetabular cavity. Stiffening of the cup was shown to reduce the cup deformation **(IIb/B)**. The authors have emphasised the importance of ensuring that the cup deformation does not significantly affect the clearance and tribological performance of the resurfacing system [147, 148].

Results

There is a paucity of long-term results in the literature, including analysis of cost-effectiveness [149-151]. Several review articles are available. Short to medium-term results of modern MoM RHA have been reported from the originators, as well as independently. We could identify one randomised controlled trial comparing RHA to cemented THR, which had to be discontinued [110]. In general, there has been good predictable pain relief, improved range of motion and return to activity, with high levels of patient satisfaction from MoM RHA, with satisfactory early outcomes (Table 3).

Howie reported a randomised clinical trial in patients 55 years of age or younger, comparing MoM cemented RHA with Exeter cemented THA. The trial was stopped after two years of recruitment, because of a high incidence of failure (eight of 11 hips revised at eight to ten years, one radiographically unstable) of the cemented resurfacing acetabular component, femoral neck fracture and early femoral component loosening **(Ib/A)**. They emphasised the need for longer-term results from clinical trials to establish the success of RHA [110].

A prospective randomised study found no significant difference in early clinical scores, but a significantly higher activity level in the RHA group, one-year postoperatively, compared to uncemented MoM THA, demonstrating better functional recovery in the short term **(Ib/A)** [152]. The one definite advantage identified was preservation of femoral bone stock.

McMinn reported a survivorship of 99.8% at a follow-up of one to eight years for 446 RHA (43 McMinn, 403 BHR) in patients with osteoarthritis (<55 years) at a mean follow-up of 3.3 years (1.1-8.2 years). One patient was revised for avascular necrosis at eight months, and the majority returned to a high level of activity **(III/B)**. The survivorship of RHA was superior to that for THA in a similar cohort from the Swedish Hip Register [92].

Treacy *et al* reported the survivorship of 144 consecutive BHR cases, with a five-year overall survival of 98% and 99% for aseptic revisions only. There were three failures of femoral components: two deep infections and one femoral neck fracture which had avascular necrosis confirmed on histology. There was no osteolysis or pedestal at the tip of the stem. Twenty-eight percent showed heterotopic bone formation [103] **(III/B)**.

Shimmin reported a 99.14% survivorship at a mean follow-up of three years with the first 230 BHR cases in an independent prospective study. There was one revision of a loose acetabulum, and one femoral neck fracture. Ninety-seven percent of patients considered the outcome to be good or excellent. No osteolysis or radiolucent lines were noticed around the acetabulum or the femoral component. Four patients had pain within one year of surgery, due to a possible stress fracture, which healed with protected weight-bearing [104] **(III/B)**.

Amstutz reported a survival of 94.4% at four years in 400 hybrid MoM RHA with an average follow-up 3.5 years (survivorship was 89% at four years in patients with SARI >3, versus 97% with SARI <3). Risk factors for femoral loosening and substantial radiolucencies were large femoral head cysts, patient height, female gender, and small component size in male patients. The stem shaft angle in hips revised for femoral loosening was significantly lower than the rest. Acetabular radiolucencies were noted in 32% of hips and around 16 uncemented metaphyseal femoral stems. Heterotopic ossification was noted in 106/400 hips (26.5%) [94] **(III/B)**.

Beaulé reported on 42 all-cemented McMinn prostheses with overall seven-year survivorship of 93% and 80% for the femoral and acetabular components, respectively, with aseptic failures as the endpoint. Using failure of any component and conversion to THA as the endpoint, the seven-year survivorship figures were 79% (95% CI 65%-92%) and 87% (95% CI 76%-98%). Nine of 14 revisions were for loosening of a cemented acetabulum, which had significantly worse results than cementless fixation at seven years (66% versus 95%). The authors recommended that cement fixation be discontinued on the acetabular side [111]. Watanabe mentioned three failures among 11 cases of cemented McMinn RHA at short-term follow-up, two due to femoral neck fractures and one acetabular loosening [138] **(III/B)**.

De Smet reported an independent series of 252 patients with a follow-up of two to five years using the BHR. Of these patients, 97.8% had no pain at the latest follow-up and 61% performed strenuous activities. Abnormal radiological findings were noted only in the revisions. Failures included one each of deep infection, avascular necrosis, and femoral neck fracture [105] **(III/B)**.

Villar reported results of 70 uncemented RHA with a mean follow-up of 28.5 months. The survivorship of the uncemented femoral component was 98.6% and the mean survival time was 37.3 months. There was no migration, radiolucency or neck fracture around the hydroxyapatite coated femoral implant [95]. The same group also reported no difference in operating time, blood loss or modified Harris hip score at 12 months postoperatively in a comparative study of hybrid RHA versus THA. They found no significant difference in postoperative pain, mean rehabilitation score, length of hospitalisation or in the speed of rehabilitation at any stage after surgery between RHA and THA [153]. The authors found no evidence to back the claimed additional benefits of RHA [154] **(III/B)**.

Grigoris reported on 200 Durom resurfacing hips with mean follow-up of 26 months (12-41) with excellent short-term results. There were no failures, impending failures, dislocations, deep infection, migration or osteolysis [35] **(III/B)**.

Beaulé reported the results of 94 hybrid MoM RHA in patients 40 years old, or younger, at a mean follow-up of 4.2 years. Thirteen hips had an adverse outcome, and this group had a significantly lower mean stem shaft angle (133°) in the coronal plane, compared to the rest of the cohort [123] **(III/B)**.

Amstutz reported 92% survivorship at 4.7 years for 25 resurfacings for hip arthritis due to childhood Perthes' disease (14 hips), and a slipped capital femoral epiphysis (11 hips), with a mean age 38.1 years. There was one case of bilateral femoral loosening. Despite the increased technical difficulty (aberrant geometry, short neck length), patients were pleased with normalisation of their hips **(III/B)**. Extra care is needed to avoid notching of the neck [155].

Siebel et al have reported their experience with 300 resurfacing hip endoprostheses at a mean follow-up of 202 days. The authors have identified this as a 'fourth generation' implant based on design modifications such as a 3° internal taper and a thinner stem on the femoral component, 2mm increments in implant sizes, 110μm diametral clearance between the head and cup, and a finger-packing cement technique. There were eight revisions (2.7%), of which five were neck fractures (1.66%) and three were cup revisions (1%). They observed a significantly higher failure rate for patients with previous proximal femoral osteosynthesis, and a significantly greater body mass index. The importance of learning curve has been emphasised **(III/B)** [156].

Pollard et al reported significantly better Oxford hip scores in male patients younger than 50 years who underwent RHA for osteoarthritis in comparison to a matched group treated with hybrid THA. Thirty-seven percent undertook sports or heavy manual activity [157]. The same group reported higher activity and quality of life scores with RHA in the medium term compared to hybrid THA. The RHA group had a 6% revision rate, 8% showed femoral component migration, and 66% had radiological changes of unknown significance **(III/B)** [145].

A small case series recommended RHA in comparison to current alternatives in patients with abnormal geometry, due to previous proximal femoral osteotomy on the basis of satisfactory short-term results [158] **(III/B)**.

The short to mid-term results of BHR in patients with primary or secondary osteoarthritis due to higher-grade dysplasia have not shown clinically relevant functional differences in the two groups [159] **(III/B)**.

Resurfacing for osteonecrosis

Overall failure rates of 32%-64% have been reported for femoral head hemiresurfacing (FHR) for osteonecrosis at short to medium-term follow-up. Others have reported 62% good to excellent results at 10.5 years and 45% survivorship at 15 years. Longer pre-operative symptoms correlated with early failure. Failures were due to femoral neck fractures, severe groin pain or conversion to THA. It offered less reliable pain relief or longevity in comparison to THA, and was not recommended as a treatment option for post-collapse AVN due to its unpredictability [160-166].

Pain relief, function, and activity after MoM total resurfacing are better than hemiresurfacing, and similar to the results of THA, especially with acetabular cartilage degeneration. Femoral-side failure is higher than for hemiresurfacing, due to the smaller size of the femoral component and smaller fixation area [167, 168] **(III/B)**.

Little et al reported a presence of osteonecrosis in bone from the femoral head remnant in the majority of revisions for failed femoral components in a series of 377 patients with RHA. None had histological evidence of osteonecrosis at initial implantation. They concluded that osteonecrosis was a common finding

Table 4. Failures and complications.

Author	Number of hips	Femoral neck fracture	Instability/ dislocation	AVN femoral remnant	Acetabular loosening	Femoral loosening	Deep infection
Howie 2005	8/11	2	-	-	5	1	-
McMinn 2004	1/446	-	0	1	-	-	-
Treacy 2005	3/144	1	0	0	0	0	2
Amstutz 2004	13/400	3 (0.75%)	3 (0.75%) (1 recurrent)	0	1 acute protrusio and infection	7 (+1 lost to follow-up)	1
Beaulé 2004	-	1	0	0	10	2	1
Shimmin 2005	-	1	0	0	1	0	
De Smet 2005	-	1	1	1	0	Same case as AVN	1
Villar 2005	-	-	1 intra-operative	-	-	-	-
Grigoris 2005	-	-	0	-	-	-	0

in failed resurfaced hips and was likely to play a role in the causation of femoral neck fractures [169] **(III/B)**.

Complications

Some unique complications have been reported for RHA (Table 4). A series of 3497 hip resurfacing operations reported from Australia performed by 89 surgeons, has identified 50 revisions for femoral fractures, 12 for cup malposition, four for aseptic loosening, two for infection, and one for presumed metal hypersensitivity [170].

Bohm *et al* have reported that 17 out of 54 Wagner MoM resurfacing prostheses have required revision at an average follow-up of nine years [171]. A retrospective review of 65 RHA procedures found a 22% revision rate at a mean follow-up of 51 months. The commonest mechanism of failure was a fractured neck of the femur (six cases). Four of these occurred in females over the age of 60 and none was associated with trauma. There were four cases of loose acetabular components and one case of progressive avascular necrosis. Two patients required revision surgery for ongoing hip pain and one required a two-stage revision for early deep infection [172].

Femoral neck fracture

This is the most common complication in the Australian National Joint Registry and may occur during or after surgery [170, 173, 174]. The overall incidence ranges from 0%-1.5%. Plain radiography and radioisotope bone scans may be useful in the diagnosis of subtle presentations. Women are twice as likely to fracture as men. Notching of the superior neck, varus component placement and failure to cover all reamed femoral bone with the component are

Table 5. Preventing femoral neck fractures.

- Accurate sizing of the femoral component
- Accurate positioning of the femoral component in neutral or slight valgus
- Cylindrical reaming at an angle of 140°
- Stop reaming before the reamer touches the lateral cortex
- Judicious removal of the impinging anterior osteophyte from the neck
- Allowing controlled cement extrusion from underneath the femoral component
- Avoiding excess force during impaction
- Ensuring complete coverage of all reamed femoral bone by the prosthesis

important risk factors **(III/B)**. Technical difficulties during surgery arising from poor exposure due to obesity, change in the intra-operative alignment and poor impaction of the femoral component were noted in cases that fractured [170, 173, 175] **(III/B)**.

Important steps in preventing femoral neck fractures are mentioned in Table 5.

Large cysts medially and inferiorly in the neck may be a contraindication for RHA [175]. Preservation of femoral head vascularity may be important to avoid osteonecrosis, which may play a role in causation. If notching is noted and resurfacing carried out, protected weight-bearing after surgery is recommended.

Non-operative management has been successful in treating incomplete and even complete fractures. Surgical treatment consists of revising the femoral component to a stemmed prosthesis with a compatible large diameter metal head, which matches the retained socket, based on the manufacturer's recommendation [170, 174, 176, 177].

Osteonecrosis

Osteonecrosis of the femoral head remnant remains a controversial issue. Many retrieval studies have shown good blood supply within the head remnant. Although not inevitable, it was often a feature underneath failed femoral components [178-181]. A recent study found a high incidence of osteonecrosis of bone beneath femoral components after failed RHA. It was

noted even under well-fixed femoral components in cases of neck fracture and was implicated as a causative factor [169]. In general, the reported incidence of osteonecrosis of the femoral head remnant in currently available studies has been low **(III/B)**. Use of a soft tissue-sparing surgical approach, controlled cement extrusion, and suction venting during femoral cementation may be protective **(IV/C)**.

Dislocation

MoM bearings have demonstrated a significantly lower dislocation rate (0.9%) compared to ceramic on polyethylene bearings (6.2%). Dislocation rates for MoM RHA have been significantly lower (about 0.75% at a mean of three years) than the published rates for conventional THA **(III/B)**. This is probably due to higher interfacial retaining forces and suction fit created by the lubricating fluid film, larger diameter heads, and better restoration of biomechanics and proprioception. MoM bearings generate significant resistance to separation at all velocities [92, 94, 95, 103, 105, 182, 183] **(IIb/B)**.

Aseptic loosening

Femoral component failure and loosening may result from avascular necrosis or fracture of the neck. A higher loosening rate has been reported for cemented McMinn acetabular components. Hydroxyapatite-coated acetabular components have given excellent results in terms of fixation. Amstutz reported a 32% incidence of radiolucency around the acetabular component, the long-term significance of which remains uncertain **(III/B)**. The overall incidence has been low [92, 94, 95, 103-105, 111, 154].

Clicking and squeaking

Many patients describe clicking (22.9%) and squeaking (3.9%) after metal-on-metal RHA without pain or functional deficit **(III/B)**. Clicking could be due to psoas tendon impingement on an oversized acetabular component, or decoaptation of the components, and usually settles down after soft tissue healing. Isolated episodes of squeaking within the first six months after surgery at the limit of flexion may be due to disruption of the fluid film between the bearing surfaces, and temporary dry running **(IV/C)**. The episode lasts for about 20-30 minutes without any obvious adverse effects [105].

Heterotopic ossification (HO)

The prevalence of heterotopic ossification after RHA is 1.6%-59.5%. Women undergoing MoM RHA had a lower incidence than men, and also when compared to women undergoing MoM THA. There was no difference in the incidence of HO in men undergoing either MoM RHA or MoM THA. In another study, 59.5% patients developed HO with the majority having lower grades of severity. There was no effect on the ultimate outcome **(III/B)**. It is important to inform patients of the risk of heterotopic ossification as a common complication after RHA [92, 94, 95, 103-105, 111, 184].

Neck thinning

This phenomenon has been reported with cemented and uncemented femoral components with an incidence as high as 27% in one series. It usually occurs in the inferomedial cortex and less commonly superolaterally. Increased height and reduced weight seem to be protective **(III/B)**. Although it was not associated with poor outcome in association with uncemented components, it may put the femoral neck at risk of fracture, especially if located superolaterally. Possible causative factors seem to be avascular necrosis or stress shielding [32, 95] **(IV/C)**.

Other rare complications such as stem fracture [185] and ischaemic optic neuropathy have been reported [186].

Biological concerns

MoM bearings produce significantly higher systemic release of cobalt and chromium ions (ng/ml) when compared with levels found in metal-on-polyethylene, ceramic-on-polyethylene, presurgery and reference groups [187-192] **(Ib/A, III/B)**. There is concern about long-term biological effects arising thereof, such as cellular toxicity, metal sensitivity and carcinogenicity. This becomes especially important in younger age groups who are expected to outlive the long latency of these effects in humans [193-196].

The levels exceed those defined by various occupational health authorities [197, 198]. Persistent elevation of levels for four to five years after implantation has been reported [188-190, 199]. The serum concentrations have not always reflected the so called run-in period of wear, possibly due to corrosion of already released particles. A recent prospective study demonstrated an initial peak at six to nine months, followed by declining levels at 24 months, with no adverse effect on the renal function and no radiographic loosening [200] **(III/B)**. Others have also reported a decline in levels to a steady state concentration, prompting calls for the possible use of metal ion analysis as a surrogate marker [201] of *in vivo* wear performance of MoM joints **(IV/C)**.

Higher levels are reported in large diameter surface replacements compared to smaller diameter implants, and in bilateral cases compared to unilateral [202, 203] **(III/B)**. A more recent study has found no significant difference between the metal ion levels following either a large diameter (50-54mm BHR) or a smaller 28mm diameter Metasul THA [204].

No significant relationship has been established between ion level increase and any demographic or surgical data, including activity level [48-50], except anteversion of the cup of more than 25°. Individual patients with higher cup inclination demonstrated significantly elevated levels compared to the median for the groups [205] **(III/B)**. Accurate cup placement is particularly recommended for MoM articulations.

No change has been found in serum ion levels in patients with well-functioning MoM implants regardless of activity, while others have reported increased levels in a patient training to run a marathon, which returned to typical levels after rest [205]. Fast jogging has been shown to generate increased volumetric wear, mean wear particle size and number of large needle-shaped particles compared to walking in hip joint simulation tests **(IIb/B)** [206, 207].

Metal particles can be ingested by macrophages and widely disseminated via the lymphatics throughout the body, including lymph nodes and distant organs, such as the liver, spleen and marrow [208, 209] **(III/B)**. Electrochemical corrosion of metal particles in body solutions can form charged metal ions. These can be concentrated inside erythrocytes, and excreted via the kidneys [63].

Evidence of cytotoxicity has been seen in patients in association with failed MoM implants, including a reduction in myeloid cells, lymphocytes and natural killer cells. Metal ions may have toxic effects upon lymphatic tissues in proximity to the implants [68]. An elevation of metal ions in asymptomatic patients with radiologically well-fixed MoM RHA was associated with reduced CD8(+) T-cell counts, but the long-term significance of this observation is not understood [210] **(III/B)**. They can induce cell death in cultures by mechanisms such as apoptosis and necrosis at higher concentrations [211] **(IIb/B)**. A statistically significant increase in cobalt and chromium concentrations and of both chromosomal translocations and aneuploidy in peripheral blood lymphocytes has been reported at 6, 12 and 24 months after surgery. These changes were progessive with time and indicate exposure to mutagens and genomic instability [195, 196, 212-214, **(III/B)**.

A small case series found no evidence yet to demonstrate passage of cobalt and chromium ions from MoM articulations in mothers across the placenta at the time of delivery [215] **(III/B)**. However, caution still needs to be exercised until longer postoperative studies with larger numbers of patients and robust evidence becomes available in this regard.

Metal sensitivity

In vivo metal ions can activate the immune system by forming protein complexes [216]. Elevated serum metal concentrations showed positive linear correlation with elevated lymphocyte reactivity in patients with MoM bearings compared to controls with MoP implants [217]. Metal sensitivity, although uncommon, has nevertheless been reported in well-functioning and failed or poorly-functioning joint replacements [218-220], and also in patients with loose surface replacement prostheses [221] **(III/B)**. However, a cause and effect relationship has not been established between metal sensitivity and loosening. Since metal particles can be generated from malfunctioning or loose implants, it is not certain whether metal hypersensitivity causes implant failure or vice versa [63]. It could be one of the causes of unexplained pain leading to revision, but this is not proven [76, 222-224].

An immunological basis has been proposed to explain early osteolysis in patients with failed MoM THA and RHA [77, 225]. Presence of ulcerated tissue surfaces and perivascular lymphocytic infiltrates around MoM articulations at the time of revision surgery could possibly be due to delayed type hypersensitivity reactions to metal. Recurrence of symptoms after revision performed for persistent pain, often with joint effusion, to a MoM bearing and healing of osteolytic lesions after changing the articulation, may hint towards an immunological basis to the radiological changes **(III/B)**. Metal-induced lymphocytes may participate in aseptic loosening, by releasing cytokines, which can promote osteoclast activity, and may represent a mechanism of biological failure [76, 223, 224, 226].

Risk of cancer

The overall risk of cancer following joint replacement is low **(III/B)**. Evidence of a carcinogenic effect of cobalt chromium metals from animal studies has been inconclusive [227, 228]. Direct extrapolation may be inaccurate due to differences in interspecies' susceptibility to carcinogens and routes of exposure. Epidemiological studies too, have provided conflicting information, which could be due to reasons such as short follow-up, long latency of cancer in humans, statistical heterogeneity, or biologic reasons [229-232].

Although a trend towards an increase in haematopoietic cancers has been observed in some cohort studies, other contributory factors were thought to be more important in the causation of cancer. The annual incidence of cancer in patients after McKee-Farrar prostheses did not deviate from the general population for a follow-up time of 28 years (III/B) [233, 234].

One study found the standardised incidence ratio for all cancers in the MoP group (0.76) to be lower than that in the MoM group (0.95), but the overall cancer incidence in both groups was lower than the general population [235, 236] (III/B).

All clinical studies have been significantly underpowered to demonstrate small differences between groups that could be clinically relevant in practice and cannot provide data on these rare outcome measures [193, 197, 198]. To date there is no conclusive evidence supporting a causal link between prolonged exposure to elevated levels of metal ions and an increased risk of cancer [235], although neither is there any evidence to the contrary. Rigorous long-term international prospective cohort studies are needed to determine if the benefits of MoM bearings outweigh the associated risks. Nevertheless, it is important that patients understand the potential long-term theoretical risks involved before consenting to the procedure. It is clear that further research is required to fully understand the effects of metal particles *in vivo*.

Future developments

There are early reports about the relative effectiveness of minimally invasive approaches for hip resurfacing. In a retrospective cohort study, RHA performed using a single mini-incision posterior approach and modified instrumentation by an experienced surgeon, there was no difference in operating time, a slightly reduced hospital stay and satisfactory component positioning compared to the

group with a more traditional posterior approach. Patients seemed to subjectively prefer the mini-incision approach for reasons such as reduced pain, faster recovery rate, and better cosmesis. The author noted that mini-incision RHA is technically more difficult and has a significant learning curve (III/B).

Another study using the anterolateral minimally invasive approach, but with standard instruments, found a reduction in blood loss, a longer operating time, and a shorter mean hospital stay in the small incision group, compared with the standard length anterolateral approach, but the differences were not significant. Component placement, and clinical and radiographic outcomes were similar in both groups at short-term follow-up (III/B). The authors recommend a gradual reduction in the size of the incision as the surgeon gains experience in the use of this technique [237, 238].

In order to reduce variability in implant placement and surgical time in a technically demanding procedure such as RHA, a computer-assisted surgical (CAS) technique used in a cadaver study of five paired femurs in the hands of a novice surgeon was shown to markedly reduce the varus / valgus variability of the implant relative to the pre-operative plan. On the other hand a mechanical jig resulted in significantly retroverted implant placement. There was no significant difference in operative time between the two techniques [239] (III/B).

Intra-operative fluoroscopic navigation systems have allowed accurate positioning of the femoral component without notching at the cost of a slightly increased operating time. Whether this translates into improved long-term outcomes remains to be seen [240, 241].

Conclusions

Recent reports on metal-on-metal hip resurfacing have demonstrated good early to medium-term results, but long-term results are awaited. The dramatic failures due to osteolysis seen with earlier metal-on-polyethylene resurfacing operations have not been observed, but some early reports of osteolysis of uncertain origin suggest caution. The appearance of femoral radiolucent lines and neck narrowing is of concern. The ease and outcome of revisions for failed resurfacing, especially on the acetabular side, remains unknown. The theoretical advantages in terms of activity and function remain to be conclusively proven in the long term. The rapid spread of this technique has not yet been fully justified by the availability of robust evidence and long-term results. The exact place of RHA in modern reconstructive hip surgery remains to be determined.

In line with NICE (UK) guidelines, the procedure should be performed only by surgeons with specific training, in the context of ongoing data collection on its clinical and cost-effectiveness, and as part of a national joint registry. Patients should understand all risks and benefits associated with it. Uncertainty of long-term outcomes should be weighed against the potential benefits claimed for MoM devices.

Further long-term independent studies, especially prospective, randomised trials with follow-up in excess of 15 years are needed to evaluate long-term performance, and biological effects of elevated metal ions in hip resurfacing, before this can be considered as a universally applicable viable alternative to THA.

Recommendations	Evidence level
♦ Modern MoM bearings have lower wear rates than metal-on-polyethylene.	IIa/B, III/B
♦ High carbon wrought or cast alloys have low wear rates.	IIa/B, III/B
♦ Larger diameter metal heads may promote existence of fluid films.	IIa/B, III/B
♦ Diametral clearance should be low enough to achieve polar bearing and large enough to prevent clamping.	IIa/B, III/B
♦ Heat treatment has not been shown to adversely affect wear behaviour.	IIa/B, III/B
♦ The effect of surgical approach on outcome is uncertain, but preservation of blood supply should be attempted.	III/B, IV/C
♦ Neutral or slightly valgus femoral component alignment is optimal.	III/B, IV/C
♦ Cementless socket fixation has superior results.	III/B
♦ Cemented and cementless femoral fixation are both successful.	III/B
♦ The notching of the superior neck is to be avoided to prevent neck fractures.	III/B
♦ Large femoral cysts and varus femoral alignment are related to early failure.	III/B
♦ The restoration of femoral offset and leg length are better with RHA, but there is disagreement between the studies.	Ib/A, III/B
♦ Proximal femoral bone stock is preserved with resurfacing.	III/B
♦ Acetabular bone stock is probably not preserved.	IIb/B, III/B
♦ RSA studies confirm early stability of resurfacing components.	III/B
♦ *In vivo* separation of MoM bearings is less than MoP.	III/B
♦ There are satisfactory short to medium-term clinical results.	III/B
♦ Femoral osteonecrosis and neck fractures are issues of concern.	III/B
♦ Dislocation rates are lower than for conventional THA.	III/B
♦ There is no published evidence linking elevated ion levels to cancer.	III/B
♦ There is evidence of metal sensitivity in association with MoM RHA, but there is no proof yet of a causal link to loosening.	III/B

References

1. White SP, Beard DJ, Smith EJ. Resurfacing hip replacement - an audit of activity in the United Kingdom 2002-2003. *Hip* 2004; 14: 163-8.

2. Curtin P, Harty J, Sheehan E, *et al*. Primary total hip replacement - a survey of current practice and identifying changing trends. *Ir Med J* 2005; 98(6): 166-8.

3. Villar R. Resurfacing arthroplasty of the hip. *J Bone Joint Surg Br* 2004; 86(2): 157-8.

4. Schmalzried TP. Metal-on-metal resurfacing arthroplasty no way under the sun! - in opposition. *J Arthroplasty* 2005; 20(4 suppl 2): 70-1.

5. Hungerford DS. Metal-on-metal resurfacing arthroplasty no way under the sun! - in the affirmative. *J Arthroplasty* 2005; 20(4 suppl 2): 70-1.

6. Wagner H. Surface replacement arthroplasty of the hip. *Clin Orthop* 1978; 134: 102-30.

7. Fukuya K, Tsuchiya M, Kawachi S. Socket cup arthroplasty. *Clin Orthop* 1978; 134: 41-4.

8. Bierbaum BE, Sweet R. Complications of resurfacing arthroplasty. *Orthop Clin N Am* 1982; 13(4): 761-75.

9. Freeman MA, Bradley GW. ICLH surface replacement of the hip. An analysis of the first 10 years. *J Bone Joint Surg Br* 1983; 65(4): 405-11.

10. Mallory TH, Ballas S, VanAtta G. Total articular replacement arthroplasty. A clinical review. *Clin Orthop Relat Res* 1984; 185: 131-6.

11. Amstutz HC, Dorey F, O'Carroll PF. THARIES resurfacing arthroplasty. Evolution and long-term results. *Clin Orthop Relat Res* 1986; 213: 92-114.

12. Head WC. Total articular resurfacing arthroplasty. Analysis of component failure in sixty-seven hips. *J Bone Joint Surg Am* 1984; 66(1): 28-34.

13. Bell RS, Schatzker J, Fornasier VL, *et al*. A study of implant failure in the Wagner resurfacing arthroplasty. *J Bone Joint Surg Am* 1985; 67(8): 1165-75.

14. Howie DW, Cornish BL, Vernon-Roberts B. Resurfacing hip arthroplasty. Classification of loosening and the role of prosthesis wear particles. *Clin Orthop* 1990; 255: 144-59.

15. Capello WN, Trancik TM, Misamore G, *et al*. Analysis of revision surgery of resurfacing hip arthroplasty. *Clin Orthop* 1982; 170: 50-5.

16. Bradley GW, Freeman MA. Revision of failed hip resurfacing. *Clin Orthop* 1983; 178: 236-40.

17. Ring PA. Complete replacement arthroplasty of the hip by the Ring prosthesis. *J Bone Joint Surg Br* 1968; 50-B: 720-31.

18. Muller ME. Total hip prostheses. *Clin Orthop* 1970; 72: 46-68.

19. Dobbs HS. Survivorship of total hip replacements. *J Bone Joint Surg Br* 1980; 62(B): 168-73.

20. Amstutz HC, Grigoris P. Metal on metal bearings in hip arthroplasty. *Clin Orthop* 1996; 329(suppl): S11-S14.

21. August AC, Aldam CH, Pynsent PB. The McKee-Farrar hip arthroplasty: a long-term study. *J Bone Joint Surg Br* 1986; 68: 520-7.

22. Schmalzried TP, Peters PC, Maurer BT, *et al*. Long duration metal on metal total hip arthroplasties with low wear of the articulating surfaces. *J Arthroplasty* 1996; 11: 322-31.

23. Weightman BO, Paul IL, Rose RM, *et al*. A comparative study of total hip replacement prostheses. *J Biomech* 1973; 6: 299-311.

24. Jacobsson SA, Djerf K, Wahlstrom O. Twenty-year results of McKee-Farrar versus Charnley prosthesis. *Clin Orthop* 1996; 329(suppl): s60-s68.

25. Long WT, Dorr LW, Gendelman V. An American experience with metal-on-metal total hip arthroplasties: a 7-year follow-up study. *J Arthroplasty* 2004; 19(8 Suppl 3): 29-34.

26. Dorr LD, Wan Z, Sirianni LE, *et al*. Fixation and osteolysis with Metasul metal-on-metal articulation. *J Arthroplasty* 2004; 19(8): 951-5.

27. Weber BG. Experience with the Metasul total hip-bearing system. *Clin Orthop* 1996; 329(suppl): s69-s77.

28. Muller ME. The benefits of metal on metal total hip replacements. *Clin Orthop* 1995; 311: 54-9.

29. Black J. Metal on metal bearings. A practical alternative to metal on polyethylene total joints? *Clin Orthop* 1996; 329(suppl): S244-S255.

30. Schmidt M, Weber H, Schon R. Cobalt chromium molybdenum metal combinations for modular hip prostheses. *Clin Orthop* 1996; 329(suppl); s35-s47.

31. Schmalzried TP, Fowble VA, Ure KJ, *et al*. Metal on metal surface replacement of the hip: technique, fixation and early results. *Clin Orthop* 1996; 329(suppl): S106-S114.

32. McMinn D, Treacy R, Lin K, *et al*. Metal on metal surface replacement of the hip: experience with the McMinn prosthesis. *Clin Orthop* 1996; 329(suppl): S89-S98.

33. McMinn DW. Development of metal/metal hip resurfacing. *Hip* 2003; 13(suppl 2): S41-53.

34. Wagner M, Wagner H Preliminary results of uncemented metal on metal stemmed and resurfacing hip replacement arthroplasty. *Clin Orthop Relat Res* 1996; (329 Suppl): S78-88.

35. Grigoris P, Roberts P, Panousis K, Bosch H. The evolution of hip resurfacing arthroplasty. *Orthop Clin North Am* 2005; 36(2): 125-34.

36. De Smet KA, Pattyn C, Verdonk R. Early results of primary Birmingham hip resurfacing using a hybrid metal on metal couple. *Hip* 2002; 12: 158-62.

37. Naudie D, Roeder CP, Parvizi J, *et al*. Metal-on-metal versus metal-on-polyethylene bearings in total hip arthroplasty: a matched case-control study. *J Arthroplasty* 2004; 19(7 Suppl 2): 35-41.

38. Lombardi AV, Mallory TH, Cuckler JM, *et al*. Mid-term results of a polyethylene-free metal on metal articulation. *J Arthroplasty* 2004; 19(7) suppl 2: 42-8.

39. Jacobs M, Gorab R, Mattingly D, *et al*. Three to six-year results with the Ultima metal-on-metal hip articulation for primary total hip arthroplasty. *J Arthroplasty* 2004; 19(7) suppl 2: 48-53.

40. Delaunay CP. Metal-on-metal bearings in cementless primary total hip arthroplasty. *J Arthroplasty* 2004; 19(8 Suppl 3): 35-40.

41. Silva M, Heisel C, Schmalzried TP. Metal-on-metal total hip replacement. *Clin Orthop* 2005; 430: 53-61.

42. McMinn D, Daniel J. History and modern concepts in surface replacement. *Proc Inst Mech Eng [H]* 2006; 220(2): 239-51.

43. Amstutz H, Le Duff M. Background of metal-on-metal resurfacing. *Proc Inst Mech Eng [H]* 2006; 220(2): 85-94.

44. Grigoris P, Roberts P, Panousis K, *et al.* Hip resurfacing arthroplasty: the evolution of contemporary designs. *Proc Inst Mech Eng [H]* 2006; 220(2): 95-105.

45. Isaac G, Siebel T, Schmalzried T, *et al.* Development rationale for an articular surface replacement: a science-based evolution. *Proc Inst Mech Eng [H]* 2006; 220(2): 253-68.

46. Shetty V, Villar R. Development and problems of metal-on-metal hip arthroplasty. *Proc Inst Mech Eng [H]* 2006; 220(2): 371-7.

47. Amstutz HC, Campbell P, McKellop H, *et al.* Metal on metal total hip replacement workshop consensus document. *Clin Orthop* 1996; 329(suppl): S297-S303.

48. Campbell P, Fu-Wen S, McKellop HC. Biological and tribologic considerations of alternative bearing surfaces. *Clin Orthop* 2004; 418: 98-111.

49. Dumbleton JH, Manley MT. Metal-on-metal total hip replacement: what does the literature say? *J Arthroplasty* 2005; 20(2): 174-88.

50. Heisel C, Silva M, Schmalzried TP. Bearing surface options for total hip replacement in young patients. *Instr Course Lect* 2004; 53: 49-65.

51. Delaunay C. Clinique de l'Yvette, Article in French. Can metal-on-metal bearings improve the longevity of total hip prostheses? *Rev Chir Orthop Reparatrice Appar Mot* 2005; 91(1): 70-8.

52. Mont MA. Michael Mont on metal-on-metal hip resurfacing arthroplasty. *Orthopedics* 2004; 27(10): 1047-8.

53. Knecht A, Witzleb WC, Gunther KP. Resurfacing arthroplasty of the hip. *Orthopade* 2005; 34(1): 79-90.

54. Witzleb WC, Knecht A, Beichler T, *et al.* Hip resurfacing arthroplasty. *Orthopade* 2004; 33(11): 1236-42.

55. Archibek MJ, Jacobs JJ, Black J. Alternate bearing surfaces in total joint arthroplasty: biological considerations. *Clin Orthop* 2000; 379: 12-21.

56. National Institute for Clinical Excellence. Hip disease - metal on metal resurfacing. The clinical effectiveness and cost effectiveness of metal on metal hip resurfacing. London: National Institute for Clinical Excellence, 2002; No. 44.

57. Kothari M, Bartel DL, Booker JF. Surface geometry of retrieved McKee Farrar total hip replacements. *Clin Orthop* 1996; 329(suppl): S141-147.

58. Walker PS, Gold BL. The Tribology (frictions, lubrication, and wear) of all metal artificial hip joints. *Wear* 1971; 17: 285-99.

59. McKellop H, Park SH, Cjiesa R, *et al. In vivo* wear of three types of metal on metal hip prostheses during two decades of use. *Clin Orthop* 1996; 329(suppl): s128-s140.

60. Rieker C, Kottig P. *In vivo* tribological performance of 231 metal-on-metal hip articulations. *Hip Int* 2002; 12: 73-6.

61. Sieber HB, Rieker CB, Kottig P. Analysis of 118 second generation metal on metal retrieved hip implants. *J Bone J Surg Br* 1999; 81: 46-50.

62. Rieker CB, Schön R, Köttig P. Development and validation of a second-generation metal-on-metal bearing: laboratory studies and analysis of retrievals. *J Arthroplasty* 2004; 19(8 Suppl 3): 5-11.

63. Cobb A, Schmalzreid T. The clinical significance of metal ion release from cobalt-chromium metal-on-metal hip joint arthroplasty. *Proc Inst Mech Eng [H]* 2006; 220(2): 385-98.

64. Anissian HL, Stark A, Gustafson A, *et al.* Metal-on-metal bearing in hip prosthesis generates 100-fold less wear debris than metal-on-polyethylene. *Acta Orthop Scand* 1999; 70(6): 578-82.

65. Clark I C, Good V, William P, *et al.* Ultra-low wear rates for rigid on rigid bearings in total hip replacements. *Proc Inst Mech Eng [H]* 2000; 21: 331-47.

66. Vassiliou K, D Elfick A, Scholes S, *et al.* The effect of 'running-in' on the tribology and surface morphology of metal-on-metal Birmingham hip resurfacing device in simulator studies. *Proc Inst Mech Eng [H]* 2006; 220(2): 269-77.

67. Hardaker C, Dowson D, Isaac G. Head replacement, head rotation, and surface damage effects on metal-on-metal total hip replacements: a hip simulator study. *Proc Inst Mech Eng [H]* 2006; 220(2): 209-17.

68. Brown C, Fisher J, Ingham E. Biological effects of clinically relevant wear particles from metal-on-metal hip prostheses. *Proc Inst Mech Eng [H]* 2006; 220(2): 355-69.

69. Catelas I, Campbell P, Bobyn J, *et al.* Wear particles from metal-on-metal total hip replacements: effects of implant design and implantation time. *Proc Inst Mech Eng [H]* 2006; 220(2): 195-208.

70. Willert HG, Buchhorn GH, Gobel D, *et al.* Wear behaviour and histopathology of classic cemented metal on metal hip endoprostheses. *Clin Orthop* 1996; 329(suppl): s160-s186.

71. Doorn PF, Campbell PA, Worrall J, Benya PD, McKellp HA, Amstutz HC. Metal wear particle characterization from metal on metal total hip replacements: transmission electron microscopy study of periprosthetic tissues and isolated particles. *J Biomed Mater Res* 1998; 42: 103-11.

72. Doorn PF, Mirra JM, Campbell PA, Amstutz HC. Tissue reaction to metal on metal total hip prostheses. *Clin Orthop* 1996; 329(suppl): s187-s205.

73. Doorn PF, Campbell PA, Amstutz HC. Metal versus polyethylene wear particles in total hip replacements. *Clin Orthop* 1996; 329(suppl): S206-S216.

74. Firkins PJ, Tipper JL, Ingham E, *et al.* Quantitative analysis of wear and wear debris from metal on metal hip prosthesis tested in a physiological hip joint simulator. *Biomed Mater Eng* 2001; 11: 143-57.

75. Tipper JL, Firkins PJ, Ingham E, *et al.* Quantitative analysis of the wear and wear debris from low and high carbon content cobalt chrome alloys used in metal on metal total hip replacements. *J Mater Sci: Materials in Medicine* 1999; 10: 353-62.

76. Davies AP, Willert HG, Campbell PA, *et al.* An unusual lymphocytic perivascular infiltration in tissues around contemporary metal-on-metal joint replacements. *J Bone Joint Surg Am* 2005; 87(1): 18-27.

77. Beaulé PE, Campbell P, Mirra J, Hooper JC, Schmalzried TP. Osteolysis in a cementless second-generation metal on metal hip replacement. *Clin Orthop* 2001; 386: 159-65.

78. Nevelos J, Shelton JC, Fisher J. Metallurgical considerations in the wear of metal-on-metal hip bearings. *Hip Int* 2004; 14: 1-10.

79. Dowson D, Jin Z. Metal-on-metal hip joint tribology. *Proc Inst Mech Eng [H]* 2006; 220(2): 107-18.

80. Scholes S, Unsworth A. The tribology of metal-on-metal total hip replacements. *Proc Inst Mech Eng [H]* 2006; 220(2): 183-94.

81. Dowson D. Tribological principles in metal-on-metal hip joint design. *Proc Inst Mech Eng [H]* 2006; 220(2): 161-71.

82. Streicher RM, Semlitsch M, Schon R, *et al.* Metal on metal articulation for artificial hip joints: laboratory study and clinical results. *Proc Inst Mech Eng (H)* 1996; 210: 223-32.

83. Smith SL, Dowson D, Goldsmith AA. The effect of femoral head diameter upon lubrication and wear of metal on metal total hip replacements. *Proc Inst Mech Eng* 2001; 215: 161-70.

84. Dowson D, Hardaker C, Flett M, *et al.* A hip joint simulator study of the performance of metal-on-metal joints: Part I: The role of materials. *J Arthroplasty* 2004; 19(8 Suppl 3): 118-23.

85. Dowson D, Hardaker C, Flett M, *et al.* A hip joint simulator study of the performance of metal-on-metal joints: Part II: Design. *J Arthroplasty* 2004; 19(8 Suppl 3): 124-30.

86. Rieker CB, Schon R, Konrad R, *et al.* Influence of the clearance on *in vitro* tribology of large diameter metal-on-metal articulations pertaining to resurfacing hip implants. *Orthop Clin N Am* 2005; 36: 135-42.

87. Medley JB, Chan FW, Krygier JJ, Bobyn JD. Comparison of alloys and designs in a hip simulator study of metal on metal implants. *Clin Orthop* 1996; 319(suppl): s148-s159.

88. Chan FW, Bobyn JD, Medley JB, *et al.* The Otto Aufranc Award: wear and lubrication of metal on metal hip implants. *Clin Orthop* 1999; 369: 10-24.

89. Chan FW, Bobyn JD, Medley JB, *et al.* Engineering issues and wear performance of metal on metal hip implants. *Clin Orthop* 1996; 333: 96-107.

90. Varano R, Bobyn J, Medley J, *et al.* The effect of microstructure on the wear of cobalt-based alloys used in metal-on-metal hip implants. *Proc Inst Mech Eng [H]* 2006; 220(2): 145-59.

91. Yan Y, Neville A, Dowson D. Understanding the role of corrosion in the degradation of metal-on-metal implants. *Proc Inst Mech Eng [H]* 2006; 220(2): 173-80.

92. Daniel J, Pynsent PB, McMinn DJ. Metal-on-metal resurfacing of the hip in patients under the age of 55 years with osteoarthritis. *J Bone Joint Surg Br* 2004; 86(2): 177-84.

93. Bowsher JG, Shelton JC. Influence of heat treatments on large diameter metal-metal hip joint wear. Abstract. Orthopaedic Proceedings. *J Bone Joint Surg Br* 2004; 86(suppl): 7.

94. Amstutz HC, Beaulé PE, Dorey FJ, *et al.* Metal on metal hybrid surface arthroplasty: two to six-year follow-up study. *J Bone Joint Surg Am* 2004; 86-A: 28-39.

95. Lilikakis AK, Vowler SL, Villar RN. Hydroxyapatite-coated femoral implant in metal-on-metal resurfacing hip arthroplasty: minimum of two years follow-up. *Orthop Clin North Am* 2005; 36(2): 215-22.

96. Bowsher J, Nevelos J, Williams P, *et al.* 'Severe' wear challenge to 'as-cast' and 'double heat-treated' large-diameter metal-on-metal hip bearings. *Proc Inst Mech Eng [H]* 2006; 220(2): 135-43.

97. Bowsher JG, Hussain A, Williams P, *et al.* Effect of ion implantation on the tribology of metal-on-metal hip prostheses. *J Arthroplasty* 2004; 19(8 Suppl 3): 107-11.

98. Williams S, Isaac G, Hatto P, *et al.* Comparative wear under different conditions of surface-engineered metal-on-metal bearings for total hip arthroplasty. *J Arthroplasty* 2004; 19(8 Suppl 3): 112-7.

99. Isaac G, Thompson J, Williams S, *et al.* Metal-on-metal bearings surfaces: materials, manufacture, design, optimization, and alternatives. *Proc Inst Mech Eng [H]* 2006; 220(2): 119-33.

100. Cuckler JM, Moore KD, Lombardi AV Jr, *et al.* Large versus small femoral heads in metal-on-metal total hip arthroplasty. *J Arthroplasty* 2004; 19(8 Suppl 3): 41-4.

101. Udofia IJ, Jin ZM. Elastohydrodynamic lubrication analysis of metal-on-metal hip resurfacing prostheses. *J Biomech* 2003; 36: 537-44.

102. Wimmer M, Nassutt R, Sprecher C, *et al.* An investigation on stick phenomena in metal-on-metal hip joints after resting periods. *Proc Inst Mech Eng [H]* 2006; 220(2): 219-27.

103. Treacy RB, McBryde CW, Pynsent PB. Birmingham hip resurfacing arthroplasty. A minimum follow-up of five years. *J Bone Joint Surg Br* 2005; 87(2): 167-70.

104. Back DL, Dalziel R, Young D, Shimmin A. Early results of primary Birmingham hip resurfacings: an independent prospective study of the first 230 hips. *J Bone Joint Surg Br* 2005; 87(3): 324.

105. De Smet KA. Belgian experience with metal on metal surface arthroplasty. *Orthop Clin North Am* 2005; 36: 203-13.

106. Chandler MZ, Kowalski R, Watkins N, *et al.* Cementing techniques in hip resurfacing. *Proc Inst Mech Eng [H]* 2006; 220(2): 321-31.

107. Howald R, Kesteris U, Klabunde R, *et al.* Factors affecting the cement penetration of a hip resurfacing implant: an *in vitro* study. *Hip Int* 2006; 16: 82-9.

108. Morlock M, Bishop N. Rüther W, *et al.* Biomechanical, morphological, and histological analysis of early failures in hip resurfacing arthroplasty. *Proc Inst Mech Eng [H]* 2006; 220(2): 333-44.

109. Beaulé PE, Antoniades J. Patient selection and surgical technique for surface arthroplasty of the hip. *Orthop Clin N Am* 2005; 36: 177-85.

110. Howie DW, McGee MA, Costi K, Graves SE. Metal-on-metal resurfacing versus total hip replacement - the value of a randomized clinical trial. *Orthop Clin N Am* 2005; 36(2): 195-201.

111. Beaulé P, Le Duff M, Campbell P, Dorey F, Park SH, Amstutz HC. Metal-on-metal surface arthroplasty with a cemented femoral component: a 7-10 year follow-up study. *J Arthroplasty* 2004; 19(8 Suppl 3): 17-22.

112. Hendrikson RP, Keggi KJ. Anterior approach to resurfacing arthroplasty of the hip: a preliminary experience. *Conn Med* 1983; 47(3): 131-5.

113. Stulberg D. Surgical approaches for the performance of surface replacement arthroplasties. *Orthop Clin N Am* 1982; 13(4): 13-4.

114. Hedley AK. Technical considerations with surface replacement. *Orthop Clin N Am* 1982; 13(4): 747-60.

115. Nork SE, Schar M, Pfander G, *et al.* Anatomic considerations for the choice of surgical approach for hip resurfacing arthroplasty. *Orthop Clin N Am* 2005; 36(2): 163-70.

116. Gautier E, Ganz K, Krugel N, *et al.* Anatomy of the medial circumflex artery and its surgical implications. *J Bone Joint Surg Br* 2000; 82(5): 679-83.

117. Freeman MAR. Some anatomical and mechanical considerations relevant to the surface replacement of the femoral head. *Clin Orthop* 1978; 134: 19-24.

118. Beaulé PE, Campbell PA, Hoke R, *et al.* Notching of the femoral neck during resurfacing arthroplasty of the hip. *J Bone Joint Surg Br* 2006; 88(1): 35-9.

119. Steffen RT, Smith SR, Urban JP, *et al.* The effect of hip resurfacing on oxygen concentration in the femoral head. *J Bone Joint Surg Br* 2005; 87(11): 1468-74.

120. Beaulé PE. A soft tissue-sparing approach for surface arthroplasty of the hip. *Oper Tech Ortho* 2004; 14(4): 16-8.

121. McMahon SJ, Young D, Ballok Z, *et al.* Vascularity of the femoral head after Birmingham hip resurfacing. A technetium tc 99m bone scan/single photon emission computed tomography study. *J Arthroplasty* 2006; 21(4): 514-21.

122. Beaulé PE, lee JL, Le Duff MJ, *et al.* Orientation of the femoral component in surface arthroplasty of the hip: a biomechanical and clinical analysis. *J Bone Joint Surg Am* 2004; 86(9): 2015-21.

123. Beaulé P, Dorey F, Le Duff M, *et al.* Risk factors affecting early outcome of metal on metal surface arthroplasty of the hip in patients 40 years old and younger. *Clin Orthop* 2004; 418: 80-7.

124. Schmalzried TP, Silva M, de la Rosa MA, *et al.* Optimizing patient selection and outcomes with total hip resurfacing. *Clin Orthop Relat Res* 2005; 441: 200-4.

125. Field RE, Kavanagh TG, Singh PJ. Birmingham Hip Resurfacing - conserving or sacrificing for acetabular bone stock? Orthop Proceedings. *J Bone Joint Surg Br* 2004; 8-B(suppl): 76.

126. Palmer SJ, Wimhurst JA, Villar RN. Does hip resurfacing really conserve bone? Orthop Proceedings. *J Bone Joint Surg Br* 2001; 83-B; (suppl I): S70.

127. Crawford JR, Palmer SJ, Wimhurst JA, *et al.* Bone loss at hip resurfacing: a comparison with total hip arthroplasty. *Hip Int* 2005; 15: 195-8.

128. Loughead JM, Starks I, Chesney D, *et al.* Removal of acetabular bone in resurfacing arthroplasty of the hip. *J Bone Joint Surg Br* 2006; 88(1): 31-4.

129. Loughead JM, Chesney D, Holland JP, *et al.* Comparison of offset in Birmingham hip resurfacing and hybrid total hip arthroplasty. *J Bone Joint Surg Br* 2005; 87(2): 163-6.

130. Silva M, Lee KH, Heisel C, *et al.* The biomechanical results of total hip resurfacing arthroplasty. *J Bone Joint Surg Am* 2004; 86-A(1): 40-6.

131. Girard J, Lavigne M, Vendittoli PA, *et al.* Biomechanical reconstruction of the hip: a randomised study comparing total hip resurfacing and total hip arthroplasty. *J Bone Joint Surg Br* 2006; 88(6): 721-6.

132. Murray JR, Cooke NJ, Rawlings D, *et al.* A reliable DEXA measurement technique for metal-on-metal hip resurfacing. *Acta Orthop* 2005; 76(2): 177-81.

133. Kishida Y, Sugano N, Nishii T, *et al.* Preservation of the bone mineral density of the femur after surface replacement of the hip. *J Bone Joint Surg Br* 2004; 86(2): 185-9.

134. Amstutz HC, Ebramzadeh E, Sarkany A, *et al.* Preservation of bone mineral density of the proximal femur following hemiresurface arthroplasty. *Orthopedics* 2004; 27(12): 1266-71.

135. Harty JA, Devitt B, Harty LC, *et al.* Dual energy X-ray absorptiometry analysis of periprosthetic stress shielding in the Birmingham resurfacing hip replacement. *Arch Orthop Trauma Surg* 2005; 20: 1-3.

136. De Waal Malefijt MC, Huiskes R. A clinical, radiological and biomechanical study of the TARA hip prosthesis. *Arch Orthop Trauma Surg* 1993; 112(5): 220-5

137. Huiskes R, Sterns PHGE, Heck JV, *et al.* Interface stresses in the resurfaced hip. *Acta Orthop Scand* 1985; 56: 74.

138. Watanabe Y, Shiba N, Matsuo S, *et al.* Biomechanical study of the resurfacing hip arthroplasty: finite element analysis of the femoral component. *J Arthroplasty* 2000; 15(4): 505-11.

139. Taylor M. Finite element analysis of the resurfaced femoral head. *Proc Inst Mech Eng [H]* 2006; 220(2): 289-97.

140. Gupta S, New AM, Taylor M. Bone remodelling inside a cemented resurfaced femoral head. *Clin Biomech* (Bristol, Avon) 2006; 21(6): 594-602.

141. Itayem R, Arndt A, Nistor L, *et al.* Stability of the Birmingham hip resurfacing arthroplasty at two years. A radiostereophotogrammetric analysis study. *J Bone Joint Surg Br* 2005; 87(2): 158-62

142. Glyn-Jones S, Gill HS, McLardy-Smith P, *et al.* Roentgen stereophotogrammetric analysis of the Birmingham hip resurfacing arthroplasty. A two-year study. *J Bone Joint Surg Br* 2004; 86(2): 172-6.

143. Fowble VA, Schuh A, Hoke R, *et al.* Clinical correlation of femoral component migration in hip resurfacing arthroplasty analyzed by einzel-bild-rontgen-analyze-femoral component analysis. *Orthop Clin North Am* 2005; 36(2): 243-50.

144. Beaulé PE, Krismer M, Mayrhofer P, *et al.* EBRA-FCA for measurement of migration of the femoral component in surface arthroplasty of the hip. *J Bone Joint Surg Br* 2005; 87(5): 741-4.

145. Pollard TC, Baker RP, Eastaugh-Waring SJ, *et al.* Treatment of the young active patient with osteoarthritis of the hip: a five- to seven-year comparison of hybrid total hip arthroplasty and metal-on-metal resurfacing. *J Bone Joint Surg Br* 2006; 88(5): 592-600.

146. Komistek RD, Dennis DA, Ochoa JA, *et al. In vivo* comparison of hip separation after metal-on-metal or metal-on-polyethylene total hip arthroplasty. *J Bone Joint Surg Am* 2002; 84-A: 1836-41.

147. Jin ZM, Meakins S, Morlock M, *et al.* Deformation of press-fitted metallic resurfacing cups. Part 1: experimental simulation. *Proc Inst Mech Eng [H]* 2006; 220(2): 299-309.

148. Yew A, Jin ZM, Donn A, *et al.* Deformation of press-fitted metallic resurfacing cups. Part 2: finite element simulation. *Proc Inst Mech Eng [H]* 2006; 220(2): 311-9.

149. Wyness L, Vale L, McCormack K, *et al.* The effectiveness of metal on metal hip resurfacing: a systematic review of the

available evidence published before 2002. *BMC Health Serv Res* 2004; 4(1): 39.

150. Vale L, Wyness L, McCormack K, *et al*. A systematic review of the effectiveness and cost-effectiveness of metal-on-metal hip resurfacing arthroplasty for treatment of hip disease. *Health Technol Assess* 2002; 6(15): 1-109.

151. McKenzie L, Vale L, Stearns S, *et al*. Metal on metal hip resurfacing arthroplasty. An economic analysis. *Eur J Health Econ* 2003; 4(2): 122-9.

152. Vendittoli PA, Lavigne M, Roy AG, *et al*. A prospective randomized clinical trial comparing metal-on-metal total hip arthroplasty and metal-on-metal total hip resurfacing in patients less than 65 years old. *Hip Int* 2006; 16: 73-81.

153. Lilikakis AK, Arora A, Villar RN. Early rehabilitation comparing hip resurfacing and total hip replacement. *Hip Int* 2005; 15: 189-94.

154. Chirodian N, Saw T, Villar R. Results of hybrid total hip replacement and resurfacing - is there a difference? *Hip Int* 2004; 14: 169-73.

155. Amstutz HC, Su EP, Le Duff MJ. Surface arthroplasty in young patients with hip arthritis secondary to childhood disorders. *Orthop Clin North Am* 2005; 36(2): 223-30.

156. Siebel T, Maubach S, Morlock MM. Lessons learned from early clinical experience and results of 300 ASR® hip resurfacing implantations. *Proc Inst Mech Eng [H]* 2006; 220(2): 345-53.

157. Pollard TCB, Basu C, Ainsworth R, *et al*. Is the Birmingham hip resurfacing worthwhile? *Hip* 2003; 13: 26-8.

158. Hart AJ, Scott G. Hip resurfacing following previous proximal femoral osteotomy. *Hip Int* 2005; 15: 119-122.

159. Knecht A, Witzleb WC, Beichler T, *et al*. Functional results after surface replacement of the hip: comparison between dysplasia and idiopathic osteoarthritis. *Z Orthop Ihre Grenzgeb* 2004; 142(3): 279-85.

160. Cuckler JM, Moore KD, Estrada. Outcome of hemiresurfacing in osteonecrosis of the femoral head. *Clin Orthop* 2004; 429: 146-50.

161. Calder PR, Hynes MC, Scott G. Short-term results of hemi-resurfacing for osteonecrosis of the femoral head. *Hip Int* 2004; 14: 174-81

162. Squire M, Fehring TK, Odum S, *et al*. Failure of surface replacement for femoral head avascular necrosis. *J Arthroplasty* 2005; 20(6 Suppl 3): 108-14.

163. Hungerford MW, Mont MA, Scott R, *et al*. Surface replacement hemiarthroplasty for the treatment of osteonecrosis of the femoral head. *J Bone Joint Surg Am* 1998; 80(11): 1656-64.

164. Mont MA, Rajadhyaksha AD, Hungerford DS. Outcomes of limited femoral resurfacing arthroplasty compared with total hip arthroplasty for osteonecrosis of the femoral head. *J Arthroplasty* 2001; 16(8 Suppl 1): 134-9.

165. Beaulé PE, Schmalzried TP, Campbell P, *et al*. Duration of symptoms and outcome of hemiresurfacing for hip osteonecrosis. *Clin Orthop* 2001; 385: 104-17.

166. Beaulé PE, Amstutz HC, Le Duff M, *et al*. Surface arthroplasty for osteonecrosis of the hip: hemiresurfacing versus metal-on-metal hybrid resurfacing. *J Arthroplasty* 2004; 19(8 Suppl 3): 54-8.

167. Schmalzried TP. Total resurfacing for osteonecrosis of the hip. *Clin Orthop* 2004; 429: 151-6.

168. Grecula MJ. Resurfacing arthroplasty in osteonecrosis of the hip. *Orthop Clin N Am* 2005; 36(2): 231-42.

169. Little CP, Ruiz AL, Harding IJ, *et al*. Osteonecrosis in retrieved femoral heads after failed resurfacing arthroplasty of the hip. *J Bone Joint Surg Br* 2005; 87(3): 320-3.

170. Shimmin AJ, Back DL. Femoral neck fractures associated with hip resurfacing: a national review of 50 cases. *J Bone Joint Surg Br* 2005; 87(4): 463-4.

171. Bohm R, Schraml A, Schuh A. Long-term results with the Wagner metal-on-metal hip resurfacing prosthesis. *Hip Int* 2006; 16: 58-64.

172. Cutts S, Datta A, Ayoub K, *et al*. Early failure modalities in hip resurfacing? *Hip Int* 2005; 15: 155-8.

173. Shimmin AJ, Bare J, Back DL. Complications associated with hip resurfacing arthroplasty. *Orthop Clin North Am* 2005; 36(2): 187-93.

174. Cossey AJ, Back DL, Shimmin A, *et al*. The nonoperative management of periprosthetic fractures associated with the Birmingham hip resurfacing procedure. *J Arthroplasty* 2005; 20(3): 358-61.

175. Amstutz HC, Campbell PA, Le Duff MJ. Fracture of the neck of the femur after surface arthroplasty of the hip. *J Bone Joint Surg Am* 2004; 86(9): 1874-7.

176. Cumming D, Fordyce MJ. Non-operative management of a peri-prosthetic subcapital fracture after metal-on-metal Birmingham hip resurfacing. *J Bone Joint Surg Br* 2003; 85(7): 1055-6.

177. Sharma H, Rana B, Watson C, Campbell AC, Singh BJ. Femoral neck fractures complicating metal-on-metal resurfaced hips: a report of 2 cases. *J Orthop Surg (Hong Kong)* 2005; 13(1): 69-72.

178. Bogoch ER, Fornasier VL, Capello WN. The femoral head remnant in resurfacing arthroplasty. *Clin Orthop* 1982; 167: 92-105.

179. Bradley GW, Freeman MA, Revell PA. Resurfacing arthroplasty. Femoral head viability. *Clin Orthop* 1987; 220: 137-41.

180. Howie DW, Cornish BL, Vernon-Roberts B. The viability of the femoral head after resurfacing hip arthroplasty in humans. *Clin Orthop* 1993; 291: 171-84.

181. Campbell P, Mirra J, Amstutz HC. Viability of femoral heads treated with resurfacing arthroplasty. *J Arthroplasty* 2000; 15(1): 120-2.

182. Clarke MT, Lee PTH, Villar RN. Dislocation after total hip replacement in relation to metal-on-metal bearing surfaces. *J Bone Joint Surg Br* 2003; 85-B(5): 650-4.

183. Lee PTH, Clarke MT, Villar RN. Bearing surface in total hip replacement as a potential risk factor for dislocation. Orthop Proceedings. *J Bone Joint Surg Br* 2004; 86-B: 16.

184. Norrish AR, Rao J, Villar RN. Heterotopic ossification: a prospective comparison between hip resurfacing and total hip replacement. Orthop Proceedings. *J Bone Joint Surg Br* 2004; 86-B(suppl): 81.

185. Stem E, Duffy G, Blasser K, O'Connor MI. Stem fracture of conserve hemiarthroplasty. *J Arthroplasty* 2004; 19(7): 923-6.

186. Arbuthnot JE, Journeaux SF, Clark DI. The Birmingham hip resurfacing procedure: a rare complication. *J Arthroplasty* 2003; 18(5): 666-7.

187. Skipor AK, Campbell P, Patterson LM, *et al.* Serum and urine levels in patients with metal-on-metal surface arthroplasty. *J Mater Sci Mater Med* 2002; 13: 1227-34.

188. Brodner W, Bitzan P, Meisinger V, *et al.* Serum cobalt levels after metal on metal total hip arthroplasty. *J Bone Joint Surg Am* 2003; 85A: 2168-73.

189. Lhotka C, Szekeres T, Steffan I, *et al.* Four-year study of cobalt and chromium blood levels in patients managed with two different metal-on-metal total hip replacements. *J Orthop Res* 2003; 21(2): 189-95.

190. MacDonald SJ, McCalden RW, Chess DG. The John Charnley Award: metal on metal versus polyethylene in total hip arthroplasty: a randomized clinical trial. *Clin Orthop* 2003; 406: 282-96.

191. Savarino L, Granchi D, Ciapetti G, *et al.* Ion release in patients with metal-on-metal hip bearings in total joint replacement: a comparison with metal-on-polyethylene bearings. *J Biomed Mater Res* 2002; 63: 467.

192. Saikko V, Nevalainen J, Revitzer H, *et al.* Metal release in total hip articulations *in vitro*: substantial from CoCr/CoCr, negligible from CoCr/PE and alumina/PE. *Acta Orthop Scand* 1998; 69(5): 449-54.

193. MacDonald SJ. Metal-on-metal total hip arthroplasty: the concerns. *Clin Orthop Relat Res* 2004; 429: 86-93.

194. Jacobs JJ, Hallab NJ, Skipor AK, *et al.* Metal degradation products. A cause for concern in metal metal bearings? *Clin Orthop* 2003; 417: 139.

195. Bhamra M, Case C. Biological effects of metal-on-metal hip replacements. *Proc Inst Mech Eng [H]* 2006; 220(2): 379-84.

196. Learmonth I, Gheduzzi S, Vail T. Clinical experience with metal-on-metal total joint replacements: indications and results. *Proc Inst Mech Eng [H]* 2006; 220(2): 229-37.

197. MacDonald SJ. Can a safe level for metal ions in patients with metal-on-metal total hip arthroplasties be determined? *J Arthroplasty* 2004; 19(8 Suppl 3): 71-7.

198. MacDonald SJ, Brodner W, Jacobs J. A consensus paper on metal ions in metal-on-metal hip arthroplasties. *J Arthroplasty* 2004; 19(8 Suppl 3): 12-6.

199. Savarino L, Granchi D, Ciapetti G, *et al.* Ion release in stable hip arthroplasties using metal on metal articulating surfaces: a comparison between short- and medium-term results. *J Biomed Mater Res* 2003; 66-A: 450-6.

200. Back DL, Young DA, Shimmin AJ. How do serum cobalt and chromium levels change after metal-on-metal hip resurfacing? *Clin Orthop* 2005; 438: 177-81.

201. Jacobs JJ, Skipor AK, Campbell PA, Hallab NJ, Urban RA, Amstutz HC. Can metal levels be used to monitor metal-on-metal hip arthroplasties? *J Arthroplasty* 2004; 19(8 Suppl 3): 59-65.

202. Clarke MT, Lee PT, Arora A, *et al.* Levels of metal ions after small- and large-diameter metal-on-metal hip arthroplasty. *J Bone Joint Surg Br* 2003; 85(6): 913-7.

203. Lee PTH, Clarke MT, Arora A, *et al.* Serum cobalt and chromium levels in patients with unilateral versus bilateral metal-on-metal total hip repacement. Orthop Proceedings. *J Bone Joint Surg Br* 2004; 86-B: 76.

204. Daniel J, Ziaee H, Salama A, *et al.* The effect of the diameter of metal-on-metal bearings on systemic exposure to cobalt and chromium. *J Bone Joint Surg Br* 2006; 88(4): 443-8.

205. Brodner W, Grübl A, Jankovsky R, *et al.* Cup inclination and serum concentration of cobalt and chromium after metal-on-metal total hip arthroplasty. *J Arthroplasty* 2004; 19(8 Suppl 3): 66-70.

206. Heisel C, Silva M, Skipor AK, *et al.* The relationship between activity and ions in patients with metal-on-metal bearing hip prostheses. *J Bone Joint Surg Am* 2005; 87(4): 781-7.

207. Bowsher J, Hussain A, Williams P, *et al.* Metal-on-metal hip simulator study of increased wear particle surface area due to 'severe' patient activity. *Proc Inst Mech Eng [H]* 2006; 220(2): 279-87.

208. Urban RM, Tomlinson MJ, Hall DJ, *et al.* Accumulation in liver and spleen of metal particles generated at nonbearing surfaces in hip arthroplasty. *J Arthroplasty* 2004; 19(8 Suppl 3): 94-101.

209. Merrit K, Brown SA. Distribution of cobalt chromium wear and corrosion products and biologic reactions. *Clin Orthop* 1996; 329(suppl): S233-S243.

210. Hart AJ, Hester T, Sinclair K, *et al.* The association between metal ions from hip resurfacing and reduced T-cell counts. *J Bone Joint Surg Br* 2006; 88(4): 449-54

211. Huk OL, Catelas I, Mwale F, *et al.* Induction of apoptosis and necrosis by metal ions *in vitro*. *J Arthroplasty* 2004; 19(8 Suppl 3): 84-7.

212. Case CP, Langkamer VG, Howell RT, *et al.* Preliminary observations on possible premalignant changes to bone marrow adjacent to worn total hip arthroplasty implants. *Clin Orthop* 1996; 329(suppl): s269-s279.

213. Ladon D, Doherty A, Newson R, *et al.* Changes in metal levels and chromosome aberrations in the peripheral blood of patients after metal-on-metal hip arthroplasty. *J Arthroplasty* 2004; 19(8 Suppl 3): 78-83.

214. Howie DW, Rogers SD, McGee MA, *et al.* Biological effects of cobalt chrome in cell and animal models. *Clin Orthop* 1996; 329(suppl): S217-232.

215. Brodner W, Grohs JG, Bancher-Todesca D, *et al.* Does the placenta inhibit the passage of chromium and cobalt after metal-on-metal total hip arthroplasty? *J Arthroplasty* 2004; 19(8 Suppl 3): 102-6.

216. Hallab NJ, Merrit K, Jacobs JJ. Metal sensitivity in patients with orthopaedic implants. *J Bone Joint Surg Am* 2001; 83: 428-36.

217. Hallab NJ, Anderson S, Caicedo M, *et al.* Immune responses correlate with serum-metal in metal-on-metal hip arthroplasty. *J Arthroplasty* 2004; 19(8 Suppl 3): 88-93.

218. Benson MK, Goodwin PG, Brostoff J. Metal sensitivity in patients with joint replacement arthroplasties. *Br Med J* 1975; 4: 374-5.

219. Evans EM, Freeman MAR, Miller AJ, *et al.* Metal sensitivity as a cause of bone necrosis and loosening in total joint replacement. *J Bone Joint Surg Br* 1974; 56: 626-42.

Chapter 17

220. Jones DA, Lucas HK, O'Driscoll M, *et al.* Cobalt toxicity after McKee hip arthroplasty. *J Bone Joint Surg* 1975; 57-B: 289-96.

221. Antony FC, Holden CA. Metal allergy resurfaces in failed hip endoprostheses. *Contact Dermatitis* 2003; 48: 49-50.

222. Long WT. The clinical performance of metal-on-metal as an articulation surface in total hip replacement. *Iowa Orthop J* 2005; 25: 10-6.

223. Willert H, Buchorn G, Fayyazi A, *et al.* Histological changes around metal / metal joint indicate delayed type hypersensitivity. Preliminary results of 14 cases. *Ostoelogie* 2000; 0: 2-16.

224. Willert H, Buchorn G, Fayyazi A, *et al.* Metal-on-metal bearings and hypersensitivity in patients with artificial hip joints. A clinical and histomorphological study. *J Bone Joint Surg Am* 2005; 87(1): 28-36.

225. Park Y, Moon Y, Lim S, Yang J. Early osteolysis following second generation metal on metal hip replacement. *J Bone Joint Surg Am* 2005; 87 (7): 1515-21.

226. Baur W, Honle W, Willert HG. Pathological findings in tissues surrounding revised metal/metal articulations. *Orthopade* 2005; 34(3): 225-33.

227. Heath JC, Freeman MA, Swanson SA. Carcinogenic properties of wear particles from prostheses made in cobalt-chromium alloy. *Lancet* 1971; 1: 564-6.

228. Lewis CG, Sunderman FW. Metal carcinogenesis in total hip arthroplasty. Animal models. *Clin Orthop* 1996; 329(suppl): S264-S268.

229. Gillespie WJ, Frampton CM, Henderson RJ, Ryan PM. The incidence of cancer following total hip replacement. *J Bone H Surg Br* 1988; 70: 539-42.

230. Gillespie WJ, Henry DA, O'Connell DL, *et al.* Development of haematopoietic cancers after implantation of total joint replacement. *Clin Orthop* 1996; 329(suppl): s290-296.

231. Visuri T, Koskenvuo M. Cancer risk after McKee-Farrar total hip replacement. *Orthopaedics* 1991; 14: 137-42.

232. Mathiesen EB, Ahlbom A, Bergmann G, *et al.* Total hip replacement and cancer. A cohort study. *J Bone Joint Surg Br* 1995; 77(3): 345.

233. Visuri TI, Pukkala E, Pulkkinen P, *et al.* Cancer incidence and causes of death among total hip replacement patients: a review based on Nordic cohorts with a special emphasis on metal-on-metal bearings. *Proc Inst Mech Eng [H]* 2006; 220(2): 399-407.

234. Visuri TI, Pukkala E. Does metal-on-metal total hip prosthesis have influence on cancer? A long-term follow-up study. In: *World Tribology Forum in Arthroplasty.* Rieker C, Oberholzer S, Weiss U, Eds. Bern: Hans Huber, 2001: 181-7.

235. Tharani R, Dorey FJ, Schmalzried TP. The risk of cancer following total hip or knee arthroplasty. *J Bone Joint Surg Am* 2001; 83: 774-80.

236. Visuri T, Pukkala E, Paavolainen P, *et al.* Cancer risk following metal on metal and polytheylene on metal total hip arthroplasty. *Clin Orthop* 1996; 329(suppl): s280-289.

237. McMinn DJ, Daniel J, Pynsent PB, *et al.* Mini-incision resurfacing arthroplasty of hip through the posterior approach. *Clin Orthop Relat Res* 2005; 441: 91-8.

238. Mont MA, Ragland PS, Marker D. Resurfacing hip arthroplasty: comparison of a minimally invasive versus standard approach. *Clin Orthop Relat Res* 2005; 441: 125-31.

239. Hodgson AJ, Inkpen KB, Shekhman M, *et al.* Computer-assisted femoral head resurfacing. *Comput Aided Surg* 2005; 10(5-6): 337-43.

240. Hess T, Gampe T, Kottgen C, *et al.* Intraoperative navigation for hip resurfacing. Methods and first results. *Orthopade* 2004; 33(10): 1183-93.

241. Allison C. Minimally invasive hip resurfacing. *Issues Emerg Health Technol* 2005; 65: 1-4.

Chapter 18

Minimally invasive hip replacement

Ajay Malviya MS (Orth/Traum) MRCS
Specialist Registrar, Orthopaedic Surgery
Andrew McCaskie MD FRCS FRCS (Orth)
Professor of Trauma and Orthopaedic Surgery

THE FREEMAN HOSPITAL, NEWCASTLE UPON TYNE, UK

Introduction

Over recent years minimally invasive and minimal access surgical techniques have become popular, e.g. laparoscopic surgery of the abdomen [1], gynaecology [2], urology [3] and arthroscopic joint surgery. More recently such descriptions have been applied to patients undergoing joint replacement. Development of a minimal-incision approach to total hip replacement is not a new concept. Cameron [4] suggested that Scotty Law in England (1976), Robert Judet in France (1974) and Kris Keggi in the United States (1972) were early proponents of this technique. There are several different types of procedures that might come under such a heading and the definition is not clear. However, a common aim is to improve short-term outcomes, such as blood loss, analgesic requirements, functional restoration and length of stay in hospital.

The most important goals of joint replacement are to relieve pain and restore function with minimal complications and optimum long-term survival of the implant. This must not be jeopardised by new techniques but rather maintained or even further improved.

Minimally invasive hip replacement

What is the definition?

There is no single definition of what constitutes minimally invasive surgery (MIS) in total hip replacement (THR). Hart *et al* [5] define it as a "procedure performed through a smaller incision (arbitrarily defined as ≤10 cm) or two smaller incisions (each defined as ≤8cm)". Howell *et al* [6] have defined it as "any hip replacement procedure in which the length of the wound and the surgical access are deliberately modified in an attempt to reduce the tissue trauma associated with hip replacement, with most investigators reporting wounds of 10cm length or less". Furthermore, as the length of incision is related to the implant size, Howell *et al* [6] also propose that "the length of the incision must be equal to or at least more than half the length of the cup circumference" for the cup to be inserted without touching or stretching the skin. Others have said that the incision is 25% longer than the estimated acetabular diameter [7]. Based on this Goldstein *et al* [8] have estimated that for an acetabular component of 56mm diameter, a 4-inch incision would be required to avoid contact between the cup and the subcutaneous fat. It is also thought that a smaller incision with excessive retraction would cause undermining and devascularisation of the skin and create a dead space, retarding the healing ability of the skin [9]. The relevance of definition based on skin incision will be discussed throughout the chapter.

What types are there?

The MIS approach may be divided into two main categories: the single-incision approach or the two-incision approach. In general, the two factors that are important to success using a less-invasive THR technique are the location of the incision and using the concept of a 'mobile window' [10].

The single-incision approaches are modifications to conventional approaches e.g. posterior [10-18], posterolateral [5, 7-9, 19], lateral [20], anterolateral [21-24] or anterior [25] approaches. Single-incision MIS is generally a familiar area of anatomy to the surgeon (when based on the surgeon's routine approach) and, if required, is extensile to a standard approach and allows complete and continuous visualisation [26].

The two-incision technique [26, 27] constitutes a novel pairing of approaches, using intermuscular planes to gain access to the hip joint and minimising the dissection of muscles and tendons. This usually requires image intensification to achieve accurate component positioning. The visualisation is complete but intermittent [26].

Methodology

Search

A Medline search (1951 to date MEZZ) was done using 'Dialog Datastar'. The keyword 'mini' or 'MIS' for title search revealed 6983 relevant articles. Further title search with the keyword 'hip' revealed 30,611 articles. Thesaurus mapping was used to explode the search for 'hip'. On selection of 'arthroplasty-replacement-hip.De' a total of 5729 searches were revealed. Combining the two searches with 'and' revealed a total of 24 relevant publications in the

Medline. Further manual search during the study revealed a few more relevant publications.

Classification of papers

Several studies with variable levels of evidence (Table 1) have been published looking into the key issues surrounding minimally invasive hip replacement. Table 1 also summarises the approach and the strength of each study. Apart from these studies there have been several published reports that are comments and opinions of respected authorities on MIS THR.

Clinical relevance of results

Length of incision

Most authors report a mean incision length of less than 10cm for the single-incision approach, with Goldstein et al [8] (IIb/B) reporting a mean of as little as 5cm. DiGioia et al [10] (IIa/B) on the other hand report a mean of 11.7cm. Chung et al [7] (IIa/B) found that the incision was approximately 25% longer than the acetabular diameter, as estimated from templating the X-rays. Archibeck et al [29] (III/B) reporting on the two-incision technique found a mean incision size of 5.8cm for the anterior incision (acetabulum) and a mean of 3.7cm for the posterior incision (femur). Chimento et al [15] (Ib/A) showed that the mean length of the incision for the MIS group was 8cm as compared to 15cm for the control. Ogonda et al [13] (Ib/A) similarly report a smaller incision size of 9.21cm for the MIS group as compared to 16cm for the control.

Blood loss

MIS techniques have been associated with reports of reduced peri-operative blood loss [7, 8, 10, 13, 15-17, 20-22, 24]. However, some [12, 14] have found no significant difference in the amount of blood loss. Most studies [8, 13, 15, 20, 22] have shown that this has not translated into an increased requirement for blood transfusion in the peri and postoperative period.

Table 1. Studies on minimally invasive hip replacement.

Authors	Level of evidence	Number	Approach
Hartzband MA [19]	III/B	100 (MIS)	Posterolateral (MIS)
Wright *et al* [14]	IIa/B	42 (MIS) vs 42 (Standard)	Posterior (MIS & Standard)
Berger [21]	IIa/B	99 (MIS) vs 100 (Standard)	Anterolateral (MIS & Standard)
Howell *et al* [22]	IIa/B	50 (MIS) vs 57 (Standard)	Anterolateral (MIS & Standard)
Berger *et al* [28]	III/B	100 (MIS)	2 incision (MIS)
Irving *et al* [27]	III/B	192 (MIS)	2 incision (MIS)
Woolson *et al* [12]	IIb/B	50 (MIS) vs 85 (Standard)	Posterior (MIS & Standard)
Archibeck *et al* [29]	III/B	851 (MIS)	2 incision (MIS)
DiGioia *et al* [10]	IIa/B	33 (MIS) vs 33 (Standard)	Posterior (MIS & Standard)
Ogonda *et al* [13]	Ib/A	109 (MIS) vs 110 (Standard)	Posterior (MIS & Standard)
Goldstein *et al* [8]	IIb/B	85 (MIS) vs 85 (Standard)	Posterolateral (MIS & Standard)
Chung *et al* [7]	IIa/B	60 (MIS) vs 60 (Standard)	Posterolateral (MIS & Standard)
de Beer *et al* [20]	IIa/B	30 (MIS) vs 30 (Standard)	Lateral (MIS & Standard)
Chimento *et al* [15]	Ib/A	28 (MIS) vs 32 (Standard)	Posterior (MIS & Standard)
Higuchi *et al* [24]	IIb/B	115 (MIS) vs 70 (Short 10-15cm) vs 27 (Standard)	Anterolateral (MIS, Short & Standard)
Nakamura *et al* [17]	IIa/B	50 (MIS) vs 42 (Standard)	Posterior (MIS & Standard)
Siguier *et al* [25]	III/B	1037 (MIS)	Anterior (MIS)
Wenz *et al* [16]	IIb/B	124 (MIS) vs 65 (Standard)	Posterior (MIS) vs Lateral (Standard)
Hart *et al* [5]	IIa/B	60 (MIS) vs 60 (Standard)	Posterolateral (MIS & Standard)
Dorr [18]	III/B	105 (MIS)	Posterior (MIS)
Fehring *et al* [30]	IV/C	3 (MIS)	-

Chapter 18

Chimento *et al* [15] **(Ib/A)** have demonstrated that the mean estimated intra-operative blood loss and the total blood loss was significantly less (p=0.003 and p=0.009 respectively) in the MIS group but there was no significant difference in the transfusion rate (p=0.4). Ogonda *et al* [13] **(Ib/A)** found a significant difference (p=0.03) in the estimated intra-operative blood loss in the MIS group (314ml) as compared to the control (366ml). However, they reported no significant difference in the postoperative blood transfusion rate (p=0.27), the haematocrit at eight hours following surgery (p=0.34) or the haematocrit at discharge (p=0.75).

Goldstein *et al* [8] **(IIb/B)**, de Beer *et al* [20] **(IIa/B)** and Howell *et al* [22] **(IIa/B)** similarly report a significant decrease in estimated blood loss but no significant difference in the need for transfusion. Nakamura *et al* [17] **(IIa/B)**, Chung *et al* [7] **(IIa/B)**, Berger [21] **(IIa/B)** and Higuchi *et al* [24] **(IIb/B)** reported a decreased estimated blood loss in the MIS group but did not comment on the transfusion requirement.

Wenz *et al* [16] **(IIb/B)** and DiGioia *et al* [10] **(IIa/B)** have, however, reported that the transfusion requirement is significantly reduced (p=0.006 and p<0.05 respectively) following single-incision MIS THR.

Postoperative pain

Use of narcotic analgesia in the postoperative period is routine after a THR. Less tissue dissection would be expected to cause less postoperative pain; however, it has been shown that narcotic usage may not be necessarily decreased in MIS [7, 13, 15, 20].

Ogonda et al [13] (Ib/A) noted no significant difference between the MIS and the standard-incision group in terms of pain scores (immediate up to 36 hours). Similarly, there was no difference in the volume of morphine used with the patient-controlled analgesia. After correction for the variation in the length of stay they found no significant difference in the mean pain score in the first seven days following discharge. Chimento et al [15] (Ib/A) routinely use patient-controlled epidural analgesia (PCEA) for postoperative pain control and they did not find any significant difference in the volume of PCEA used (p=0.3) or in the amount of oral narcotic used per day (p=0.5) following discontinuation of the epidural analgesia.

Chung et al [7] (IIa/B) and de Beer et al [20] (IIa/B) also reported no significant difference in the narcotic use after MIS THR. Berger et al [28] (III/B) have reported that after two-incision MIS THR the patients stopped using oral narcotics at a mean of six days postoperatively.

Duration of operation

Surgical time for MIS is expected to increase because of limited visualisation and increased time spent in obtaining an accurate placement, especially during the initial learning phase [6]. Howell et al [22] (IIa/B) reported a significant (p=0.0001) increase in the mean operation time for MIS THR (97 minutes) as compared to the control (84 minutes). DiGioia et al [10] (IIa/B) reported a longer surgical time (two hours) for the mini-incision group, as compared to the control (one hour 40 minutes) without stating whether this difference was significant.

Ogonda et al [13] (Ib/A) found that the mean operative time for the standard-incision group was 5.6 minutes longer than that for the mini-incision group. They reported that the difference in the initial and the last phase of surgery was significantly higher (p=0.001 and p<0.001 respectively) in the standard-incision group. They felt that the difference in the first phase was related to the fact that the arthroplasty fellow performed 15% of the exposure in the standard-incision group.

Chimento et al [15] (Ib/A), Goldstein et al [8] (IIb/B), Woolson et al [12] (IIb/B), Berger [21] (IIa/B), Chung et al [7] (IIa/B) and de Beer et al [20] (IIa/B) found no significant difference in the surgical time between the conventional and MIS approach. Wright et al [14] (IIa/B), Wenz et al [16] (IIb/B), Nakamura et al [17] (IIa/B) and Higuchi et al [24] (IIb/B), however, found that the operative time significantly decreased in the MIS group.

Intra-operative complications

Limited exposure has obvious implications on adequate visualisation and thus has an inherent risk of intra-operative fractures [12, 21, 22, 26, 27, 29] and nerve injuries [12, 25, 27, 29]. Archibeck et al [29] (III/B) have looked into the learning curve associated with minimally invasive two-incision hip replacement and have noted the complications and problems in the first ten cases of 159 surgeons. They report a rate of 3.2% for neurological injuries and 7.3% for intra-operative fractures. Woolson et al [12] (IIb/B) reported a higher risk of wound complications (p=0.02) in patients undergoing MIS THR.

Fehring et al [30] (IV/C) reported three cases of catastrophic intra-operative complications following minimally invasive hip surgery: in the first, a segmental defect of superior aspect of acetabulum was created during surgery; in the second, poor orientation of the acetabulum led to recurrent dislocation, leading to further surgeries ending up in a large posterior wall defect and pelvic dissociation; in the third, a two-incision technique resulted in a comminuted fracture of the greater trochanter with the operative time being nine hours and 13 minutes.

Siguier et al [25] (III/B) in a series of 1037 MIS hip replacements reported a dislocation rate of 0.96% with the time of dislocation being between two weeks and eight months. They noted two cases of postoperative femoral nerve palsies that resolved completely by one year.

Irving [27] (III/B), during two-incision MIS THR without the use of navigation, reported intra-operative proximal femoral fractures during implant insertion in five of 192 patients. All were managed by cerclage wiring without extending the incision and this did not interfere with the rehabilitation.

Woolson et al [12] (IIb/B) have found a significantly higher risk of wound complications in the MIS group. Ogonda et al [13] (Ib/A) and Chimento et al [15] (Ib/A) have found no significant difference in the complication rates between the two groups.

Postoperative recovery

One of the purported advantages of MIS THR is the early rehabilitation and improvement in limp [6].

Ogonda et al [13] (Ib/A) have shown no significant difference in the walking time and stair climbing at day two after MIS THR. Chimento et al [15] (Ib/A) using a posterior approach MIS, noted a significant decrease in limp at six weeks but could not find any difference in the number of days required to independently transfer, ambulate with a walker, ambulate with a cane, and negotiate stairs. Chung et al [7] (IIa/B) found that the requirement for walking aids was significantly less (p<0.05) in the MIS group (21.4 days) as compared to the standard-incision group (24.8 days).

Dorr [18] (III/B) performed a gait analysis on ten patients undergoing MIS THR and showed a 12.6% increase in velocity, 8.9% increase in cadence and 9.4% increase in stride length, which they suggested is better than the patients with standard-incision hip replacement. Ogonda et al [13] (Ib/A) on the other hand revealed no significant difference between the MIS group and the standard-incision group with respect to the mean step length, mean stride length, mean cadence or mean walking speed in the postoperative period.

Wenz et al [16] (IIb/B) who compared a posterior approach MIS THR with a lateral approach standard THR, reported that the patients in the mini-incision group ambulated significantly sooner than the control and significantly fewer patients needed assistance for supine-to-sit, sit-to-stand, and bed-to-chair transfers.

Berger et al [28] (III/B) reported a rapid recovery in a series of 100 consecutive two-incision MIS THR. Their mean time to discontinue using crutches was six days, the mean time to return to work was eight days and the average time to walk ½ mile was 16 days.

DiGioia et al [10] (IIa/B) reported a significant improvement in Harris Hip Score (HHS), limp and ability to climb stairs at three months and six months, but no significant difference at one year. De Beer et al [20] (IIa/B) on the other hand found no significant difference between the two groups in terms of HHS, Oxford Hip Score and range of motion at six weeks and this was reproduced in the studies by Goldstein et al [8] (IIb/B) and Nakamura et al [17] (IIa/B) who reported no significant difference in the HHS at six weeks.

Length of hospital stay

It might be expected that faster recovery time would lead to an earlier discharge of patients after a MIS hip replacement. The time for hospital stay obviously varies between centres. While Berger et al [28] after two-incision surgery have been able to mobilise and discharge all patients within 23 hours, no other published result reflects a similar rapid recovery process.

Wenz et al [16] (IIb/B), Chung et al [7] (IIa/B), Howell et al [22] (IIa/B) and Berger [21] (IIa/B) have shown that the length of stay is reduced after MIS THR. Chimento et al [15] (Ib/A), Ogonda et al [13] (Ib/A), Woolson et al [12] (IIb/B), Wright et al [14] (IIa/B), and de Beer et al [20] (IIa/B) found no significant difference in the length of hospital stay between the MIS and the standard-incision group. DiGioia et al [10] (IIa/B), despite reporting better recovery at the three-month and six-month stage, did not find any difference in the duration of hospital stay.

Heterotopic ossification

It has been proposed that less dissection and soft tissue damage would lead to less heterotopic ossification. DiGioia et al [10] (IIa/B) have reported a higher incidence of heterotopic ossification in the control group (9.1%), as compared to none for the study group. However, the sample size was too small to detect a statistically significant difference. Irving et al [27] (III/B), in a series of 192 MIS THR through a two-incision approach, reported one case of heterotopic ossification.

Component alignment

Ogonda et al [13] (Ib/A) and Chimento et al [15] (Ib/A) reported no significant difference in the cup or stem alignment and cement grading in the two groups. Hart et al [5] (IIa/B) on the other hand specifically looked at component alignment following posterolateral MIS THR and found no significant difference in the alignment of both the cup and the femoral stem in comparison to the control group. Similarly, de Beer et al [20] (IIa/B), Chung et al [7] (IIa/B) and Wright et al [14] (IIa/B) have reported no difference in component alignment in the control and the MIS group.

Woolson et al [12] (IIb/B) during posterior approach MIS THR reported a higher percentage of acetabular malposition (p=0.04), a higher number of stems in varus alignment (p=0.056), a higher percentage of hips with poor fixation grade or in varus alignment (p=0.02) and a higher percentage with poor fit and fill of femoral components inserted without cement.

Chimento et al [15] (Ib/A), using a posterior approach MIS THR, have noted a higher dislocation rate in the study group (2/28), as compared to the control group (0/32) in their randomised controlled trial. This difference was, however, not statistically significant. Siguier et al [25] (III/B), in a retrospective analysis of 1037 cases of MIS THR through an anterior approach, have reported a dislocation rate of 0.96%.

Patient selection

The technique is difficult in obese patients (Body Mass Index or BMI >30kg/m^2) with a distribution of body fat around thighs and buttocks and even in those with heavily built musculature in these regions [11].

Goldstein et al [8] (IIb/B), Wright et al [14] (IIa/B), Woolson et al [12] (IIb/B), Higuchi et al [24] (IIb/B) and Wenz et al [16] (IIb/B) reported a significantly lower BMI in the MIS group, as compared to the standard approach.

Ogonda et al [13] (Ib/A), Chimento et al [15] (Ib/A), DiGioia et al [10] (IIa/B), de Beer et al [20] (IIa/B) and Nakamura et al [17] (IIa/B) reported no significant difference in the BMI of the two groups. However, Chimento et al [15] (Ib/A) in their randomised controlled trial had excluded patients with a BMI of more than 30kg/m^2.

Wenz et al [16] (IIb/B) have found that a BMI more than and equal to 30kg/m^2 is associated with a significantly higher operative time and estimated blood loss but no significant difference in incision length and component alignment. Archibeck et al [29] (III/B) reported a higher incidence of key complications (p=0.05) in patients with a BMI more than and equal to 30kg/m^2. Goldstein et al [8] (IIb/B) carried out further analysis of 23 MIS THR with a BMI more than and equal to 28kg/m^2 and found that the operative time, postoperative blood loss, the need for transfusion or component position of this group did not differ with the MIS group as a whole or with the standard-incision group.

Another consideration is the nature and degree of hip pathology. A severely dysplastic acetabulum with superior migration of the femoral head, those undergoing revision procedures and those with retained metalwork need more extensive surgery [11]. Wider exposure may again be required for soft tissue release in hips stiffened by contractures [11].

Pre-operative planning

Visualisation of extra-articular landmarks is quite limited in MIS and therefore the importance of pre-operative planning and templating is paramount [21]. The aim is to gather anatomical parameters that would guide accurate placement of femoral and acetabular components and allow restoration of the normal anatomy with correction of any leg length discrepancy [21].

Thornhill [31] suggests that MIS THR should not only focus on a minimal dissection of soft tissues but also other aspects of care "including pre-operative patient teaching and education, use of short-acting anaesthetic agents, and proper patient selection".

Learning curve

Any new procedure carries with it risks during the learning phase and MIS THR is no exception. Surgeons performing a larger volume of THR would be expected to have a shorter learning curve with less complication rates than low volume units.

Archibeck *et al* [29] **(III/B)** looked into the learning curve for the first ten cases of 159 surgeons. Between the first to the tenth case they noted a decrease in operative time ($p<0.05$), fluoroscopy time ($p<0.05$) and blood loss ($p>0.05$). However, the prevalence of key complications in the 49 surgeons who completed an index of ten cases did not show a systematic change. They did report that the complication rate was significantly less for surgeons performing more than 50 THR annually.

While the results of MIS are expected to be reproducible and satisfactory for high volume experienced surgeons, the same may not be true for lower volume and less experienced surgeons [13].

Instrumentation and fluoroscopy

Specialised lighted retractors, low profile acetabular reamers and fluoroscopy have attempted to improve the visualisation during the procedure and help in the performance of MIS safely [32]. Endoscopic light sources temporarily fixed to conventional retractors have been proposed to facilitate illumination and visualisation during surgery, especially for difficult cases in extremely obese patients [33]. Combining the computer-assisted techniques with minimally invasive surgery may help in accurate placement of the components and reduce the need for fluoroscopy [32]. It could increase the accuracy and reproducibility of a number of crucial steps like cup alignment, leg length, femoral offset and anteversion, and femoral stem position and alignment.

A number of single-incision techniques do not require the use of fluoroscopy [8, 13, 15, 16, 20]; however, some have routinely used fluoroscopy to guide the accurate placement of the stem and cup [10]. The two-incision technique, although thought to need imaging routinely [28, 29], has been performed without fluoroscopy by Irving *et al* [27] **(III/B)**.

Conclusions

The informed patient is influencing healthcare by requesting minimally invasive surgical techniques in all areas, including joint replacement surgery [34]. The impetus for minimally invasive hip replacement is multifactorial and includes more rapid patient rehabilitation and patient demand for the newest techniques. Minimally invasive THR is technically possible and the results reproducible, but this may not necessarily translate into an improved outcome in the short or long term. The potential benefit of a smaller incision and possibly somewhat quicker rehabilitation needs to be balanced against the added operative difficulty due to reduced visualisation with the drawbacks of a learning curve. It would appear that further evidence of benefit is needed before MIS techniques are universally adopted.

Recommendations	Evidence level

What is MIS hip replacement?

- There is no single definition but at the current time MIS THR is the insertion of standard prosthetic designs through a modified approach, designed to minimise soft tissue trauma. — Ib/A
- Further aspects of definition involve the length of skin incision, and typically quote length from 6-10cm. — Ib/A
- The approach can be:
  - o a modification of a standard single-incision approach; — Ib/A
  - o or involve two separate incisions. — III/B

Differences between MIS surgery and conventional surgery

- MIS hip replacement is associated with a significantly shorter length of incision. — Ib/A
- Whilst the effect on duration of surgery can vary from an increase to a decrease, the strongest level of evidence relates to a single-incision posterior approach MIS technique and there is no difference with conventional surgery. — Ib/A
- The estimated blood loss is reduced with MIS surgery. — Ib/A
- Concerning the blood transfusion rate in the peri and postoperative period, the strongest level of evidence relates to a single-incision posterior approach and there is no significant difference. — Ib/A
- There have been reports that after a single-incision posterior approach MIS, there may be a reduction in blood transfusion requirement. — IIa/B
- There are various reports of an increase in intra-operative complication rates linked to the learning curve and type of procedure. — III/B
- The strongest level of evidence is that in experienced hands with the single-incision posterior approach MIS technique, there is no increased complication rate. — Ib/A
- There appears to be no significant difference between MIS surgery and conventional surgery in terms of the level of pain or narcotic use after the operation and the strongest level of evidence relates to a single-incision posterior approach MIS technique. — Ib/A
- In terms of length of stay there are various reports and this outcome is influenced by other factors. The strongest level of evidence relates to a single-incision posterior approach MIS technique and it supports that there is no difference in the length of hospital stay. — Ib/A
- After two-incision MIS THR, a single report has suggested that all patients may be discharged within 23 hours. — III/B
- There are variable reports as to improved early rehabilitation after MIS THR, but the strongest evidence is that there is no significant difference in walking and stair climbing after single-incision MIS THR using a posterior approach. — Ib/A

Recommendations *continued:*   **Evidence level**

- The strongest evidence in studies that specifically looked for limp noted a   Ib/A
  significant decrease in the MIS group at six weeks, but not at one year.
- Component alignment and cement grading is an issue and the strongest level   Ib/A
  of evidence relates to a single-incision posterior approach MIS technique,
  suggesting that in experienced hands there is no significant difference in the
  two groups.
- Poor component alignment and fixation grade has been reported after a   IIb/B
  single-incision posterior approach MIS technique.
- The learning curve significantly influences results in terms of the level of   III/B
  experience with the MIS technique and the volume of THRs performed
  annually.

Conclusions reported in the literature:

- Various generalised opinions exist, including the suggestion that MIS   IV/C
  "should not be used to benefit an individual surgeon, a manufacturing
  company, or a hospital" and that "until we have sufficient scientific evidence
  to support its universality, minimally invasive surgery should be performed
  only by surgeons who can evaluate the procedure and thus compare it with
  the conventional technique". [35]
- Rapid rehabilitation after THA using a minimally invasive approach can be   III/B
  done safely in selected patients with excellent results [28].
- It remains our conclusion that for primary THA performed through a direct   IIa/B
  lateral exposure, the length of the skin incision is clinically and functionally
  irrelevant [20].
- THA performed through a minimally invasive approach results in decreased   Ib/A
  measured blood loss at 24 hours and less patients limped at six weeks. At one-
  and two-year follow-up, there is no difference between the two groups [15].
- Minimally invasive total hip arthroplasty performed through a single-   Ib/A
  incision posterior approach by a high-volume hip surgeon with extensive
  experience, is a safe and reproducible procedure, but it offers no significant
  benefit in the early postoperative period compared with a standard incision
  of 16cm [13].

References

1. Abraham NS, Young JM, Solomon MJ. Meta-analysis of short-term outcomes after laparoscopic resection for colorectal cancer. *Br J Surg* 2004; 91(9): 1111-24.
2. Johnson N, Barlow D, Lethaby A, Tavender E, Curr L, Garry R. Methods of hysterectomy: systematic review and meta-analysis of randomised controlled trials. *Br Med J* 2005; 330(7506): 1478.
3. Abbou CC, Hoznek A, Salomon L, Ben Slama MR, Chopin D. Is open surgery for partial nephrectomy an obsolete surgical procedure? *Curr Opin Urol* 1999; 9(5): 383-9.
4. Cameron HU. Mini-incisions: visualisation is the key. *Orthopaedics* 2004; 25(5): 473.
5. Hart R, Stipcak V, Janecek M, Visna P. Component position following total hip arthroplasty through a mini-invasive posterolateral approach. *Acta Orthop Belg* 2005; 71(1): 60-4.
6. Howell JR, Garbuz DS, Duncan PC. Minimally invasive hip replacement: rationale, applied anatomy, and instrumentation. *Orthop Clin N Am* 2004; 35(2): 107-18.
7. Chung WB, Liu D, Foo LSS. Mini-incision total hip replacement - surgical technique and early results. *J Orthop Surg* 2004; 12(1): 19-24.

Chapter 18

8. Goldstein WM, Branson JJ, Berland KA, Gordon AC. Minimal-incision total hip arthroplasty. *J Bone Joint Surg Am* 2003; 85(4): 33-8.

9. Goldstein WM, Branson JJ. Posterior-lateral approach to minimal incision total hip arthroplasty. *Orthop Clin N Am* 2004; 35(2): 131-6.

10. DiGioia AM, Plakseychuk AY, Levison TJ, Jaramaz B. Mini-incision technique for total hip arthroplasty with navigation. *J Arthroplasty* 2003; 18(2): 123-8.

11. Sculco TP, Jordan LC, Walter W. Minimally invasive total hip arthroplasty: the hospital for special surgery experience. *Orthop Clin N Am* 2004; 35(2): 137-42

12. Woolson ST, Mow CS, Syquila JF, Lannin JV, Schurmann DJ. Total hip replacement performed with a standard incision or a mini incision. *J Bone Joint Surg Am* 2004; 86(7): 1353-8.

13. Ogonda L, Wilson R, Archbold P, Lawlor M, Humphreys P, O'Brien S, Beverland D. A minimal-incision technique in total hip arthroplasty does not improve early postoperative outcomes. A prospective, randomized, controlled trial. *J Bone Joint Surg Am* 2005; 87(4): 701-10.

14. Wright JM, Crockett HC, Delgado S, Lyman S, Madsen M, Sculco TP. Mini-incision for total hip arthroplasty: a prospective, controlled investigation with 5-year follow-up. *J Arthroplasty* 2004; 19(5): 538-45.

15. Chimento GF, Pavone V, Sharrock N, Kahn B, Cahill J, Sculco TP. Mini-incision total hip arthroplasty: a comparative assessment of perioperative outcomes. *J Arthroplasty* 2005; 20(2): 139-44.

16. Wenz JF, Gurkan I, Jibodh SR. Mini-incision total hip arthroplasty: a comparative assessment of perioperative outcomes. *Orthopedics* 2002; 25(10): 1031-43.

17. Nakamura S, Matsuda K, Arai N, Wakimoto N, Matsushita T. Mini-incision posterior approach for total hip arthroplasty. *Int Orthop* 2004; 28(4): 214-7.

18. Dorr LD. The mini-incision hip: building a ship in a bottle. *Orthopedics* 2004; 27(2): 192-3.

19. Hartzband MA. Posterolateral minimal incision for total hip replacement: technique and early results. *Orthop Clin N Am* 2004; 35(2): 119-29.

20. de Beer J, Petruccelli D, Zalzal P, Winemaker MJ. Single-incision, minimally invasive total hip arthroplasty: length doesn't matter. *J Arthroplasty* 2004; 19(8): 945-50.

21. Berger RA. Mini-incision total hip replacement using an anterolateral approach: technique and results. *Orthop Clin N Am* 2004; 35(2): 143-51.

22. Howell JR, Masri BA, Duncan CP. Minimally invasive versus standard-incision anterolateral hip replacement: a comparative study. *Orthop Clin N Am* 2004; 35(2): 153-62.

23. Bertin KC, Rottinger H. Anterolateral mini-incision hip replacement surgery: a modified Watson-Jones approach. *Clin Orthop Relat Res* 2004; 429: 248-55.

24. Higuchi F, Gotoh M, Yamaguchi N, Suzuki R, Kunou Y, Ooishi K, Nagata K. Minimally invasive uncemented total hip arthroplasty through an anterolateral approach with a shorter skin incision. *J Orthop Sci* 2003; 8(6): 812-7.

25. Siguier T, Siguier M, Brumpt B. Mini-incision anterior approach does not increase dislocation rate: a study of 1037 total hip replacements. *Clin Orthop Relat Res* 2004; 426: 164-73.

26. Berger RA, Duwelius PJ. The two-incision minimally invasive total hip arthroplasty: technique and results. *Orthop Clin N Am* 2004; 35(2): 163-72.

27. Irving JF. Direct two-incision total hip replacement without fluoroscopy. *Orthop Clin N Am* 2004; 35(2): 173-81.

28. Berger RA, Jacobs JJ, Meneghini RM, Valle CD, Paprosky W, Rosenberg AG. Rapid rehabilitation and recovery with minimally invasive total hip arthroplasty. *Clin Orthop Relat Res* 2004; 429: 239-47.

29. Archibeck MJ, White RE. Learning curve for the two-incision total hip replacement. *Clin Orthop Relat Res* 2004; 429: 232-8.

30. Fehring TK, Mason JB. Catastrophic complications of minimally invasive hip surgery. *J Bone Joint Surg Am* 2005; 87(4): 711-4.

31. Thornhill TS. The mini-incision hip: proceed with caution. *Orthopaedics* 2004; 27(2): 193-4.

32. Stulberg SD. The rationale for using computer navigation with minimally invasive THA. *Orthopedics* 2004; 27(9): 942-6.

33. Suarez-Suarez MA, Murcia-Mazon A. A simple method to facilitate mini-incision in total hip arthroplasty. *J Arthroplasty* 2004; 19(3): 395-6.

34. Rodrigo JJ. Minimally invasive hip surgery. *Orthopaedics* 2002; 25(10): 1016-28.

35. Ranawat CS, Ranawat AS. Minimally invasive total joint arthroplasty: where are we going? *J Bone Joint Surg Am* 2003; 85(11): 2070-1.

Chapter 19

Surgical management of the infected hip prosthesis

Matthew Revell BSc MB BS FRCS (Tr & Orth)
5th Cavendish Hip Fellow [1]
Ian Stockley MD FRCS
Consultant Orthopaedic Surgeon [1]
Paul Norman MA MSc MB FRCPath
Consultant Microbiologist [2]

1 LOWER LIMB ARTHROPLASTY UNIT, DEPARTMENT OF ORTHOPAEDICS
2 DEPARTMENT OF MICROBIOLOGY
THE NORTHERN GENERAL HOSPITAL, SHEFFIELD, UK

Introduction

The treatment of patients with prosthetic hip infection is a challenging area of reconstructive joint surgery. In this chapter we outline our approach to management with reference to the evidence base in the orthopaedic literature. There are many aspects of the subject that are controversial: the best method for diagnosis; the role of debridement and washout; the relative merits of one-stage or two-stage revision; and the efficacy of locally delivered or systemically administered antibiotics.

It is essential that the care of these patients should be multidisciplinary. Interpretation of the microbiological data requires experience and a sound knowledge of surgical principles. Treatment should be tailored to the needs of the individual, taking into account the surgical expertise and experience available in the arthroplasty unit. There are some cases where suppression of infection with antibiotics is more appropriate than further surgery, such as when patient comorbidity would mean a significant risk to life if an operation were to be undertaken [1, 2]. If this kind of management regime is being considered, it is essential that the prosthesis be soundly fixed, that the infective organism has been identified and its antibiotic sensitivity profile is known.

Our recommendations, as well as areas of current controversy, are summarised in tabular form at the end of this chapter.

Methodology

Citations were searched using the Endnote (Thomson Corporation, Stamford, Conneticut, USA) reference manager to run a text-based search of the PubMed bibliographic database (National Library of Medicine, National Institutes of Health, USA). Individual searches were carried out corresponding to each subheading of this chapter, as well as a catch-all search; 'infection' and 'hip replacement' or 'hip arthroplasty'.

The pathophysiology of prosthetic joint infection

Some bacteria will enter the operative field at the time of surgery. There is a broad base of literature regarding bacterial counts in theatre [3] **(IIb/B)** and the need for minimising them, in order to bring infection rates down to the lowest possible level [4] **(III/B)**.

Bacteria may also reach the hip through haematogenous seeding from a separate site of primary sepsis. It is difficult to say why some patients become infected and others do not, considering the degree of bacterial contamination identified at surgery [5]. It seems safe to assume that, as well as surgical and environmental influences, patient factors play an important role (especially those relating to immune function) in the development of clinical infection. Bacteria approach the surface of an artificial joint through an interaction of physical and chemical forces. Once bacteria have a hold near the prosthesis, it will provide no protection against colonisation because of its relative immunological inertness [6, 7]. The bacteria bind and multiply. Specific bonds between bacteria and biomaterial vary with species and the composition of the implant: *Staphylococcus aureus* (*S. aureus*), for example, is thought to have an affinity for metal alloys; *Pseudomonas* for polymers. Antibiotics can also interact with the surface of the implant to inhibit bacterial adherence [8]. Most infecting micro-organisms produce some form of glycocalyx (or 'slime layer') which enhances nutrition and acts as an exopolysaccharide barrier to host immunological defences, moderating susceptibility to phagocytosis and antibodies [9]. Not only are bacteria sequestered from immune response, the penetration of antibiotics is reduced and this can lead to reduced efficacy with a higher probability of developing antibiotic resistance. Best known for this behaviour are the staphylococci, including *S. aureus* and the coagulase-negative staphylococci (CNS), such as *Staphylococcus epidermidis* (*S. epidermidis*), as well as the *Pseudomonas* species.

The pre-operative diagnosis of deep infection

History (IV/C)

Many patients will report that the joint has never, in fact, felt quite right. The commonest presentation is groin or thigh pain. The pain may be mechanical, occurring when the joint is moved or loaded, or non-mechanical and unrelated to physical activity. Early onset following the index procedure is suggestive of peri-operative inoculation. When looking back, it is often possible to see that some patients who develop infection have had a prolonged hospital stay, early wound problems, or repeated courses of antibiotic from their general practitioner. Onset of pain after a problem-free interval and an episode of sepsis is suggestive of haematogenous seeding of infective organisms from elsewhere. In these cases it is sensible to attempt to identify the source of bacteraemia (e.g. skin, dentition, urinary tract).

Examination (IV/C)

In the early stages, clinical examination may be of little value. Range of motion may be limited. The hip may be irritable. A frank abscess or sinus leaves little doubt over the diagnosis. More commonly, there is subtle induration, discolouration or no external sign of an underlying problem, meaning that further investigation is necessary to confirm the diagnosis.

Investigations

Further tests, based on clinical suspicion, are required to confirm the diagnosis of infection and establish the identity and sensitivities of the organism(s) causing it. If these are to help refine clinical information, it is important that they are sensitive (able to pick up truly infected cases) and specific (able to exclude appropriately those cases which are not infected) (Table 1). When evaluating such tests, authors may also refer to the positive predictive value (the probability that a patient with a positive result genuinely has infection - PPV) and the negative predictive value (the probability that a patient with a negative test result has genuinely avoided infection - NPV). Combining investigations often improves the accuracy of diagnosis.

Blood tests (IIb/B)

In the UK, it is normal practice, when infection is suspected, to measure the 'inflammatory markers' in the blood: the C-Reactive Protein (CRP) and the Erythrocyte Sedimentation Rate (ESR), as well as the white cell count (WCC). We would regard an ESR of

Table 1. Assessing the accuracy of investigations for infected hip replacement.

	Test positive	Test negative	
Truly infected cases	True positives = a	False negatives = b	Sensitivity = a/(a+b)
Truly uninfected cases	False positives = c	True negatives = d	Specificity = d/(c+d)
	Positive predictive value = a/(a+c)	Negative predictive value = b/(b+d)	Accuracy = (a+c)/(a+b+c+d)

30mm/hour or greater as being grounds for suspicion of present infection, mindful of the fact that the ESR may take up to a year to return to its normal value after the index operation [10]. The negative predictive value of a low ESR (approximately 95%) is often of more use than a raised ESR (positive predictive value 58%) [11] (Table 2). A cut-off value of 10mg/litre is the upper end of normality for CRP. The usual pattern after surgery is for the CRP to rise acutely for about 48 hours and then to decline fairly rapidly over two to three weeks in the absence of continuing infection; it is therefore more useful in gauging the success of surgical intervention in the early postoperative period [12, 13]. The accuracy improves if the results of both tests are considered together and the highest rewards come from monitoring their change over time. Typically, when a hip is infected, they will remain chronically raised. The WCC, although always checked, is seldom raised except in cases of obvious systemic sepsis. Patients with longstanding infection may develop anaemia and raised platelet counts are also seen.

Imaging (IIb/B)

Plain radiographs are obligatory, but unfortunately can be normal. Infection is suggested by radiolucent lines, osteolysis and scalloping around the infected prosthesis, or a periosteal reaction [14], but the appearances in aseptic loosening can be very similar. It is most helpful to look at the evolution of any changes over time by assessing serial radiographs. The speed of progression is important; infective loosening tends to be more rapidly progressive than aseptic loosening.

A radio-isotope scan may be a useful adjunct, but results are open to variable interpretation. The reported

Table 2. The accuracy of diagnostic interventions in the diagnosis of peri-prosthetic hip infection [11].

	Sensitivity	Specificity	PPV	NPV
ESR (>30)	0.82	0.85	0.58	0.95
CRP (>10)	0.96	0.92	0.74	0.99
Aspiration	0.86	0.94	0.67	0.98
Frozen section	0.80	0.94	0.74	0.96
ESR and CRP			0.83	1.00 (0.96-1.00)
ESR, CRP and aspiration			0.89	1.00 (0.96-1.00)

Chapter 19

accuracy varies greatly [15, 16]. We consider it to be a sensitive investigation, but it is often not specific enough to help diagnose infection routinely [17]. Technetium-99m scanning will show increased isotope uptake, even in an uninfected hip, for up to 18 months after joint replacement. False negative investigations may result when the infective process interferes with local blood supply (e.g. by a soft tissue swelling or collection causing pressure). Gallium 67 citrate scanning has been added to improve accuracy [18]. Indium 111-labelled white cell scans have also been employed. Their usefulness is limited by cost and time constraints, but as additional investigations, they improve the sensitivity and specificity of technetium scanning used alone [19].

Magnetic resonance imaging, computed tomograpy [20] and ultrasound [17] are rarely used, except to demonstrate the extent of soft tissue involvement.

Aspiration or biopsy (IIb/B)

Hip aspiration offers the only possibility of pre-operatively determining the infective micro-organism and learning its antibiotic sensitivity profile (Table 3). Here, again, the evidence should be interpreted with caution. The often-cited paper by Barrack and Harris suggests that given the low incidence of hip infection, the low detection rate for true infection should deter its use in all revision cases [21]. The incidence of infection in this series was only 2%, leading other authors to question the extent to which these results should be extrapolated to patients where the index of suspicion for infection is high [22]. Aspiration has a high PPV, but is less useful when the implant has been *in situ* for a long period (e.g. five years or more) [23] or in the absence of

Table 3. Sensitivity and specificity of hip aspiration for infection.

Author	Specificity %	Sensitivity %
Elson 1991 [22]	87	84
Roberts 1992 [26]	95	87
Lachiewicz 1996 [25]	97	92
Spangehl 1999 [11]	94	86
Williams 2004 [27]	94	80

raised inflammatory markers [24, 25]. Accuracy is improved by ensuring that any course of antibiotics is discontinued two to three weeks before the procedure, by immediate inoculation of samples to appropriate culture media and rapid transfer to the laboratory. Williams *et al* examined 273 consecutive hip revisions that underwent aspiration and tissue biopsy, comparing the investigation results with those from specimens obtained ultimately at operation. Twenty-six percent (71) were infected. The sensitivity of aspiration was found to be 80% and the specificity 94%. These figures are in broad agreement with the findings of other authors (Table 1) [11, 25-27]. In the Williams study, the sensitivity of biopsy was 83% with a specificity of 90% and, therefore, the authors found little to support the more invasive biopsy procedure over aspiration alone.

Frozen section (IIb/B)

This investigation can only be performed at operation and therefore does not help with pre-operative diagnosis. With the interpretation of an experienced pathologist it can supplement the information obtained from surgical specimens. If ten polymorphs per high-powered field are used to define infection, the investigation may have a specificity as high as 99% with a sensitivity of 84% [28]. The recommended thresholds for identification and the number of high-power fields that should be inspected vary greatly between major centres [29-31].

Polymerase chain reaction (PCR) (IIb/B)

Amplification of microbial DNA using appropriate primers in a polymerase chain reaction allows the detection of bacteria in small numbers. The method therefore promises improved sensitivity in diagnosing infection [32]. There are a few drawbacks that currently limit its potential. It cannot offer knowledge of bacterial sensitivities directly. It has been found in at least one study to give positive results in what otherwise would have been regarded as cases of aseptic loosening [33]. In cases where more than one organism is detected, it does not identify a primary agent. We regard it as a possible aid to diagnosis in the future. More refinement of PCR techniques and experience in interpreting the results are required before it comes into routine practice.

Multiple investigations

As a general rule, the more investigation modalities that are used, the better the accuracy in diagnosis. Cost and practicality limit the number of tests and most cases can be diagnosed on the basis of clinical history, examination, blood investigations and hip aspiration, where indicated.

The range of surgical interventions

Surgical debridement

Debridement and washout with retention of the original prosthesis is a less aggressive surgical procedure than prosthesis removal. In the first three weeks after the initial operation, it offers success rates of up to 84%. Lower success rates (56%) are reported between three and six weeks [34]. In haematogenous infection, the diagnosis and referral are often delayed, as the onset of symptoms can be insidious. Debridement remains an option here, particularly for the infirm. The success rate here is probably not greater than one in three of those treated within the first month [34-36]. Gustilo reported a 71% success rate in the treatment of early postoperative infections and a 50% success rate treating haematogenous infection. The clinical picture with hips can be ambiguous for some time, leading to a tendency to make the diagnosis later than, for example, with an infected total knee replacement, where signs and symptoms are usually apparent at an earlier stage. Provided there is no radiological evidence of loosening and the time from onset of infection is thought to be short, we regard debridement as a safe surgical option.

Surgical exchange of hip prosthesis

While debridement alone can be helpful under special conditions, a more effective approach in established infection is to remove the infected implant and re-implant a new prosthesis. This offers the best chance of maximising function at the same time as clearing the infection. The two stages can be done separately or at the same time. The same underlying principles hold good for both. With either method, it is vital that the microbiological information obtained is as accurate and comprehensive as possible. We recommend taking at least five tissue specimens as soon as the joint is entered, using a new scalpel and forceps. Early transfer of specimens to the laboratory improves results. Intra-operative antibiotics are withheld until the samples have been obtained [37, 38].

The use of antibiotics (III/B)

Antibiotics can be given systemically or delivered to the infected area by adding them to bone cement. Where possible, we prefer to use the latter, local delivery method, because it produces far higher antibiotic levels in the area they are required [39].

We know that local levels of antibiotic are enhanced by increasing the concentration of antibiotic within the cement and that elution is improved if more than one antibiotic is used, raising the porosity of the cement [40, 41]. The choice of any additional agent is made either with knowledge of the extended sensitivity profile of the organism from culture, or by knowledge of the typical sensitivity profile of similar organisms based on local experience, if the precise sensitivities are not yet known. Common supplementary antibiotics include the amino-glycosides (e.g. gentamicin, tobramycin and amikacin) and the glycopeptides (e.g. vancomycin and teicoplanin) (Table 4). If cement beads are being used to clear infection following implant removal, the mechanical properties of the bone cement are unimportant. When antibiotics are added to cement at the time of re-implantation, *in vitro* studies suggest that the addition of antibiotics to cement carries a theoretical risk of lowering its mechanical strength [42]. *In vivo* studies, however, suggest that up to 10% of the cement can be substituted with antibiotic at the time of re-implantation with no difference in mechanical survival at 13 years (this would translate to up to 4g vancomycin per 40g mix of Palacos R® cement in our unit, for example) [22]. The main aim of infected arthroplasty surgery is to eradicate infection and if mechanical failure occurs in a sterile arthroplasty, this is preferable to failure due to infection. Some antibiotics are not suitable for addition

Table 4. Antibiotics added to polymethylmethacrylate cement.

	Typical organism sensitivities	
	Often effective	**Not usually effective**
Antibiotics in common use		
Gentamicin	Enterobacteriaceae Pseudomonas Many *S. aureus* (including some MRSA in the UK) Some *S. epidermidis sp*	Streptococci Enterococci
Tobramycin	Similar to gentamicin with improved efficacy against *Pseudomonas sp*	Similar to gentamicin
Vancomycin	Most gram-positive organisms	Some enterococci (e.g. vancomycin-resistant enterococcus - VRE)
Antibiotics used with reported success		
Clindamycin	*S. aureus* (MSSA and some MRSA) Streptococci Certain anaerobes	
Ciprofloxacin	Enterobacteriaceae Pseudomonas MSSA Some CNS	
Penicillins and cephalosporins	Variable heat degradation properties and local tissue levels	

Chapter 19

to bone cement. The heat from the exothermic polymerisation of cement inactivates chloramphenicol and tetracycline, as well as some penicillins, while other antibiotics (e.g. rifampicin) interfere with the polymerisation process itself [43]. In the rare case of fungal infection, both amphotericin and fluconozole have been used with success [22, 44].

Direct exchange (III/B)

Removal of the infected prosthesis, debridement and re-implantation of a new prosthesis offers improved efficacy over debridement alone. For the patient, it offers the potential of eradicating the infection with only one operation and therefore avoids the morbidity of a temporary pseudarthrosis and a second major surgical procedure. There is no opportunity for limb and muscle to shorten or scar, making re-implantation technically more straightforward. The outlook is improved if the condition of the soft tissues and the femoral bone stock, in particular, are favourable. It is generally accepted that single-stage revision is less successful in clearing infection than a two-stage revision, particularly with virulent or resistant micro-organisms [45, 46]. Nevertheless, the reported success rates of direct exchange are good in some centres [47, 48], if appropriate antibiotics are added in powdered form to bone cement mix. It is a very reasonable option, particularly when the organism is known to be of low virulence and the bone stock is good [49].

Staged exchange (III/B)

Two-staged exchange is often regarded as the gold standard treatment for the surgical eradication of peri-prosthetic infection. Radical debridement along with insertion of depot antibiotic is the first part of a staged revision. We make polymethylmethacrylate (PMMA) beads (Palacos R®) during surgery and mix in further antibiotic powders as required. There has been some research into alternative antibiotic carriers with superior elution profiles [50]. At present, the convenience and cost of PMMA, as well as its ease of preparation, lead us to continue to recommend its use. Adverse effects from systemic absorption have not been reported [43]. Many centres advocate the use of a four to six-week course of systemic antibiotic in addition, but the evidence for any particular length of systemic treatment is patchy. We may use systemic antibiotics when the intra-operative cultures suggest that the organism is not fully sensitive to the antibiotic we have added to the beads. Two-staged exchange with the use of an antibiotic spacer has a success rate thought to exceed 90% [34].

The role of antibiotic carrier may be combined with that of a spacer device, designed to preserve, as far as possible, normal length and relative position [51, 52]. The aim is to facilitate exposure at the reconstruction stage and thereby reduce morbidity. If used, the spacer should aim to preserve the normal relationship between structures, allow reasonable attempts at mobilisation on the affected limb, be relatively straightforward to remove and it should be a suitable vector for local antibiotic delivery. We have little experience of such spacers, as we have not found soft tissue shortening to be a major cause for concern.

The timing of re-implantation is guided by the clinical progress of the patient. Monitoring the ESR and CRP as they fall, following successful clearance of the infective organism is helpful. Those who treat patients with systemic antibiotic require the patient to complete a full course prior to reconstruction. Some prefer the added reassurance of obtaining a negative joint aspirate after a short period without antibiotic treatment. In our centre, we rely largely on clinical and blood markers, as we feel the technical difficulties of aspirating a pseudarthrosis potentially undermine its accuracy. Most centres delay the second stage by a minimum of six weeks, but it may be three to six months, or even longer. There is no absolute indication for proceeding with reconstruction if the health or preferences of the patient prohibit it. The patient may choose to continue without re-implantation if the functional outcome is thought to be acceptable when considered against the risks of proceeding to re-implantation. Almost all such patients will require a walking aid of some description and a shoe-raise.

Excision arthroplasty (III/B)

While it remains an option after a first-stage revision, excision arthroplasty is rarely used as a first-line treatment method. It is reserved for those patients where limited mobility is expected in the light of pre-morbid function or is acceptable because of anticipated operative risks. The reported results in terms of pain relief from this procedure are variable. Independent ambulation with a walking aid is achieved in many patients but by no means all [53-55].

Surgical choices at re-implantation

There are a wide variety of implants available. This reflects the divergent preferences of individual surgeons, as well as the different requirements for reconstruction. It is important that the surgeon is using a prosthesis with which he is comfortable.

Cemented or uncemented prosthesis (III/B)

While we recommend that antibiotic-impregnated cement should be used at the time of re-implantation in single-stage exchange for infection, its use is not mandatory in the two-stage model. On occasions the pattern of femoral bone loss prohibits a cemented

Table 5. Comparison of success rates for staged revision results and the use of antibiotic-loaded cement in 1641 patients collated from a number of individual studies [34].

% Success	Direct exchange	Two-stage revision
Antibiotic-loaded cement	86	93
No antibiotic	59	86

prosthesis. There are strong advocates of uncemented stem designs in these cases. Langlais has reviewed 29 articles, relating to 1641 patients. He found that higher cure rates were associated with a two-staged exchange and antibiotic-loaded cement (93%) than with a direct exchange and no antibiotic cement (59%) (Table 5). These findings are in broad agreement with other authors [56]. Our approach with the two-stage technique is that the choice of prosthesis is made on the basis of the mechanical environment, the surgeon's preference, and his familiarity with various prosthesis types. One must assume, if the inflammatory markers and the clinical and intra-operative findings agree, that the first stage of the procedure has been successful in eradicating infection as planned. We believe that, in serial procedures, each use of antibiotic-loaded cement increases the chance of clearing the infection [57].

The use of allograft and massive endoprostheses (III/B)

During reconstruction, we may use allograft or massive endoprosthetic replacement. The choice relates to the individual needs of the patient and the quality of the bone stock. It will often be the case that younger patients will receive allograft in an attempt to reconstitute bony architecture, while older patients may be better served with a massive endoprosthesis, which is expected to involve a shorter operation. The level of difficulty in obtaining consistent good results under such end-stage conditions should not be underestimated [58], but results in experienced hands are encouraging, as long as patients are monitored closely [59]. Studies have suggested that there is not a increased re-infection rate [5, 60].

Conclusions

A complex series of choices lies before an arthroplasty surgeon when embarking on the treatment of an infected hip replacement. The tremendous delay before meaningful feedback data can be retrieved after the initial management decisions have been made mean that evidence above level III (a retrospective review) is hard to come by.

With the added value of experience, sensible schemes of treatment can be based around the evidence available. We regard a two-staged revision of the infected implant, with the use of antibiotic-impregnated cement beads between the procedures and a cemented second-stage prosthesis as being currently the most efficacious method of clearing infection in the hands of most surgeons. Other methods are acceptable in certain circumstances. At the time of re-implantation, the choice of prosthesis is decided primarily by the mechanical environment, the quality of the remaining bone stock and surgeon preference.

Recommendations	Evidence level

Not controversial

- ◆ A multidisciplinary approach is the successful model. — IV/C
- ◆ Accurate culture and sensitivity reports by a microbiologist with a special interest in joint infections is highly desirable. — IV/C
- ◆ Antibiotics should be tailored to the sensitivities of the infecting organism. — IV/C
- ◆ Properly performed surgical debridement is the pre-requisite of any other treatment method. — IV/C
- ◆ Always take cultures of tissue for microbiology if a surgical procedure is carried out (we recommend an odd number of cultures). — IV/C
- ◆ Whether or not systemic antibiotics are given, local antibiotic delivery from beads or cement improves clearance. The aims of treatment are: — III/B
  - o eradication of infection;
  - o alleviation of pain;
  - o restoration of function.

Areas of ongoing debate

- ◆ The limitations of debridement and washout.
- ◆ The role for direct exchange of the infected prosthesis.
- ◆ The acceptability of any extra morbidity associated with a two-stage exchange.
- ◆ The number of times attempts to clear infection surgically may be carried out before clearance of the micro-organism is deemed unobtainable.

References

1. Rao N, *et al*. Long-term suppression of infection in total joint arthroplasty. *Clin Orthop Relat Res* 2003; 414: 55-60.

2. Widmer A, *et al*. Antimicrobial treatment of orthopedic implant-related infections with rifampicin combinations. *Clin Infect Dis* 1992; 14: 1251-3.

3. Davis N, *et al*. Intraoperative bacterial contamination in operations for joint replacement. *J Bone Joint Surg Br* 1999; 81-B(Sep): 886-9.

4. Lidwell OM. Clean air at operation and subsequent sepsis in the joint. *Clin Orthop Relat Res* 1986; 211: 91-102.

5. Ammon P, Stockley I. Allograft bone in two-stage revision of the hip for infection. Is it safe? *J Bone Joint Surg Br* 2004; 86(7): 962-5.

6. Gristina AG, Naylor PT, Webb LX. Molecular mechanisms in musculoskeletal sepsis: the race for the surface. *Instr Course Lect* 1990; 39: 471-82.

7. Gristina A, Norman P, Myrvik Q. Molecular mechanisms of musculoskeletal sepsis. In: *Musculoskeletal Infection*. Esterjhai J, Gristina A, Poss R, Eds. American Academy of Orthopaedic Surgeons Symposium, 1992.

8. Oga M, Arizono T, Sugioka Y. Inhibition of bacterial adhesion by tobramycin-impregnated PMMA bone cement. *Acta Orthop Scand* 1992; 63(3): 301-4.

9. McAuley JP, Moreau G. Sepsis: Etiology, Prophylaxis and Diagnosis. In: *The Adult Hip*. Callaghan JJ, Rosenberg AG, Rubash HE, Eds. Philadelphia: Lippincot-Raven, 1998: 1295-306.

10. Forster IW, Crawford R. Sedimentation rate in infected and uninfected total hip arthroplasty. *Clin Orthop* 1982; 168: 48.

11. Spangehl MJ, *et al*. Prospective analysis of preoperative and intraoperative investigations for the diagnosis of infection at the sites of two hundred and two revision total hip arthroplasties. *J Bone Joint Surg Am* 1999; 81(5): 672-83.

12. Aalto K, *et al*. Changes in erythrocyte sedimentation rate and C-reactive protein after total hip arthroplasty. *Clin Orthop Relat Res* 1984; 184: 118-20.

13. Choudhry RR, *et al*. Plasma viscosity and C-reactive protein after total hip and knee arthroplasty. *J Bone Joint Surg Br* 1992; 74(4): 523-4.

14. Fitzgerald RH, Jr. Infected total hip arthroplasty: diagnosis and treatment. *J Am Acad Orthop Surg* 1995; 3(5): 249.

15. Della Valle CJ, Zuckerman JD, Di Cesare PE. Periprosthetic sepsis. *Clin Orthop Relat Res* 2004; 420: 26-31.

16. Kraemer WJ, *et al*. Bone scan, gallium scan, and hip aspiration in the diagnosis of infected total hip arthroplasty. *J Arthroplasty* 1993; 8(6): 611-6.

17. Spangehl MJ, *et al*. Diagnosis of infection following total hip arthroplasty. *Instr Course Lect* 1998; 47: 285-95.

18. Itasaka T, *et al*. Diagnosis of infection after total hip arthroplasty. *J Orthop Sci* 2001; 6(4): 320-6.

19. Merkel KD, *et al*. Comparison of indium-labeled-leukocyte imaging with sequential technetium-gallium scanning in the diagnosis of low-grade musculoskeletal sepsis. A prospective study. *J Bone Joint Surg Am* 1985; 67(3): 465-76.

20. Cyteval C, *et al*. Painful infection at the site of hip prosthesis: CT imaging. *Radiology* 2002; 224(2): 477-83.

21. Barrack RL, Harris WH. The value of aspiration of the hip joint before revision total hip arthroplasty. *J Bone Joint Surg Am* 1993; 75(1): 66-76.

22. Elson RA. Sepsis: one-stage exchange. *The Adult Hip*. Callaghan JJ, Rosenberg AG, Rubash HE, Eds. Philadelphia: Lippincot-Raven, 1998: 1307-16.

23. Somme D, *et al*. Contribution of routine joint aspiration to the diagnosis of infection before hip revision surgery. *Joint Bone Spine* 2003; 70(6): 489-95.

24. Fehring TK, Cohen B. Aspiration as a guide to sepsis in revision total hip arthroplasty. *J Arthroplasty* 1996; 11(5): 543-7.

25. Lachiewicz PF, Rogers GD, Thomason HC. Aspiration of the hip joint before revision total hip arthroplasty. Clinical and laboratory factors influencing attainment of a positive culture. *J Bone Joint Surg Am* 1996; 78(5): 749-54.

26. Roberts P, Walters AJ, McMinn DJ. Diagnosing infection in hip replacements. The use of fine-needle aspiration and radiometric culture. *J Bone Joint Surg Br* 1992; 74(2): 265-9.

27. Williams JL, Norman P, Stockley I. The value of hip aspiration versus tissue biopsy in diagnosing infection before exchange hip arthroplasty surgery. *J Arthroplasty* 2004; 19(5): 582-6.

28. Lonner JH, *et al*. The reliability of analysis of intraoperative frozen sections for identifying active infection during revision hip or knee arthroplasty. *J Bone Joint Surg Am* 1996; 78(10): 1553-8.

29. Athanasou NA, *et al*. Diagnosis of infection by frozen section during revision arthroplasty. *J Bone Joint Surg Br* 1995; 77(1): 28-33.

30. Feldman DS, *et al*. The role of intraoperative frozen sections in revision total joint arthroplasty. *J Bone Joint Surg Am* 1995; 77(12): 1807-13.

31. Athanasou N, *et al*. Correspondence. *J Bone Joint Surg Am* 1997; 79: 1433-4.

32. Mariani BD, *et al*. The Coventry Award. Polymerase chain reaction detection of bacterial infection in total knee arthroplasty. *Clin Orthop Relat Res* 1996; 331: 11-22.

33. Clarke MT, *et al*. Polymerase chain reaction can detect bacterial DNA in aseptically loose total hip arthroplasties. *Clin Orthop Relat Res* 2004; 427: 132-7.

34. Langlais F, Lambotte JC, Thomazeau H. Treatment of Infected Total Hip Replacement. *In: EFORT - European Instructional Course Lectures*. Lemaire R, *et al*, Eds. London: British Editorial Society of Bone and Joint Surgery, 2003.

35. Tattevin P, *et al*. Prosthetic joint infection: when can prosthesis salvage be considered? *Clin Infect Dis* 1999; 29(2): 292-5.

36. Crockarell JR, *et al*. Treatment of infection with debridement and retention of the components following hip arthroplasty. *J Bone Joint Surg Am* 1998; 80(9): 1306-13.

37. Atkins BL, *et al*. Prospective evaluation of criteria for microbiological diagnosis of prosthetic-joint infection at revision arthroplasty. The OSIRIS Collaborative Study Group. *J Clin Microbiol* 1998; 36(10): 2932-9.

38. Atkins BL, Bowler IC. The diagnosis of large joint sepsis. *J Hosp Infect* 1998; 40(4): 263-74.

39. Salvati EA, *et al*. Reimplantation in infection. A 12-year experience. *Clin Orthop* 1982; 170(62): 62-75.

40. Wahlig H, *et al*. Pharmacokinetic study of gentamicin-loaded cement in total hip replacements. Comparative effects of varying dosage. *J Bone Joint Surg Br* 1984; 66(2): 175-9.

41. Murray WR. Use of antibiotic-containing bone cement. *Clin Orthop Relat Res* 1984; 190: 89-95.

42. Lee A, Ling R, Vangala S. The mechanical properties of bone cements. *J Med Eng Tech* 1977; 1: 137-40.

43. Youngman JR, Ridgway GL, Haddad FS, Antibiotic-loaded cement in revision joint replacement. *Hosp Med* 2003; 64(10): 613-6.

44. Marra F, *et al*. Amphotericin B loaded bone cement to treat osteomyelitis caused by *Candida albicans*. *Can J Surg* 2001; 444: 383-6.

45. Hanssen AD, Osmon DR. Assessment of patient selection criteria for treatment of the infected hip arthroplasty. *Clin Orthop Relat Res* 2000; 381: 91-100.

46. Ure KJ, *et al*. Direct-exchange arthroplasty for the treatment of infection after total hip replacement. An average ten-year follow-up. *J Bone Joint Surg Am* 1998; 80(7): 961-8.

47. Wroblewski BM. One-stage revision of infected cemented total hip arthroplasty. *Clin Orthop Relat Res* 1986; 211: 103-7.

48. Steinbrink K, Frommelt L. Treatment of periprosthetic infection of the hip using one-stage exchange surgery. *Orthopade* 1995; 24(4): 335-43.

49. Hanssen AD, Rand JA. Evaluation and treatment of infection at the site of a total hip or knee arthroplasty. *Instr Course Lect* 1999; 48: 111-22.

50. Penner MJ, Duncan CP, Masri BA. The *in vitro* elution characteristics of antibiotic-loaded CMW and Palacos-R bone cements. *J Arthroplasty* 1999; 14(2): 209-14.

51. Younger AS, Duncan CP, Masri BA. Treatment of infection associated with segmental bone loss in the proximal part of the femur in two stages with use of an antibiotic-loaded interval prosthesis. *J Bone Joint Surg Am* 1998; 80(1): 60-9.

52. Younger AS, *et al*. The outcome of two-stage arthroplasty using a custom-made interval spacer to treat the infected hip. *J Arthroplasty* 1997; 12(6): 615-23.

53. Bittar ES, Petty W. Girdlestone arthroplasty for infected total hip arthroplasty. *Clin Orthop Relat Res* 1982; 170: 83-7.

Chapter 19

54. Girdlestone GR. Acute pyogenic arthritis of the hip. *Lancet* 1943; 1: 419.

55. Lieberman JR, *et al*. Treatment of infected total hip arthroplasty with a two-stage reimplantation protocol. *Clin Orthop Relat Res* 1994; 301: 205-12.

56. Langlais F. Can we improve the results of revision arthroplasty for infected total hip replacement? *J Bone Joint Surg Br* 2003; 85(5): 637-40.

57. Garvin KL, *et al*. Palacos gentamicin for the treatment of deep periprosthetic hip infections. *Clin Orthop Relat Res* 1994; 298: 97-105.

58. Clarke HD, Berry DJ, Sim FH. Salvage of failed femoral megaprostheses with allograft prosthesis composites. *Clin Orthop Relat Res* 1998; 356: 222-9.

59. Haddad FS, *et al*. Structural proximal femoral allografts for failed total hip replacements: a minimum review of five years. *J Bone Joint Surg Br* 2000; 82(6): 830-6.

60. Gross AE, *et al*. Proximal femoral allografts for reconstruction of bone stock in revision arthroplasty of the hip. *Clin Orthop Relat Res* 1995; 319: 151-8.

Chapter 19

Surgical management of the infected hip prosthesis

Chapter 20

Anterior cruciate ligament reconstruction

Vasilios Moutzouros MD

Chief Resident, Orthopaedic Surgery

John C Richmond MD

Chairman, Department of Orthopaedic Surgery

NEW ENGLAND BAPTIST HOSPITAL, BOSTON, USA

Introduction

The anterior cruciate ligament (ACL) is the primary ligamentous restraint to anterior translation of the tibia relative to the femur. Nearly half of all ligamentous knee injuries are isolated anterior cruciate ligament tears. Both recreational and competitive athletes are particularly at risk of injury to this structure. Tears can result from both contact and non-contact events. Skiing has been highlighted as an activity that places patients at particular risk for ACL injury. ACL reconstruction has become the standard of care for these injuries. Multiple prospective studies have shown that reconstruction is superior to repair or non-operative treatment with regard to return to sports, stability of the knee, and rate of future meniscal injury [1-3] **(Ib/A)**. In the USA, it is estimated that more than 100,000 anterior cruciate ligament reconstructions are performed each year [4]. Over the past three decades, techniques and fixation devices have evolved, leading to overwhelmingly successful results in reconstruction. Much debate continues on a variety of topics related to reconstruction, including the type of graft, fixation devices, and rehabilitation protocol used for treatment.

With the increasing participation of women in sports, a higher rate of ACL injury has been identified in this population. Studies have shown the rate of ACL injury is four times greater in female basketball players than in males, and two times greater in female soccer players than their male counterparts [5, 6]. Attention has been paid to explaining this great disparity. Differences in dynamic knee stabilisers, the structural characteristics of notch width and ACL size, resistance to anterior shear, and hormonal variation, have all been investigated to uncover the reasons for the increased risk to female athletes. Training regimens have been developed to emphasise proper landing mechanics, and to increase muscle strength in females in an attempt to decrease their rate of injury.

Methodology

A broad search of the literature was performed to identify studies on anterior cruciate ligament reconstruction with a particular interest in prospective randomised studies. The review of current literature was completed using Ovid, PubMed, and Cochrane databases. Multiple searches were performed using the key words Anterior Cruciate Ligament reconstruction, prospective, randomised, patellar tendon, hamstring tendon, allograft tendon, and fixation devices in a variety of combinations. Over 3,000 articles were identified with 860 being of primary interest due to their recurrence in the various searches. Focus was placed on prospective studies dealing with outcomes using various types of fixation, grafts, or rehabilitation protocols. Furthermore, expert knowledge of the research was used to place particular attention to those articles classically referenced. This chapter focuses on anterior cruciate ligament reconstruction as the gold standard for treatment of ACL injuries. It further uses the literature to give an overview of the current ongoing debates on fixation devices, graft material, and rehabilitation.

Anatomy

The anterior cruciate ligament originates from the posteromedial aspect of the intercondylar notch of the lateral femoral condyle (Figure 1). It attaches on the tibia just medial to the anterior horn of the lateral meniscus. Descriptions of the exact locations of these attachment points have varied in the literature [7, 8]. The ligament is composed of two bundles. The anteromedial bundle has been shown to lengthen

during knee flexion and the posterolateral bundle is in maximum tension at full extension. It is composed of primarily Type I collagen fibers [9, 10]. The average thickness of the anterior cruciate ligament is 5mm, with an average width of 10mm, and cross-sectional area of $50mm^2$ [8]. Both the tibial and femoral attachment sites have expansions of ligament considerably greater than the $40mm^2$ cross-sectional midsubstance thickness. The innervation is from the posterior articular nerve, a branch of the tibial nerve [11]. It receives its blood supply from the middle genicular artery [12].

Along with its primary role in preventing anterior translation of the tibia on the femur, the anterior cruciate ligament is a secondary stabiliser to tibial rotation [13]. Biomechanical studies have shown the ligament to have an ultimate tensile load of around 2160 N [14, 15]. This load value is frequently used as a standard for comparison in evaluating the strengths of various graft materials used for reconstruction. Walking produces about 400 N of force, and activities that require rapid acceleration and deceleration, typically cutting sports, produce almost 1800 N [16]. Therefore, only an atypically excessive load pattern would result in ACL failure. The ligament has also been shown to tolerate strain of up to 20%. The position of the knee and the dynamic effect of the muscles surrounding are the most critical factors in strain determination [17]. Isolated hamstring contraction produces the lowest level of strain while isolated quadriceps contraction produces the greatest. Co-contraction of these muscles during closed chain activities results in a lower level of strain than isolated quadriceps contraction. Rehabilitation protocols have used this information to develop training regimens that protect ACL reconstructions early in recovery.

Evaluation of the patient

As with any injury, a thorough history and physical examination is first performed, leading to a diagnosis and from this, a treatment regimen is determined. Basic information such as the age, gender, and activity level of the patient can alert the clinician to the possible pathology involved. Questioning on the mechanism of injury, initial symptoms, and previous

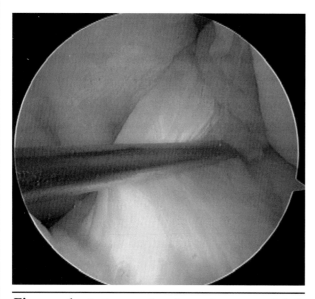

Figure 1. Arthroscopic view of a normal left ACL.

injuries will help focus the examination. Often patients will be unable to recall the exact mechanism of injury or even if contact was involved [18]. In these situations, interviewing those individuals who witnessed the event is helpful though not always possible.

Injuries to the ACL can occur by low or high-energy mechanisms. The most common mechanism is an injury occurring during an athletic event. These are typically low-energy injuries. They can be both contact or non-contact in nature. Contact injuries are often the result of a hyperextension or valgus force applied to the knee. They account for up to a third of all ACL injuries. Non-contact injuries occur during rapid acceleration and deceleration activities in such sports as skiing, basketball, and volleyball [18]. Any athletic participation that includes jumping or cutting activities puts individuals at risk for ACL injury. High-energy mechanisms, such as motor vehicle accidents, are the second subset to ACL injuries. Details of the mechanism of the injury are often lacking. Physical examination findings are often the first sign of ACL injury, as associated injuries frequently take the primary attention of those evaluating the patient.

At presentation, complaints of knee swelling, instability and pain are described. Individuals will often describe an initial 'pop' in their knee that led to pain and immobility. Swelling rapidly develops and patients are often unable to continue the activity that they were performing at the time of injury. A variety of knee injuries can present in this typical fashion that are not ACL tears. These include patellar dislocation or subluxation, medial or lateral collateral ligament tears, or meniscal injuries. A third of patients will present with this 'popping' sensation which can guide the examination and further radiographic evaluation [18]. A haemarthrosis develops rapidly after ACL injury occurs. This has been shown to be one of the most predictive signs of an ACL injury. In one study nearly 75% of patients presenting with an acute haemarthrosis following a traumatic event to the knee were shown to have an ACL tear on arthroscopic evaluation [18, 19]. Again, a number of other knee injuries can present with this finding but investigation into a possible ACL injury should be performed in these patients.

The timing of evaluation will have an impact on the quality of the physical examination. On-field examinations are often the most revealing, as they occur prior to accumulation of the acute haemarthrosis. This is also a time when patients are less prone to resist the examiner's manipulations. Evaluations that occur 12 hours after injury can be difficult due to swelling and guarding. In this setting, re-examination after a few days is helpful, as some of the swelling and pain have often improved.

The physical examination of a knee-injured patient should always begin with inspection of both knees. Malalignment can be evident and represent fracture or possibly patellar instability. Effusions are again critical to appreciate their predictive value. Palpation and manipulation of the uninjured knee is then performed. This allows for the examiner to develop an appreciation of the ligamentous laxity a patient has at baseline. It can also reassure the patient that the examiner is aware of the potential discomfort involved and help them to relax during the evaluation of the injured knee. A variety of manipulations have been shown to suggest ACL injury, including the pivot shift, Lachman, and anterior drawer tests. By comparing the 'normal' side to the affected side, the examiner can make his evaluations more objective. Attention is then turned to the injured knee. Palpation can uncover a small effusion initially missed on inspection. Joint line tenderness may suggest a meniscal tear, whilst medial and lateral collateral ligament injuries can be shown by pain along their course. The knee is then taken through both active and passive range of motion which helps assess for quadriceps and patellar tendon injuries, along with possible patellar tracking issues. Some clinicians favour aspiration of the joint to alleviate pain and allow for improved range of motion. It can also help assess for osteochondral injury or fracture if marrow contents are returned.

Finally, the injured knee is taken through manipulations suggestive of ACL injury. The anterior drawer test and Lachman examination assess for anterior translation of the tibia against the femur. It is again critical to compare the laxity of the injured to the non-injured knee. It must be noted that patients assessed weeks after injury have the opportunity to create scar and create a pseudo-endpoint leading the examiner to believe the ACL is competent. A pivot shift examination is used to assess the rotational component of the ACL. Patients often guard against this test as the subluxation and subsequent reduction often produce pain. Bach *et al* showed that the pivot shift manoeuvre is over 90% sensitive when performed under anaesthesia, as compared to 24% while awake [20].

Typically, ACL injuries can be diagnosed without the need for further radiographic evaluation when a thorough history and physical examination are performed. The common practice of MRI is reserved for the evaluation of associated injuries. It is understandable that patient pressures have led to MRI use in a majority of suspected ACL injuries. This can be justified in those occasions that meniscal or osteochondral injuries are found. Usually, meniscal tears are repairable in the ACL-injured patient [21, 22]. This information is helpful in decision making for surgery, operative planning, and in discussions concerning postoperative care with the patient.

Non-operative treatment

Anterior cruciate ligament injuries do not pose a threat to life or limb. They can be disabling and prevent patients from achieving their desired activity level. Basic activities of daily living can be accomplished by individuals with an incompetent ACL. Advances in surgical techniques and rehabilitation have allowed patients undergoing ACL reconstruction to return to pre-injury levels of activity and performance at an increased frequency. Non-operative treatment, though, has fallen out of favour largely because of later injury and pathology that can occur as a consequence of an ACL incompetency [1, 23, 24] **(Ib/A)**.

Patients with ACL-deficient knees develop secondary meniscal tears in 10%-25% of cases. Numerous studies have shown a high incidence of articular injury, and subsequent degenerative changes [24, 25] **(IIa/B)**. Maletius *et al* presented a study on patients followed 12-20 years after complete rupture of the ACL treated conservatively [26] **(IIb/B)**. Eighty-four percent of the patients evaluated had evidence of osteoarthritis on radiographs. Forty-five percent had at least one

operation after their injury, mostly for meniscal pathology. With aggressive physical therapy and strengthening, patients can maintain adequate ability to perform activities of daily living. Function typically fails to return to pre-injury levels in these patients though, even after completion of an intense physical therapy program. Therefore, if the decision to pursue non-operative management is made, patients must understand that modification of their activities is required to minimise the risk of further injury. Fithian showed that even in low-risk patients, classified using their pre-injury sports participation and knee laxity, there is an increased rate of late meniscal injury [1] **(Ib/A)**. Rehabilitation should focus on hamstring strengthening. Typically, the older, sedentary patient is the best candidate for non-operative treatment of an ACL tear.

Operative treatment

The operative management of ACL injuries has continued to develop over the past three decades. Efforts, which began with repair and augmentation, have evolved to arthroscopic anatomic reconstruction. Primary repairs of the ACL resulted in poor outcomes with laxity and functional levels equal to non-operative treatment [27]. Biological augmentation, with hamstring tendons or strips of iliotibial band, was used in both intra-articular and extra-articular procedures. Augmentation procedures have become obsolete due to advances in reconstruction. Synthetic Gore-tex and polypropylene prostheses and augmentation devices were also used in the 1980s for repairs and reconstruction of the ACL. The materials allowed for a strong ligament reconstruction that could tolerate increased loads to failure, but failed due to stiffness and a lack of biological incorporation [28, 29]. Inflammatory responses to the materials resulted in increased scar tissue formation, recurrent effusions, and limitations in motion [30, 31, 32].

Operative intervention for ACL injuries is often delayed until almost full range of movement has returned. Studies have shown that acute ACL reconstruction in the days immediately following injury leads to an increased risk of stiffness [33, 34] **(IIb/B)**. At initial evaluation, patients are often instructed to begin a therapy program to focus on regaining range of motion to the knee. Elevation, compression, cryotherapy, and anti-inflammatory medication are used in conjunction with rehabilitation to achieve this goal. A quicker return of quadriceps strength and improved range of motion have been shown postoperatively in patients whose surgery was postponed until motion was restored pre-operatively [34, 35] **(IIb/B)**. Straight leg raises, wall slides and closed chain exercises are implemented, while jumping and cutting activities are avoided. The literature does not support a specific amount of time for delay. Hunter *et al* showed that surgical timing made no statistical difference in restoration of knee range of motion or stability at 12 months if an aggressive postoperative physical therapy regimen is implemented [36] **(IIa/B)**. The importance of rehabilitation cannot be overemphasised and may be the most critical factor in restoration of knee range of motion. The benefits of delay though, have been well studied and cannot be ignored.

Graft selection

A number of graft types are available to the surgeon for reconstruction of the ACL. Prosthetic grafts are no longer used due to high failure rates and the potential for inflammatory reactions. Biologic materials are used for reconstructions and can be autograft or allograft tissue. Currently, patellar tendon and hamstring tendon autografts are the most common materials used. Quadriceps autograft and a number of different types of allograft, including achilles, anterior and posterior tibial, and patellar tendon can be used. The various tendons, whether autograft or allograft, possess different biomechanical characteristics. Ideally, the material used for reconstruction should have ultimate tensile load and stiffness that closely resembles a native ACL.

Patellar tendon grafts are often referred to as the gold standard material for ACL reconstruction (Figure 2). The structural properties of this graft type, along with the advantage of bone to bone healing, make it the preferred option for many surgeons. The average cross-sectional area of the tendon is 50mm², with an ultimate tensile load of close to 3000 N and a stiffness

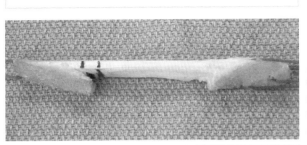

Figure 2. Autologous bone patellar tendon bone autograft as harvested and prepared for ACL reconstruction.

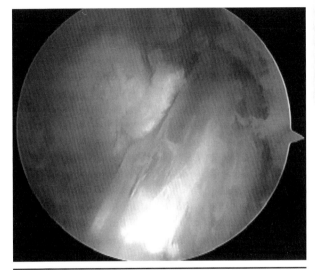

Figure 3. Arthroscopic view of a left knee at the time of autologous hamstring graft ACL reconstruction.

of 620N/mm [15, 37, 38]. This exceeds a native ACL in both stiffness and ultimate tensile load. Bone to bone healing allows the entire tendon to be functional and, therefore, maintain these structural properties. It has the longest track record with numerous studies showing a rate of return to sport close to 80% [39-41] **(Ib/A)**. Laxity has regularly been shown to be less than 3mm in comparison to the unaffected knee [40-42]. The disadvantage of patellar tendon autograft is frequent reports of anterior knee pain, but this is not a universal finding. Other complications, such as patellar fracture and patellar tendon rupture, have been reported but are infrequent.

Hamstring tendon autografts have become the main alternative to patellar tendon grafts (Figures 3

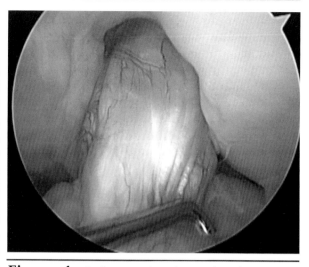

Figure 4. Arthroscopic view of a hamstring autograft two years following implantation showing excellent incorporation and revascularisation.

and 4). The semitendinosus and gracilis tendons have an increased collagen mass as compared to the patellar tendon. They have been used in a variety of combinations including double and quadrupled constructs. The most popular of the constructs, and not coincidentally the strongest, is the quadrupled semitendinosus-gracilis graft. The ultimate tensile load of this graft has been shown to be up to 4600 N [15, 38, 43]. Tensioning of the graft at the time of implantation impacts on the final ultimate tensile strength of the graft. Hamner *et al* presented a range of tensile load from 4590 N to 1831 N depending on this tensioning [43]. This wide discrepancy is of concern, as the native ACL has an ultimate tensile load of 2160 N [14]. When typical tensioning techniques are used, the average ultimate tensile load is 2831 N with a stiffness of 456N/mm [43]. Other concerns with hamstring use revolve around the security of fixation and the healing of soft tissue to bone. Postoperative hamstring recovery has also caused some concern. Newer fixation techniques have blurred the differences between patellar tendon and hamstring grafts.

Allografts have increasingly been used due to reduced surgical time, decreased surgical morbidity, and rapid rehabilitation. They have been used in revision surgery after previous autograft surgery has failed. Fears of disease transmission have developed as transmission of HIV, hepatitis C, and bacterial infections have been reported. Review of harvesting techniques, processing, and terminal sterilisation have led to new guidelines. In the USA, the American Association of Tissue Banks now accredits tissue banks. This has led to hospitals choosing to use companies that have been evaluated and accredited. Sterilisation techniques in the past used ethylene oxide or high-dose radiation, which led to a loss of structural integrity and post-surgical reactions [44, 45]. A variety of tendons have been used for reconstruction including bone-patellar-bone, quadriceps, and hamstring tendons. They serve as a valuable graft source in multiple ligament reconstructions and revision surgery. Allografts have shown a delay in incorporation as compared to autografts [46]. Their use in primary surgery appears to be favoured in older patients, with less athletic demands.

Graft fixation

The choice of graft fixation is a critical decision in ACL reconstruction. Without stable fixation, the newly placed construct can slip, leading to unacceptable laxity or complete detachment. Fixation strength over the initial 12 weeks after reconstruction is crucial in allowing biological healing to occur while rehabilitation begins. Two types of fixation have been recognised: aperture and suspensory. Aperture fixation places a construct in direct contact with the graft near the entry to the joint. Suspensory fixation secures the graft at a point distant from the entry point into the joint. The perfect construct would limit graft motion at the joint line and resist loosening with cyclic loading.

Patellar tendon grafts, both allografts and autografts, have the advantage of bone to bone healing. With the incorporation of graft bone, the entire ligament is recruited for functionality with a strong bone-tendon interface that has not been violated. Most of our knowledge on fixation strength and incorporation is derived from *in vitro* studies. Nonetheless, investigations have produced useful information regarding pull-out strength, time to incorporation, and mechanisms of loosening. Brown *et al* reported that bone-patellar-bone grafts are securely fixed by incorporation at six weeks [47]. The bone to bone contact also allows for more resistance to slippage and failure.

Interference screw fixation has become the standard method of fixation of these grafts. The strength and stiffness of the construct has been demonstrated to be superior to other forms of fixation for bone-patellar-bone grafts [48]. An additional advantage is the posterior translation of the graft on the femoral side, which closely resembles the native anatomy. Their ultimate failure load approaches 600 N [48, 49]. The importance of screw size and divergence cannot be ignored. The space between the bone block and interference screw dictates the size of the screw to be used. A gap of less than 2mm has been shown to be most effective in avoiding pull-out [50]. Divergence of greater than 30° can also negatively affect pull-out strength [51]. Both metal and bioabsorbable screws are used with no difference in ultimate failure loads [49].

Fixation strength for soft tissue grafts varies considerably depending on the type of construct chosen. Unlike bone-patellar-bone fixation, femoral and tibial side fixation techniques can differ. Femoral methods include EndoButton, suture posts, anchors, cross-pins, and interference screws. Tibial side fixation includes interference screws, suture posts, and screw and washer constructs. Buttons and screw posts are indirect fixation techniques, while the remaining devices are direct. Indirect methods have been questioned due to the bridging material used for fixation. This material has been shown to be the weak link in strength and stiffness. Another concern with indirect fixation is the location of fixation away from the tunnel entry. Interference screw fixation on the femoral side allows for direct contact closer to the anatomic bone-ligament interface. Indirect methods place their contact further from this area depending on the type of fixation used. Even cross-pin fixation, which has performed well in *in vivo* testing, secures the graft 2-4cm from the femoral tunnel entrance. To *et al* showed the superiority of cross-pin fixation as compared to bone anchor and EndoButton constructs [52]. The ultimate failure load of cross-pin fixation was almost three times that of the other two. Interference screws for soft tissue grafts on the femoral side do not compare to those used for patellar tendon grafts. They have been shown to have approximately 50% of the ultimate failure load strength that their patellar tendon counterparts possess [53]. The possibility of creep with early motion and soft tissue fixation has led to surgeons cycling the graft prior to tension and fixation on the tibial side [54].

Tibial side fixation is felt to be the likely weak link in soft tissue grafts. The quality of bone in this area is poorer. Clinical studies by Aglietti showed no appreciable difference in joint laxity between anatomic and non-anatomic tibial fixation [55] **(IIb/B)**. Kousa *et al* have performed *in vitro* studies of tibial fixation devices. His investigations showed tapered 35mm interference screws had the greatest pull-out strength for tibial fixation [56]. Again, previous studies quoting fixation strength are all *in vitro* investigations that are presumed to relate to *in vivo* conditions [56, 57]. No prospective long-term studies comparing the variety of soft tissue fixation devices have been published. Most prospective investigations have focused on comparing outcomes between bone-patellar-bone and hamstring reconstructions, using an assortment of soft tissue devices and graft arrangements [58-63] **(Ib/A)**.

No discussion on graft fixation is complete without mentioning graft tensioning. Regardless of the fixation used, without appropriate graft tensioning techniques, reconstructions can have unacceptable laxity or increased tightness leading to failure. The amount of tension placed on the graft at the time of fixation impacts on the future kinematics of the knee [64]. Tension is determined by the amount of force applied to the graft, the amount of knee flexion and the degree of posterior translation at the time of graft fixation [65]. Overtensioning the graft is a possibility and can lead to a limited range of motion and theoretically an increased risk of early articular degeneration. The preferred position of fixation is with the knee in full extension, as this is the position of greatest tension in the arc of motion of the knee [65]. If the graft is tensioned whilst the knee is in 30° of flexion, it is feared that the graft may then be at risk of failure, as tension increases when the knee is fully extended [66]. Studies have focused on the amount of tension to apply to a graft at the time of fixation. It has been found that different graft types require different amounts of tension to most accurately represent anatomic conditions [67]. Higher initial graft tension leads to increased stiffness of the graft. The ideal tension has yet to be clearly elucidated. Nicholas *et al* evaluated bone-patellar-bone reconstructions tensioned at 90 N or 45 N. They found a statistically significant difference in anterior side-to-side translation between the two groups evaluated at an average of 20 months postoperatively, with the low tension cohort showing greater laxity [68] **(IIb/B)**.

With new emphasis on anatomical reconstructions, debate has surfaced with regard to double-bundle reconstructions and tunnel location. Current investigations are attempting to better elucidate the proper position of both the tibial and femoral tunnels. At this time, no *in vivo* prospective studies have shown the ideal location of these tunnels. Marcacci *et al* have developed an approach to anterior cruciate ligament reconstruction that attempts to recreate the anterior and posterior bundles of the ligament [69]. Further study is needed to evaluate the outcomes of this new technique, as compared to current ligament reconstruction methods.

Rehabilitation

The proper rehabilitation program is critical in obtaining the best outcome after ACL reconstruction. Closed-kinetic chain exercises are those that focus on the co-contraction of the hamstrings and quadriceps muscles. These have been the preferred exercises, as they decrease the stress placed on the newly reconstructed ACL. Open chain exercises isolate a particular joint and allow it to move in a single rotational axis. Their use in the initial postoperative period have diminished, due to fears of unnecessary strain occurring in the graft. Closed chain exercises have been shown to result in lower KT-1000 side-to-side differences, less patellofemoral pain and improved patient satisfaction as compared to open chain programs [70]. With advances in fixation, surgeons have accelerated their rehabilitation programs. Beynnon *et al* showed no difference in anterior knee laxity between patients randomised for an accelerated versus a non-accelerated rehabilitation program after bone-patellar tendon-bone ACL reconstruction [71] **(Ib/A)**.

Full range of motion is encouraged after ACL reconstruction, with particular attention to extension. Weight-bearing is generally progressed over the first few weeks. Immediate weight-bearing has been shown to reduce muscle inhibition and decrease the incidence of anterior knee pain [72] **(Ib/A)**. When comparing weight-bearing and non-weight-bearing groups, no difference in knee laxity or range of motion is found [72]. An increase in synovitis has been noted in those patients rehabilitated aggressively [73].

A variety of treatment protocols are followed for ACL reconstructions. While most surgeons allow weight-bearing, range of motion, and closed chain exercises, there is no clear position on the use of braces, timing of resistive exercises, or advancement of activity level. Return to full activity is common within six months. Proprioceptive training is allowed when adequate quadriceps and hamstring strength returns. Athletic participation is allowed when patients increase their strength to levels approaching their uninjured side. Some practitioners favour the use of braces in the postoperative period and with the return to athletic participation. This currently has not been shown to be of any clear protective benefit.

Conclusions

The support for reconstruction of the ACL in complete injuries is clear. The risk of subsequent meniscal tears and early degenerative changes in the injured knee make surgical intervention routine in active patients. Fithian *et al* showed that patients at all levels of risk treated non-operatively had an increased incidence of late meniscal tears, potentially supporting reconstruction even in low-risk patients [1] **(Ib/A)**. Their specific findings though, did not establish an increase in radiographic degenerative changes in the non-operative group. Non-operative management with rehabilitation remains a treatment plan for selected patients who are sedentary or pose an unacceptable surgical risk.

The preferred graft choice and fixation methods remain topics for debate in ACL reconstruction. The different graft types have benefits in respect to the ease of operative technique, strength and stiffness, and rate of rehabilitative recovery. In this respect, surgeons often use multiple graft types and try to personalise the type of graft they use depending on patient factors such as age and activity level. Multiple studies have been performed comparing the results of autogenous bone-patellar tendon-bone to hamstring grafts. These prospective studies repeatedly state that knee outcome scores and patient satisfaction are equal for the two types of grafts [58-63] **(Ib/A)**. Differences do exist in morbidity, postoperative muscular strength and knee laxity on arthrometry measurement [74]. Knee walking tests continually favour hamstring reconstructions [58, 60]. Quadriceps and hamstring deficits are found depending on the type of graft harvested, with recovery in quadriceps strength by 12 months. Hamstring groups have showed active flexion deficits for up to 24 months [59]. Objective knee laxity measurements show a statistically significant difference favouring bone-patellar tendon-bone reconstructions [58, 59, 62].

With all of this information, surgeons often stratify the use of each type of graft, including allograft, depending on the activity level of the individual. Many surgeons prefer bone-patellar tendon-bone reconstructions in their elite athletes and most active patients. Hamstring reconstructions are also often used in athletes, but a preference for the recreational athlete is apparent. Allografts are often used for both recreational and low-activity level patients. They are also used in the setting of revision when autograft was previously used.

Fixation methods have been studied in *in vitro* conditions. The extrapolation of this data into *in vivo* settings is only natural. Interference fixation for bone-patellar-bone grafts is clearly preferred. Soft tissue fixation, on the other hand, continues to be controversial. Cross-pin fixation has been favoured for femoral side fixation in biomechanical studies [52]. Direct contact with the graft is preferred to indirect methods of fixation. It is also theoretically favourable to fix the graft close to the anatomical attachments of the ACL. No matter what the fixation device selected, appropriate placement of the graft may be the most critical factor in stability and longevity.

Rehabilitation protocols now focus on early advancement of weight-bearing and immediate range of motion exercises. Closed chain exercises have been shown to put less strain on the new reconstruction [70]. Improved therapy has led patients to return to sports as early as six months after reconstruction. Rates of return to the pre-injury level of function approach 80% for both bone-patellar tendon-bone and hamstring autograft reconstructions [39-41, 59]. No standard has yet been established, however, in terms of the rate of advancement of activity level. Most practitioners continue to use quadriceps and hamstring strength recovery as a gauge for advancement. Brace use is also variable and without definitive evidence of benefit [75]. With the improvements in surgical technique and fixation, rehabilitation programs have progressed and are contributing to improved outcomes.

The evaluation of evidence for graft selection and fixation remains difficult. The weight of importance of the various differences between soft tissue and bone-patellar tendon-bone autografts is not clear. Objective data support the benefits of bone-patellar tendon-bone reconstructions in relation to knee laxity. Patient satisfaction scores do not, however, correspond with this finding. Outstanding results have been shown with both types of reconstructions. After careful consideration of the patients' activity level, preferences, and future athletic goals, an appropriate graft material can be selected by the surgeon and patient.

Recommendations	**Evidence level**

Treatment option

Repair or reconstruction

- One RCT showing early phase reconstruction leads to improved knee   Ib/A
  stability and reduces the rate of meniscal tears.

Patellar or hamstring autograft

- Five RCTs showing equivalent results between the two graft types in terms of   Ia/A
  patient satisfaction and activity level. Objective knee laxity was improved in
  patellar tendon groups.

Open or closed chain exercises

- One RCT showing improved objective knee stability with improved   Ib/A
  patellofemoral pain for the closed chain group.

Accelerated or non-accelerated rehabilitation

- One RCT showing no difference in knee laxity, patient satisfaction, or   Ib/A
  functional performance at two years.

Timing of surgery

- One prospective trial showing no impact of surgical timing on knee range of   IIa/B
  motion and stability at 12 months.

References

1. Fithian DC, Paxton EW, Stone ML, *et al*. Prospective trial of a treatment algorithm for the management of the anterior cruciate ligament-injured knee. *Am J Sports Med* 2005; 33(3): 335-46.
2. Engebretsen L, Benum P, Fasting O, *et al*. A prospective, randomized study of three surgical techniques for treatment of acute ruptures of the anterior cruciate ligament. *Am J Sports Med* 1990; 18: 585-90.
3. Grontvedt T, Engebretsen L, Benum P, *et al*. A prospective, randomized study of three operations for acute rupture of the anterior cruciate ligament: five-year follow-up of one hundred and thirty-one patients. *J Bone Joint Surg Am* 1996; 78A: 159-68.
4. Graham SM, Parker RD. Anterior cruciate ligament reconstruction using hamstring tendon grafts. *Clin Orthop* 2002; 402: 64-75.

5. Messina, DF, Farney WC, DeLee JC. The incidence of injury in Texas high school basketball. *Am J Sports Med* 1999; 27: 294-9.
6. Lindenfeld TN, Schmitt DJ, Hendy MD, *et al*. Incidence of injury in indoor soccer. *Am J Sports Med* 1994; 22: 364-71.
7. Harner CD, Baek GH, Vogrin TM, *et al*. Quantitative analysis of human cruciate ligament insertions. *Arthroscopy* 1999; 15: 741-9.
8. Odensten M, Gilllquist J. Functional anatomy of the anterior cruciate ligament and a rationale for reconstruction. *J Bone Joint Surg Am* 1985; 67: 257-62
9. Amiel D, Frank C, Harwood F, *et al*. Tendons and ligaments: a morphological and biochemical comparision. *J Orthop Res* 1984; 1: 257-65.
10. Baek GH, Carlin GJ, Vogrin TM, *et al*. Quantitative analysis of collagen fibrils of human cruciate and meniscofemoral ligaments. *Clin Orthop* 1998; 357: 205-11.
11. Kennedy JC, Weinberg HW, Wilson AS. The anatomy and functions of the anterior cruciate ligament. *J Bone Joint Surg Am* 1974; 56: 223-35.

12. Arnoczky SP. Blood supply to the anterior cruciate ligament and supporting structures. *Orthop Clin North Am* 1985; 16: 15-28.

13. Markolf KL, Mensch JS, Amstutz HC. Stiffness and laxity of the knee: the contributions of the supporting structures. *J Bone Joint Surg Am* 1976; 58: 583-93.

14. Noyes FR, Butler DL, Grood ES, *et al*. Biomechanical analysis of human ligament grafts used in knee-ligament repairs and reconstructions. *J Bone Joint Surg Am* 1984; 66: 344-52.

15. Woo SL-Y, Hollis JM, Adams DJ, *et al*. Tensile properties of the human femur-anterior cruciate ligament-tibia complex: the effects of specimen age and orientation. *Am J Sports Med* 1991; 19: 217-25.

16. Markloff KL, Burchfield DM, Shapiro MM, *et al*. Biomechanical consequences of replacement of the anterior cruciate ligament with a patellar ligament allograft. Part II: Forces in the graft compared with forces in the intact ligament. *J Bone Joint Surg Am* 1996; 78: 1728-34.

17. Beynnon BD, Fleming BC. Anterior cruciate ligament strain *in vivo*: a review of previous work. *J Biomech* 1998; 31: 519-25.

18. Noyes FR, Basset RW, Grood ES, *et al*. Arthroscopy in acute traumatic hemarthrosis of the knee. *J Bone Joint Surg Am* 1980; 62: 687-95.

19. DeHaven KE. Diagnosis of acute knee injuries with hemarthrosis. *Am J Sports Med* 1980; 8: 9-13.

20. Nogalski MP, Bach BR. Acute anterior cruciate ligament injuries. In: *Knee Surgery*. Fu FH, Harner CD, Vince KG, Eds. Baltimore: Williams & Wilkins, 1994: 679-730.

21. Buseck MS, Noyes FR. Arthroscopic evaluations of meniscal repairs after anterior cruciate ligament reconstruction and immediate motion. *Am J Sports Med* 1991; 19: 489-94.

22. Cannon WD, Vittori JM. The incidence of healing in arthroscopic meniscal repair in anterior cruciate ligament reconstructed knees versus stable knees. *Am J Sports Med* 1992; 20: 176-81.

23. Odenstein M, Hamberg P, Nordin M, *et al*. Surgical or conservative treatment of the acutely torn anterior cruciate ligament. *Clin Orthop* 1985; 198: 87-93.

24. Seitz H, Schlenz I, Muller E, *et al*. Anterior instability of the knee despite an intensive rehabilitation program. *Clin Orthop* 1996; 328: 159-64.

25. Marzo JM, Warren RF. Results of treatment of anterior cruciate ligament injury: changing perspectives. *Adv Orthop Surg* 1991; 15: 59-69.

26. Maletius W, Messner K. Eighteen to twenty-four year follow-up after complete rupture of the anterior cruciate ligament. *Am J Sports Med* 1999; 27: 711-7.

27. Sherman MF, Lieber L, Bonamo JR, *et al*. The long-term follow-up of primary ACL repair: defining a role for augmentation. *Am J Sports Med* 1991; 19: 243-55.

28. Kumar K, Maffulli N. The ligament augmentation device: a historical perspective. *Arthroscopy* 1999; 15: 422-32.

29. Dahlstedt L, Dalen N, Jonsson U, *et al*. Cruciate ligament prosthesis vs. augmentation. *Acta Orthop Scand* 1993; 64: 431-3.

30. McPherson GK, Mendenhall HV, Gibbons DF, *et al*. Experimental, mechanical, and histological evaluation of the Kennedy ligament augmentation device. *Clin Orthop* 1985; 196: 186-95.

31. Roth JH, Shkrum MJ, Bray RC. Synovial reaction associated with disruption of polypropylene braid augmented intraarticular anterior cruciate ligament reconstruction. A case report. *Am J Sports Med* 1988; 16: 301-5.

32. Yamamoto H, Ishibashi T, Muneta T, *et al*. Effusions after anterior cruciate ligament reconstruction using the ligament augmentation device. *Arthroscopy* 1992; 8: 305-10.

33. Harner CD, Irrgang JJ, Paul J, *et al*. Loss of motion after anterior cruciate ligament reconstruction. *Am J Sports Med* 1992; 20: 499-506.

34. Shelbourne KD, Foulk AD. Timing of surgery in anterior cruciate ligament tears on the return of quadriceps muscle strength after reconstruction using an autogenous patellar tendon graft. *Am J Sports Med* 1995; 23: 686-89.

35. Shelbourne KD, Wilckens JH, Mollabaashy A, *et al*. Arthrofibrosis in acute anterior cruciate ligament reconstruction: the effect of timing of reconstruction and rehabilitation. *Am J Sports Med* 1991; 9: 332-6.

36. Hunter RE, Mastrangelo J, Freeman JR, *et al*. The impact of surgical timing on postoperative motion and stability following anterior cruciate ligament reconstruction. *Arthroscopy* 1996; 12(6): 667-74.

37. Cooper DE, Deng XH, Burstein AL, *et al*. The strength of the central third patellar tendon graft. A biomechanical study. *Am J Sports Med* 1993; 21: 818-24.

38. Noyes FR, Butler DL, Grood ES, *et al*. Biomechanical analysis of human ligament grafts used in knee-ligament repairs and replacements. *J Bone Joint Surg Am* 1984; 66: 344-52.

39. Aglietti P, Buzii R, D'Andria S, *et al*. Arthroscopic anterior cruciate ligament reconstruction with patellar tendon. *Arthroscopy* 1992; 8: 510-6.

40. O'Neill DB. Arthroscopically-assisted reconstruction of the anterior cruciate ligament. A prospective randomized analysis of three techniques. *J Bone Joint Surg Am* 1996; 78(6): 803-13.

41. Sgaglione NA, Schwartz RE. Arthroscopically-assisted reconstruction of the anterior cruciate ligament: initial clinical experience and minimal 2-year follow-up comparing endoscopic transtibial and two-incision techniques. *Arthroscopy* 1997; 13: 156-65.

42. Marder RA, Raskind JR, Carroll M. Prospective evaluation of arthroscopically-assisted anterior cruciate ligament reconstruction: patellar tendon versus semitendinosus and gracilis tendons. *Am J Sports Med* 1991; 19: 478-84.

43. Hamner DL, Brown CH, Steiner ME, *et al*. Hamstring tendon grafts for reconstruction of the anterior cruciate ligament: biomechanical evaluation of the use of multiple strands and tensioning techniques. *J Bone Joint Surg Am* 1999; 81: 549-57.

44. Smith CW, Young IS, Kearney JN. Mechanical properties of tendons: changes with sterilization and preservation. *J Biomech Eng* 1996; 118: 56-61.

45. Jackson DW, Windler GE, Simon TM. The intraarticular reaction associated with the use of freeze-dried, ethylene oxide-sterilized bone-patellar tendon-bone allografts in the reconstruction of the anterior cruciate ligament. *Am J Sports Med* 1990; 18: 1-11.

46. Jackson DW, Grood ES, Goldstein JD, et al. A comparison of patellar tendon autograft and allograft used for anterior cruciate ligament reconstruction in the goat model. Am J Sports Med 1993; 21: 176-85.

47. Brown CH, Hecker AT, Hipp JA, et al. The biomechanics of interference screw fixation of patellar tendon anterior cruciate ligament grafts. Am J Sports Med 1993; 21: 880-6.

48. Kurosaka M, Yoshiya S, Andrish JT. A biomechanical comparison of different surgical techniques of graft fixation in anterior cruciate ligament reconstruction. Am J Sports Med 1987; 15: 225-9.

49. Caborn DNM, Urban WP, Johnson DL, et al. Biomechanical comparison between bioscrew and titanium alloy interference screws for bone-patellar tendon-bone graft fixation in anterior cruciate ligament reconstruction. Arthroscopy 1997; 13: 229-32.

50. Butler JC, Branch TP, Hutton WC. Optimal graft fixation - the effect of gap size and screw size on bone plug fixation in ACL reconstruction. Arthroscopy 1994; 10: 524-29.

51. Lemos MJ, Jackson DW, Lee TQ. Assessment of initial fixation of endoscopic interference femoral screws with divergent and parallel placement. Arthroscopy 1995; 11: 37-41.

52. To JT, Howell SM, Hull ML. Contributions of femoral fixation methods to the stiffness of anterior cruciate ligament replacements at implantation. Arthroscopy 1999; 15: 379-87.

53. Caborn DNM, Coen M, Neef R, et al. Quadrupled semitendinosus-gracilis autograft fixation in the femoral tunnel: a comparison between a metal and a bioabsorbable interference screw. Arthroscopy 1997; 13: 229-32.

54. Kousa P, Jarvinen TN, Vihavainen M, et al. The fixation strength of six hamstring tendon graft fixation devices in anterior cruciate ligament reconstruction, Part I: Femoral site. Am J Sports Med 2003; 31: 174-81.

55. Aglietti P, Zaccherotti G, Simeone AJ, et al. Anatomic versus non-anatomic tibial fixation in anterior cruciate ligament reconstruction with bone-patellar tendon-bone graft. Knee Surg Sports Traumatol Arthrosc 1998; 6(suppl 1): S43-48.

56. Kousa P, Jarvinen TN, Vihavainen M, et al. The fixation strength of six hamstring tendon graft fixation devices in anterior cruciate ligament reconstruction: Part II: Tibial site. Am J Sports Med 2003; 31: 182-8.

57. Magen HE, Howell SM, Hull ML. Structural properties of six tibial fixation methods for anterior cruciate ligament soft tissue grafts. Am J Sports Med 1999; 27: 35-43.

58. Laxdal G, Kartus J, Hannson L, et al. A prospective randomized comparison of bone-patellar tendon-bone and hamstring grafts for anterior cruciate ligament reconstruction. Arthroscopy 2005; 21(1): 34-42.

59. Feller JA, Webster KE. A randomized comparison of patellar tendon and hamstring tendon anterior cruciate ligament reconstruction. Am J Sports Med 2003; 31(4): 564-73.

60. Ejerhed L, Kartus J, Sernert N, et al. Patellar tendon or semitendinosus autografts for anterior cruciate ligament reconstruction? A prospective randomized study with a two-year follow-up. Am J Sports Med 2003; 31(1): 19-25.

61. Jansson KA, Linko E, Sandelin J, et al. A prospective randomized study of patellar versus hamstring tendon autografts for anterior cruciate ligament reconstruction. Am J Sports Med 2003; 31(1): 12-8.

62. Beynnon BD, Johnson RJ, Fleming BC, et al. Anterior cruciate ligament replacement: comparison of bone-patellar tendon-bone grafts with two-strand hamstring grafts. A prospective, randomized study. J Bone Joint Surg Am 2002; 84-A(9): 1503-13.

63. Shaieb MD, Kan DM, Chang SK, et al. A prospective randomized comparison of patellar tendon versus semitendinosus and gracilis tendon autografts for anterior cruciate ligament reconstruction. Am J Sports Med 2002; 30(2): 214-20.

64. Nicholas SJ, D'Amato MJ, Mullaney MJ, et al. A prospectively randomized double-blind study on the effect of initial graft tension on knee stability after anterior cruciate ligament reconstruction. Am J Sports Med 2004; 32(8): 1881-6.

65. Nabors ED, Richmond JC, Vannah WM, et al. Anterior cruciate ligament graft tensioning in full extension. Am J Sports Med 1995; 23: 488-92.

66. Gertel TH, Lew WD, Lewis JL, et al. Effect of anterior cruciate ligament graft tensioning direction, magnitude, and flexion angle on knee biomechanics. Am J Sports Med 1993; 21: 572-81.

67. Burks RT, Leland R. Determination of graft tension before fixation in anterior cruciate ligament reconstruction. Arthroscopy 1988; 4: 260-66.

68. Nicholas SJ, D'Amato MJ, Mullaney MJ, et al. A prospectively randomized double-blind study on the effect of initial graft tension on knee stability after anterior cruciate ligament reconstruction. Am J Sports Med 2004; 32: 1881-6.

69. Marcacci M, Malgora AP, Zaffagnini S, et al. Anatomic double-bundle anterior cruciate ligament reconstruction with hamstrings. Arthroscopy 2003; 19: 540-6.

70. Bynum EB, Barrack RL, Alexander AH. Open versus closed chain kinetic exercises after anterior cruciate ligament reconstruction. A prospective randomized study. Am J Sports Med 1995; 23(4): 401-6.

71. Beynnon BD, Uh BS, Johnson RJ, et al. Rehabilitation after anterior cruciate ligament reconstruction: a prospective, randomized, double-blinded comparison of programs administered over 2 different time intervals. Am J Sports Med 2005; 33(3): 347-59.

72. Tyler TF, McHugh HP, Gleim GW, et al. The effect of immediate weight-bearing after anterior cruciate ligament reconstruction. Clin Orthop 1998; 357: 141-8.

73. Majima T, Yasuda K, Tago H, et al. Rehabilitation after hamstring anterior cruciate ligament reconstruction. Clin Orthop 2002; 397: 370-80.

74. Fox, JA, Nedeff DD, Bach BR, et al. Anterior cruciate ligament reconstruction with patellar autograft tendon. Clin Orthop 2002; 402: 53-63.

75. Risberg MA, Holm I, Steen H, et al. The effect of knee bracing after anterior cruciate ligament reconstruction. A prospective, randomized study with two years' follow-up. Am J Sports Med 1999; 27(1): 76-83.

Chapter 21

Posterolateral instability of the knee

Mark S Falworth FRCS (Tr & Orth)
Specialist Registrar, Orthopaedic Surgery
Robin Allum FRCS
Consultant, Orthopaedic Surgery

WEXHAM PARK HOSPITAL, SLOUGH, UK

Introduction

Posterolateral corner (PLC) instability is defined as the instability that results from injuries to the posterolateral stabilising structures of the knee. The resulting instability is of a posterior, varus and external rotation nature. However, isolated posterolateral ligamentous instability of the knee is uncommon. Instead, instability is often associated with injuries to either the anterior cruciate ligament (ACL), the posterior cruciate ligament (PCL), or both.

The recognition and adequate management of this injury pattern is crucial. Failure to do so can compromise the repair, particularly when a cruciate ligament reconstruction has been undertaken and the repair of the posterolateral corner omitted. There should always, therefore, be a high degree of suspicion when examining the knee, particularly in those patients where the mechanism of injury and symptoms are suggestive of a complex knee injury.

This chapter will provide an understanding of posterolateral corner injuries and critically review evidence regarding currently available treatment methods.

Methodology

There is an increasing amount of literature on the biomechanics and management of posterolateral corner injuries. Although no papers could be identified using the Cochrane Library database, a Medline search on the 'posterolateral corner' identified 100 publications, with 44 being published in the last two years. Despite this explosion in interest, the publications reviewed describe varying injury patterns and relatively new management techniques. As such, there is little evidence on long-term outcome.

Anatomy

The anatomy of the posterolateral corner is variable and complicated. Although the critical layers related to stability are the popliteus, popliteofibular ligament (PFL) and lateral collateral ligament (LCL) [1-5], a sound understanding of the anatomy is needed if the surgical management of these injuries is to be considered. Seebacher [6] divided the posterolateral corner into three layers (Figure 1) **(IV/C)**.

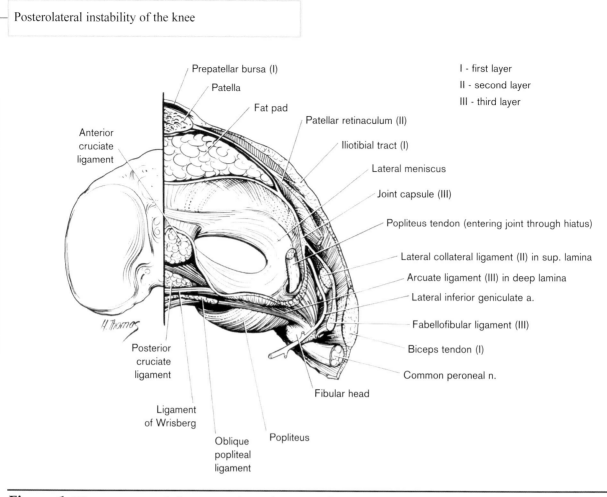

Prepatellar bursa (I)
Patella
Fat pad
Patellar retinaculum (II)
Iliotibial tract (I)
Lateral meniscus
Joint capsule (III)
Popliteus tendon (entering joint through hiatus)
Lateral collateral ligament (II) in sup. lamina
Arcuate ligament (III) in deep lamina
Lateral inferior geniculate a.
Fabellofibular ligament (III)
Biceps tendon (I)
Common peroneal n.
Fibular head
Anterior cruciate ligament
Posterior cruciate ligament
Ligament of Wrisberg
Oblique popliteal ligament
Popliteus

I - first layer
II - second layer
III - third layer

Figure 1. **The structure of the posterolateral aspect of the knee.** *Reproduced with permission from The Journal of Bone and Joint Surgery, Inc.* [6]

Layer I

Layer I consists of a fascial layer incorporating the iliotibial band (ITB) and biceps femoris.

The ITB makes up the anterior aspect of this layer. It originates from the level of the greater trochanter and extends down the lateral aspect of the thigh. The superficial layers insert into Gerdy's tubercle whilst the deeper layers insert into the lateral intermuscular septum at the distal femur.

The combined short and long heads of the biceps femoris make up the posterior aspect of layer I. The long head is made up of two tendinous components, one inserts into the posterolateral head of the fibula, whilst the other attaches to the lateral edge of the fibular head. Similarly, the short head of biceps femoris also has two tendinous insertions. One inserts into the

superior surface of the fibular head just lateral to the styloid process but medial to the LCL, whilst the other extends anteriorly, medial to the LCL, and inserts on to the posterior aspect of the tibial tuberosity. The biceps tendon, therefore, folds around the LCL at its insertion. The common peroneal nerve also runs in this layer.

Layer II

Layer II is formed by the lateral quadriceps retinaculum, the LCL and the two patellofemoral ligaments.

The LCL is a cord-like structure, approximately 6cm in length. It attaches slightly proximal and posterior to the lateral epicondyle of the femur and slopes postero-inferiorly to insert into the lateral aspect of the head of the fibula [7] **(III/B)**. It is not attached to either the capsule or lateral meniscus, and the inferior lateral genicular vessel and popliteus tendon lie deep to it preventing the ligament from attaching to either the capsule or lateral meniscus. As the LCL is attached behind the femoral condyle's axis of flexion, it becomes taut and limits extension when the knee reaches full extension.

Layer III

Layer III is composed of the joint capsule, popliteus tendon and the coronary, fabellofibular, arcuate and popliteofibular ligaments.

The coronary ligament is part of a capsuloligamentous complex that connects the lateral meniscus to the lateral tibial condyle. Its integrity determines the degree of mobility of the lateral meniscus. A hiatus in the posterolateral border of the ligament permits the passage of the popliteus tendon and bursa. This region of the lateral meniscus is referred to as the bare area.

The popliteus tendon arises from just below the lateral femoral epicondyle and anterior to the LCL insertion. It descends inferomedially, passing through the hiatus of the coronary ligament and inserting into the popliteal surface of the tibia above the soleal line. In extension, the tendon subluxes anteriorly relative to the

popliteal sulcus and only enters the sulcus in deep flexion [7]. Medial to the tendon is an aponeurotic attachment to the posterior capsule and to the posterior horn of the lateral meniscus [8, 9]. Although its presence has been questioned [10, 11], it has been termed the posterior inferior popliteomeniscal fascicle [12] and is believed to provide a protective role for the lateral meniscus. Its rupture may result in meniscal instability and subsequent injury **(III/B)**.

The PFL arises from the medial and inferior fibres of the popliteus tendon [11, 13] **(IIb/B)**. It lies deep to the lateral limb of the arcuate ligament and inserts into the most proximal and posterior projection of the fibula with smaller insertions into the lateral limb of the arcuate and the fabellofibular ligaments. The inferior lateral geniculate artery separates these two latter insertions from the fibular insertions.

The arcuate ligament is a Y-shaped structure. Its stronger lateral limb arises from the styloid process of the fibula and arches medially, superficial to the popliteus muscle and tendon where it inserts into the posterior joint capsule. The oblique popliteal ligament (Ligament of Winslow) forms the medial limb. This ligament is formed from the union of the oblique popliteal expansion of the semimembranosus and the capsular arm of the posterior oblique ligament, which originates from the medial side of the knee [9] **(III/B)**. The oblique popliteal ligament arches anteriorly to insert into the posterior joint capsule overlying the lateral femoral condyle. The arcuate ligament also forms part of the arcuate complex, which includes the LCL, popliteus and the lateral head of gastrocnemius.

The presence of the fabellofibular ligament is inconsistent [11, 14] **(IIb/B)**. It arises from the lateral aspect of the fabella, or in its absence, the posterior aspect of the supracondylar process of the femur [9] **(III/B)**. It descends distally and laterally, running parallel with the tendon of the long head of biceps femoris muscle before inserting into the posterior and lateral edge of the styloid process of the fibula just medial to the insertion of the short head of the biceps femoris.

The anatomical components of the posterolateral corner can also be classified functionally with respect to the structures that provide static and dynamic stability to the knee (Table 1).

Table 1. Dynamic and static stabilisers of the posterolateral corner.

	Structure
Dynamic stabilisers	Biceps femoris
	Lateral head of gastrocnemius *
Static stabilisers	Popliteus *
	Lateral collateral ligament *
	Popliteofibular ligament
	Arcuate ligament *
	Fabellofibular ligament
	Iliotibial band
	Lateral meniscus

* These structures make up the arcuate complex

Biomechanics

The biomechanics of the posterolateral corner can be investigated by the selective sectioning of cadaveric knee ligaments. The sequence of sectioning can also be varied.

Posterior translation

Studies demonstrate that although division of the PCL results in no increase in anterior translation, posterior translation increases with increasing knee flexion [1] **(IIb/B)**. Selective sectioning of the popliteus, LCL, and arcuate ligament complex results in no significant increase in posterior translation between 0-30° of flexion when compared to isolated PCL sectioning. However, if the PCL, and all the structures of the posterolateral corner, are divided, there is a significant increase in the posterior translation between 0-90°, when compared to selective sectioning.

Varus instability

In an intact knee, varus and valgus rotation is at its least in extension and increases with increasing flexion to 90°. Following either the collective or individual sectioning of the PCL, LCL and the arcuate complex, valgus rotation was not increased. However, varus rotation increased by 1-4° in all angles of flexion when selective sectioning of the LCL was performed. This increased to 5-9° degrees when the arcuate complex was sectioned and 14-19° when the PCL was also divided. Maximum varus rotation was noted at 60° of knee flexion when the PCL, LCL and popliteus, and the arcuate complex were divided [1] **(IIb/B)**.

Primary internal and external rotational instability

Rotational instability arises when internal or external tibial torque is applied to the knee. In an intact knee, combined internal and external rotational instability is at a maximum at 45° of flexion and a minimum at 0°. No isolated or combined sectioning of the PCL, LCL or deep lateral structures produces any increase in internal rotation; however, a 2-3° increase in external rotation is noted following isolated sectioning of the LCL at 30°, 60° and 90° of flexion.

An increase of 6° +/- 3° external rotation was recorded with isolated sectioning of the arcuate complex at 90° of flexion. When both the LCL and arcuate complex were sectioned, an increase in external rotation at all flexion angles was noted; however, it was at its greatest at 30°. Although isolated division of the PCL resulted in no change of external rotation, subsequent division of the LCL and arcuate complex caused significant increases in external rotation at 60° and 90° of flexion [1] **(IIb/B)**.

The importance of the restraining influence of the popliteal and popliteofibular ligaments during knee flexion has been reported [3]. Furthermore, Amis *et al* [15] suggests that rotatory instability is influenced by fibular head position and ligament orientation during knee flexion. The LCL was found to slacken in flexion, whereas the PFL complex did not, suggesting that the PFL is dominant in flexion. Reconstructive surgery should, therefore, address any popliteofibular deficiency, although it is possible that anatomical variations of ligament orientation may make some individuals more prone to posterolateral instability and, conversely, some to a less favourable outcome following reconstruction **(IIb/B)**.

Coupled internal and external rotational instability

Coupled movements are those in which the resultant motion is in a different direction to the applied force. This can be demonstrated by applying a posterior force to the tibia. In an intact knee the tibia will rotate externally; conversely, if an anterior force is applied, it will rotate internally.

The degree of knee flexion also affects stability. When assessing the PCL, experimental sectioning or traumatic rupture of the ligament will result in an increase in the posterior translation of the knee at all degrees of flexion, but it is maximal between 75° and 90° [1] **(IIb/B)**. The PCL is, therefore, best tested with the knee in 90° of flexion.

Chapter 21

Isolated sectioning of the LCL shows maximal varus rotation at 30° of knee flexion. Therefore, in injuries where the PCL remains intact, an isolated posterolateral corner injury results in the largest increase in posterior translation, varus rotation and external rotation at 30° of flexion. Patients should, therefore, be examined at both 30° and 90°. An increase in varus rotation and external rotation at 30°, but not 90° of flexion, suggests an isolated posterolateral corner injury. However, both a posterolateral corner and PCL injury should be considered if increases are noted at both 30° and 90°.

Although the biomechanical constraints are complicated, there is increasing evidence that the most critical layers of posterolateral corner instability include the popliteus, the PFL and LCL [1, 3, 4, 15] (IIb/B). The integrity of these structures is critical for stability of the posterolateral corner.

Injury mechanism

Posterolateral injuries commonly occur following a direct blow to the anteromedial aspect of the knee or proximal tibia, with the knee in full extension. This often occurs in injuries where the knee is forced into a varus deformity with associated hyperextension and external rotation of the tibia.

The lateral capsule, and in particular, the posterior arcuate complex, accounts for most of the restraint at 5° of flexion [2]. Posterolateral corner injuries may, therefore, also occur after a varus force is applied with the knee in varying degrees of flexion [16, 17]. Instability may also arise following knee dislocation and indirect mechanisms involving twisting injuries.

Clinical aspects

Symptoms

Posterolateral insufficiencies often result in instability during everyday activities. Hyperextension and instability whilst the knee is in extension is a common complaint and may cause difficulties whilst ascending and descending stairs. Medial joint line

pain may also result in a misdiagnosis of medial meniscal pathology [16]. Nerve injury may occur following cases involving knee dislocation.

Signs

In direct trauma, contusions and bruising may be present over the anteromedial aspect of the proximal tibia. Swelling and induration may be apparent acutely; however, in the event of a capsular disruption an effusion may not be present.

Diagnostic tests

Examination of the standing patient may show the tibia to be positioned with increased recurvatum, a varus deformity and internal rotation. Gait assessment may reveal a varus thrust. Swelling, pain and muscle guarding may, however, make acute injuries difficult to examine and a more accurate examination is often achieved in an anaesthetised patient. Generalised ligamentous laxity should be excluded.

Posterior drawer test

Anteroposterior translation should be examined at both 30° and 90° of flexion. If posterior translation is noted at 30° but not at 90°, then a posterolateral injury is likely. If posterior translation is noted at both 30° and 90°, then an isolated PCL or combined injury is present.

Quadriceps active test

This is used to demonstrate the presence of posterior tibial subluxation and is important in establishing the presence of an associated PCL injury. With a patient in a supine position, the hip and knee are flexed to 45° and 90° respectively. The foot is fixed and the quadriceps are contracted without extending the knee. In a normal knee, the patellar insertion of the patella tendon is angled slightly posteriorly with respect to the insertion at the tibial tuberosity, as such there is no resultant anterior shift of the tibia relative to the distal femur [18] **(III/B)**. If PCL-deficient, the posterior subluxation of the tibia results in the patella tendon becoming angled anteriorly relative to the tibial tuberosity. Subsequent contraction of the quadriceps will result in an anterior shift of the tibia. This is not reproduced in an isolated posterolateral corner injury.

Varus stress test

This tests lateral instability in one plane and should be performed at both 0° and 30° of flexion whilst the ankle is stabilised. Instability at 30° is due to an isolated posterolateral corner injury, whilst a positive test in full extension indicates both a posterolateral corner and cruciate injury.

External rotation recurvatum test

Whilst in a supine position the great toe of each foot is grasped and used to lift the heels and legs off the examination couch. In posterolateral instability, there will be varus and hyperextension deformities at the knee. The tibia will also fall into external rotation [19] **(IV/C)**.

Posterolateral external rotation drawer test

This is used to test the integrity of the arcuate ligament complex [19]. With the patient in a supine position, the hip and knee are flexed to 45° and 80°, respectively, and a posterior drawer test is performed with the tibia externally rotated 15° and the foot held in a fixed position. If the lateral tibial condyle externally rotates relative to the lateral femoral condyle the test is considered positive **(IV/C)**.

Although biomechanical studies [1] report that external rotation is normally coupled with posterior translation, if excessive external rotation is noted, injuries to both the posterolateral corner and the PCL should be suspected. If a positive result is found when the test is repeated in 30°, an isolated posterolateral corner injury may be considered more likely [20] **(III/B)**.

Tibial external rotation test (dial)

This test is used to determine the degree of external rotation of the tibia relative to the femur at both 30° and 90° of flexion. With the patient prone the degree of external rotation is determined by measuring the angle between the medial border of a forcibly externally rotated foot and the vertical axis. An increased degree of external rotation can be indicative of a posterolateral corner injury. However, care should be taken in the test's interpretation, as the joints of the foot and ankle can all influence the degree of external rotation [21]. Comparison with the contralateral side is therefore imperative.

Reversed pivot shift test

This is performed by extending the knee from a position of 70° to 80° whilst the foot is in external rotation and a valgus strain is applied to the knee [22]. In a posterolateral-deficient knee, the lateral tibial plateau will be subluxed posteriorly relative to the lateral femoral condyle whilst the knee is in flexion. This is recognised as a posterior sag of the proximal tibia. As the knee is extended the examiner should feel and observe the lateral tibial plateau abruptly shifting into its reduced position at approximately 20°-30° of flexion **(IV/C)**.

The movement describes the shift of the lateral tibial plateau in the opposite direction from the true pivot shift sign [23] and will reproduce the patient's discomfort and simulate the feeling of the knee giving way. The test is, however, not specific [21, 22]. The contralateral side should therefore be examined to exclude false positives.

One can also link clinical instability to anatomical injury. Injuries to the LCL are demonstrated by increased varus instability at 30°. External rotation at 30° is consistent with an injury to the popliteus, arcuate ligament, PFL and fabellofibular ligament. Hyperextension and an increased varus deformity at 0° indicates a posterolateral capsule and PCL disruption (Table 2).

Table 2. Specificity of clinical examination.

Test	PCL	PLC	PCL / PLC
Posterior drawer at 30° flexion	+/-	+	++
Posterior drawer at 90° flexion	+	-	++
Quadriceps active	+	-	+
Varus stress at 0° flexion	-	+/-	+
Varus stress at 30° flexion *	-	+	++
External rotation recurvatum *	-	+	++
Posterolateral external rotation drawer at 30° flexion *	-	+	++
Posterolateral external rotation drawer at 90° flexion	+/-	+/-	++
Tibial external rotation test (dial) at 30° flexion *	-	+	++
Tibial external rotation test (dial) at 90° flexion	+/-	+	++
Reversed pivot shift *	-	+	++

* Denotes a test specific for posterolateral injury

Investigation

Imaging

Plain long leg standing anteroposterior and varus stress films can demonstrate evidence of osteoarthritis and varus malalignment. Magnetic resonance imaging utilising T1 weighted techniques can also prove helpful [24] **(III/B)**. Associated injuries including tibial plateau fractures, Segond fractures (indicating associated ACL injury) and avulsion fractures of the head of the fibula can all indicate significant soft tissue disruption, such that a posterolateral corner injury is also evident. In such cases vascular assessment, with appropriate imaging, is essential.

Arthroscopy

Arthroscopy is beneficial prior to reconstructive surgery, especially in chronic insufficiency where associated cruciate ligament, meniscal and articular cartilage injuries may be evident. Evidence of posterolateral insufficiency includes a positive lateral compartment 'drive through sign' [25] and the presence of greater than 1cm of lateral joint laxity with the application of varus stress **(III/B)**. Cadaveric studies suggest that in knees demonstrating symptomatic rotatory instability, an avulsion or partial disruption of the femoral insertion of the popliteus may be present, resulting in its altered arthroscopic appearance. Further variations will occur depending on the integrity of the PFL [26] **(III/B)**.

Management

Management is aimed at restoring knee stability and kinematics to facilitate a pain-free return to normal activity. The indications for surgical intervention depend on the nature and extent of the injury. In patients with an old injury and no significant symptoms or functional impairment, conservative measures may prove successful [27] **(III/B)**. However, in acute injuries with clear symptoms associated with rotatory instability, surgical reconstruction should be considered. Furthermore, if reconstructive surgery is not undertaken, continued instability may predispose the knee to meniscal tears, chondral injury and late osteoarthritis.

The timing and nature of the surgery is, however, controversial. It has been suggested that acute repair of the posterolateral corner is more successful than chronic reconstruction [5, 17, 27, 28] **(III/B)**. However, surgery should usually be deferred until after the acute inflammatory phase of the injury has subsided, especially during arthroscopic procedures, as the leakage of irrigation fluid through a capsular defect may increase the risk of a compartment syndrome.

Associated injuries to the cruciate ligaments should be reconstructed prior to, or concurrently with, the posterolateral corner. Indeed, failure to recognise and repair posterior lateral corner injuries when reconstructing the ACL is a common cause of failed ACL reconstruction [29] **(III/B)**. The need for combined reconstruction has been shown to be protective in a number of biomechanical studies. Forces through ACL grafts following the sequential sectioning of structures of the posterolateral corner were shown to increase, potentially threatening the graft [4] **(IIb/B)**. Furthermore, a study investigating double-bundle PCL graft reconstruction in combined PCL and PLC-deficient knees has also shown that posterolateral reconstruction has a protective effect on the reconstructed PCL [30] **(IIb/B)**.

In the late presentation of posterolateral instability, limb alignment and pathological gait cannot be corrected with soft tissue procedures alone and hence, the assessment of limb alignment is crucial. Patients who have a varus knee deformity and demonstrate lateral thrust in the stance phase of gait should be considered for a proximal valgus tibial osteotomy [31] **(III/B)**. When performed prior to posterolateral reconstruction, some symptoms of instability may resolve such that further reconstruction is not required. However, failure to correct alignment may result in eventual failed reconstruction.

Acute repair

In acute injuries, direct repair of the posterolateral structures has been considered to be advantageous; however, this should only be attempted following assessment of the injured structures. If the tissues are of good quality, primary repair can be attempted. Direct suturing techniques with transosseous sutures, anchors, staples and screws have all been suggested [5, 27, 32].

Although acute repair has been perceived as being a satisfactory treatment option, there is little evidence regarding its success and one report documents that results may not be as good as previously considered [32] **(IIb/B)**.

Augmentation

Augmentation techniques have been proposed for injuries to the popliteus tendon, PFL and LCL [5, 33] **(III/B)**. Strips of the ITB or biceps femoris tendon can be used for augmentation, but there is no published evidence to document the success or otherwise of these procedures.

Advancement

Proximal advancement of the posterolateral structures can be considered for chronic instability where the PFL and LCL are lax but intact.

The posterolateral complex is exposed, osteotomised and advanced proximal to the LCL. It is fixed to a decorticated area using staples and/or cancellous bone screws. Short-term results of this re-tensioning procedure are, however, not ideal [34] **(III/B)**.

Reconstruction

Many techniques have been proposed, some aiming to reconstruct the lateral collateral and popliteofibular ligaments, whilst others also attempt to reconstruct the popliteus muscle/tendon complex. Success is dependent on the isometric placement of the graft. If non-isometric grafts are used, the graft will not remain tensioned during a normal range of knee movement.

Although numerous graft choices have been suggested [35], biomechanical studies comparing the failure properties of different grafts support the use of hamstrings in posterolateral corner reconstruction [36] **(IIb/B)**.

Lateral collateral ligament and popliteo-fibular ligament reconstruction

A technique which uses the biceps tendon to reconstruct the PFL and LCL has been suggested [37] **(IV/C)**. The biceps tendon is tenodesed between the isometric point on the lateral femoral epicondyle and the fibular head. However, the success of this technique is dependent on the preservation of the biceps femoris insertion into the fibular head, an intact tibiofibular joint and intact posterolateral capsular attachments to the common biceps tendon; patient selection is therefore imperative. Furthermore, *in vitro* reports suggest that this technique may over-constrain external tibial rotation throughout flexion and varus angulation at 60° and 90° of flexion [38] **(IIb/B)**.

Although there are alternative methods of achieving an anatomically similar type of reconstruction [5], a Sling technique using a free semitendinous graft to reconstruct the PFL and LCL has gained popularity [39] **(III/B)**. Based on the principle that a graft placed from the posterior aspect of the fibular head to the lateral femoral condyle is in an isometric position, an anterolateral to posteromedial drill hole is placed in the fibular head to accommodate the graft. A tunnel is drilled at the isometric point on the lateral femoral condyle and the graft is then fed through the drill hole in the head of the fibula and its ends passed beneath the biceps tendon and the ITB. The graft is delivered into the tunnel, tensioned from the medial side of the knee and fixed with a soft tissue interference screw. In this method of reconstruction the anterior band of the graft reconstructs the LCL and the posterior band the PFL, thus restoring the anatomy, biomechanics and stability of the posterolateral corner.

Popliteus, lateral collateral and popliteo-fibular ligament reconstruction

With recent biomechanical studies concluding that the three critical layers of the posterolateral corner are the popliteus, LCL and PFL, surgical techniques are now being described to reconstruct these structures [32, 40, 41].

In these anatomical reconstructions, stability is restored by using either a tibialis anterior or tibialis posterior allograft in a modified two-tailed technique [32] **(IIb/B)** or by using a split achilles tendon allograft [40] **(IV/C)** or a two-graft achilles tendon technique [41] **(IIb/B)**. In the first technique described by Stannard [32], an anterior to posterior lateral tibial tunnel is drilled, as well as proximal fibula and isometric lateral femoral condyle tunnels. A screw and spiked ligament washer is placed at the isometric point of the lateral femoral condyle and the allograft is then taken from the posterior tibia up to, and around, the anterior aspect of the isometric screw before running down to the posterior aspect of the fibula. It is passed through the fibular tunnel and then back to the screw and washer where it is tensioned and fixed.

Rehabilitation

The primary role of surgery is to provide sufficient stability for a functional rehabilitation programme to commence. However, as with the choice of surgery, there is no general consensus regarding the ideal postoperative rehabilitation regime in this group of patients. Some reports advocate an immediate range of motion rehabilitation program [35], using continuous passive motion to try to prevent arthrofibrosis in those most at risk **(III/B)**. The use of a Compass Knee Hinge (CKH, Smith & Nephew, Memphis, Tenn) has also been advocated, although its routine use is yet to be shown objectively to be of benefit [32]. Others are more cautious, restricting movement in the early postoperative period.

It is the authors' view that postoperative rehabilitation should be tailored to the type of injury and the method of repair or reconstruction. In multiple ligament injuries greater restraint will need to be shown to preserve the repair or reconstruction. In those patients undergoing an isolated reconstruction of the PLC, or in those where a late staged reconstruction is to be undertaken, a more aggressive rehabilitation programme can be followed.

Chapter 21

Results

As yet there are few reports in the literature of the results of posterolateral corner reconstruction and certainly no long-term series with large numbers of patients.

As previously mentioned, one paper has questioned the role of acute repair versus reconstruction, a concept that challenges previously considered opinion. Stannard et al [32] reported that in a series of 57 patients, where 35 patients had an acute primary repair and 22 had primary reconstructions using a modified two-tailed technique, outcome assessment showed a significantly higher failure rate in the acute repair group. They concluded that repair is indicated in their practice in the presence of a bony avulsion where the fragment can be held rigidly by screw fixation. However, the study included knees with different combinations of ligament injuries and used a uniform rehabilitation programme irrespective of the nature of the injury, such that errors in data interpretation may have occurred. This may therefore not be a true representation of the results of tailored acute repairs (IIb/B).

The biomechanics of advancement procedures can also be questioned. By advancing the posterolateral complex, its isometric position on the lateral femoral condyle will be lost, and failure, or stretching, of the tissues likely. Further instability is, therefore, probable, a view reflected in the early reported results [34] (III/B).

A split biceps femoris tendon transfer augmentation procedure in the management of ten consecutive ACL/PCL/posterolateral corner injuries and 17 PCL/posterolateral corner reconstructions has been reported [39]. It concluded that posterolateral stability was restored in 90% of the former group and 94% of the latter after a follow-up of one to six years (III/B).

An LCL reconstruction utilising an Achilles tendon allograft in 20 consecutive patients with a follow-up of 24-73 months, has also been reported with a success rate of 76% with respect to knee stability and stress radiographs [35]. Thirteen patients had concomitant ruptures of their ACL, three of their PCL and three of their medial collateral ligaments. All were treated at the same time as the index operation (III/B).

Biomechanical studies have suggested that the three most important constraints involved in the posterolateral stability of the knee include the popliteus tendon, popliteofibular ligament and the lateral collateral ligaments. If these studies are accepted then a more anatomical approach to reconstruction may prove to be successful in the long term. Although there is a paucity of objective evidence in the literature, Stannard [32] reports a technique which restores the anatomy of the deep layer of the posterolateral corner and is strong enough to permit early motion of the knee. Reported results suggest that the technique gives better results than acute repair with 20 of 22 reconstructions performed being considered successful when rated by physical examination, Lysholm and International Knee Documentation Committee (IKDC) objective scores. Only two cases were considered failures (IIb/B). No clinical data are available to assess the outcome using the alternative anatomical reconstruction techniques [40, 41].

Conclusions

The management of injuries to the posterolateral corner of the knee is both complex and challenging. A thorough understanding of the anatomy and biomechanics of the region is essential for their diagnosis and management. Instability is predominantly posterior, varus and external rotation, maximal at 30° of flexion. As these injuries rarely occur in isolation, care should be taken to determine the presence of any associated injuries, especially those involving the cruciate ligaments. Conversely, failure to recognise a posterolateral corner injury is likely to compromise reconstruction of the ACL or PCL.

Much has been written on the management of this condition but very little objective analysis of outcomes has been reported. This is largely due to difficulties in comparing patient cohorts due to the variable nature of the associated injuries and the use of different surgical techniques. Many treatment regimes are based on small patient numbers reported with limited follow-up. There, therefore, remains a lack of consensus on the best treatment options.

Early reconstruction may give more favourable results by preventing secondary injury to the knee, although there is no evidence that acute reconstruction gives any greater stability than reconstruction of a chronic injury. Recently, there has been a move to reconstruct the three prime components of the posterolateral corner: the lateral

collateral ligament, the popliteus tendon, and the popliteofibular ligament. This appears to be supported by biomechanical and *in vitro* studies; however, as yet little clinical data are available.

It is fair to say that, at present, interest and enthusiasm are not matched by experience.

Recommendations	Evidence level
◆ A thorough understanding of anatomy is needed in the management of posterolateral corner injuries. This is easiest considered in three layers.	IV/C
◆ The three most critical layers of the posterolateral corner are the popliteus, the popliteofibular ligament and the lateral collateral ligament.	IIb/B
◆ Clinical examination remains the best way to assess the presence of injury. Plain radiographs, MRI and arthroscopy may be informative.	III/B
◆ Failure to repair posterior lateral corner injuries when reconstructing the ACL is a common cause of failed ACL reconstruction.	III/B
◆ In combined injuries, posterolateral reconstruction has a protective effect on a reconstructed PCL.	IIb/B
◆ Patients who have a varus knee deformity and demonstrate lateral thrust in the stance phase of gait should be considered for a proximal valgus tibial osteotomy.	III/B
◆ In patients with a chronic injury, conservative management may prove satisfactory if there are no significant symptoms or functional impairment.	III/B
◆ Reconstruction of the posterolateral corner appears to offer better results than acute repair, unless a bony avulsion is present.	IIb/B

References

1. Gollehon DL, Torzilli PA, Warren RF. The role of the posterolateral and cruciate ligaments in the stability of the human knee. *J Bone Joint Surg Am* 1987; 69A: 233-42.
2. Grood ES, Stowers SF, Noyes FR. Limits of movement in the human knee. *J Bone Joint Surg Am* 1988; 77A: 88-97.
3. Veltri DM, Deng XH, Torzilli PA, *et al*. The role of the popliteofibular ligament in instability of the human knee. A biomechanical study. *Am J Sports Med* 1996; 24: 19-27.
4. LaParade RF, Resig S, Wetorf F, *et al*. The effects of grade III posterolateral knee complex injuries on anterior cruciate ligament graft force. A biomechanical analysis. *Am J Sports Med* 1999; 27: 469-75.
5. Veltri DM, Warren RF. Posterolateral instability of the knee. *J Bone Joint Surg Am* 1994; 76A: 460-72.
6. Seebacher JR, Inglis AE, Marshall JL, *et al*. The structure of the posterolateral aspect of the knee. *J Bone Joint Surg Am* 1982; 64A: 536-41.
7. LaParde RF, Ly TV, Wentorf FA, *et al*. A qualitative and quantitative morphologic analysis of the fibular collateral ligament, popliteus tendon, popliteofibular ligament and lateral gastrocnemius tendon. *Am J Sports Med* 2003; 31: 854-60.
8. Last RJ. The popliteus muscle and the lateral meniscus. *J Bone Joint Surg Br* 1950; 32B: 93-9.
9. Terry GC, LaPrade RF. The posterolateral aspect of the knee; anatomy and surgical approach. *Am J Sports Med* 1996; 24: 732-9.
10. Tria AJ, Johnson CD, Zawadsky JP. The popliteus tendon. *J Bone Joint Surg* 1989; 71A: 714-6.
11. Diamantopoulos A, Tokis A, Tzurbakis M, *et al*. The posterolateral corner of the knee: evaluation under microsurgical dissection. *Arthroscopy* 2005; 21: 826-33.

12. Stäubli H-U, Birrer S. The popliteus tendon and its fascicles at the popliteal hiatus: gross anatomy and functional arthroscopic evaluation with and without anterior cruciate ligament deficiency. *Arthroscopy* 1990; 6: 209-20.

13. Maynard MJ, Deng X, Wickiewicz TL, *et al.* The popliteofibular ligament. Rediscovery of a key element in posterolateral stability. *Am J Sports Med* 1996; 24: 311-6.

14. Watanabe Y, Moriya H, Takahashi K, *et al.* Functional anatomy of the posterolateral structures of the knee. *Arthroscopy* 1993; 9: 57-62.

15. Sugita T, Amis A. Anatomical and biomechanical study of the lateral collateral and popliteofibular ligaments. *Am J Sports Med* 2001; 29: 466-72.

16. Hughston JC, Jacobson KE. Chronic posterolateral rotatory instability of the knee. *J Bone Joint Surg Am* 1985; 67A: 351-9.

17. DeLee JC, Riley MB, Rockwood CA. Acute posterolateral rotatory instability of the knee. *Am J Sports Med* 1983; 11: 199-206.

18. Daniel DM, Stone M, Barnett P, *et al.* Use of the quadriceps active test to diagnose posterior cruciate-ligament disruption and measure posterior laxity of the knee. *J Bone Joint Surg Am* 1988; 70A: 386-91.

19. Hughston JC, Norwood LA. The posterolateral drawer test and external recurvatum test for posterolateral rotatory instability of the knee. *Clin Orthop Rel Res* 1980; 147: 82-7.

20. LaPrade RF, Terry GC. Injuries to the posterolateral aspect of the knee. *Am J Sports Med* 1997; 25: 433-8.

21. Cooper DE. Tests for posterolateral instability of the knee in normal subjects. *J Bone Joint Surg Am* 1991; 73A: 30-6.

22. Jakob RP, Hassler H, Stäubli HN. Observations on rotatory instability of the lateral compartment of the knee. *Acta Orthop Scand* 1981; 191: 1-32.

23. Galway RD, Beaupre A, MacIntosh DL. Pivot shift: a clinical sign of symptomatic anterior cruciate insufficiency. *J Bone Joint Surg Br* 1972; 54: 763-4.

24. LaPrade RF, Gilbert TJ, Bollom TS, *et al.* The magnetic resonance imaging appearance of individual structures of the posterolateral knee. *Am J Sports Med* 2000; 28: 191-9.

25. LaPrade RF. Arthroscopic evaluation of the lateral compartment of knees with grade 3 posterolateral knee complex injuries. *Am J Sports Med* 1997; 25: 596-602.

26. Ferrari DA. Arthroscopic evaluation of the popliteus: clues to posterolateral laxity. *Arthroscopy* 2005; 21: 721-6.

27. Baker CL, Norwood LA, Hughston JC. Acute posterolateral rotatory instability of the knee. *J Bone Joint Surg Am* 1983; 65A: 614-8.

28. Baker CL, Norwood LA, Hughston JC. Acute combined posterior cruciate and posterolateral instability of the knee. *Am J Sports Med* 1984; 12: 204-8.

29. O'Brien SJ, Warren RF, Pavlov H, *et al.* Reconstruction of the chronically insufficient anterior cruciate ligament with the central third of the patellar ligament. *J Bone Joint Surg Am* 1991; 73A: 278-86.

30. Sekiya JK, Haemmerle MJ, Stabile KJ, *et al.* Biomechanical analysis of a combined double-bundle posterior cruciate ligament and posterolateral corner reconstruction. *Am J Sports Med* 2005; 33: 360-9.

31. Noyes FR, Barber-Weistin SD, Simon R. High tibial osteotomy and ligament reconstruction in varus angulated, anterior cruciate ligament-deficient knees. *Am J Sports Med* 1993; 21: 2-12.

32. Stannard JP, Brown SL, Farris RC, *et al.* The posterolatertal corner of the knee. Repair versus reconstruction. *Am J Sports Med* 2005; 33: 881-8.

33. Maynard MJ, Warren RF. Surgical and reconstructive techniques for knee dislocations. In: *Reconstructive knee surgery.* Jackson DW, Ed. New York: Raven Press, 1995: 161-83.

34. Noyes FR, Barber-Westin SD. Surgical restoration to treat chronic deficiency of the posterolateral complex and cruciate ligaments of the knee joint. *Am J Sports Med* 1996; 24: 415-26.

35. Noyes FR, Barber-Westin SD. Surgical reconstruction of severe chronic posterolateral complex injuries of the knee using allograft tissues. *Am J Sports Med* 1995; 23: 2-12.

36. LaParade RF, Bollom, TS, Wentorf FA, *et al.* Mechanical properties of the posterolater structures of the knee. *Am J Sports Med* 2005; 33: 1-6.

37. Clancy WG, Meister K, Craythorne CB. Posterolateral corner collateral ligament reconstruction. In: *Reconstructive knee surgery.* Jackson DW, Ed. New York: Raven Press, 1995: 143-59.

38. Wascher DC, Grauer JD, Markoff KL. Biceps tendon tenodesis for posterolateral instability of the knee. An *in vitro* study. *Am J Sports Med* 1993; 21: 400-6.

39. Fanelli GC, Larson RV. Practical management of posterolateral instability of the knee. *Arthroscopy* 2002; 19: 1-8.

40. Lee MC, Park YK, Lee S, *et al.* Posterolateral reconstruction using split Achilles tendon allograft. *Arthroscopy* 2003; 19: 1043-9.

41. LaParade RF, Johansen S, Wentorf FA, *et al.* An analysis of an anatomical posterolateral knee reconstruction. An *in vitro* biomechanical study and development of a surgical technique. *Am J Sports Med* 2004; 32: 1405-14.

Chapter 21

Chapter 22

Meniscus repair

Jesus Lozano BS, Medical Student [1]
C. Benjamin Ma MD, Assistant Professor in Residence [2]
W. Dilworth Cannon MD, Professor of Clinical Orthopaedics [2]

1 UNIVERSITY OF CALIFORNIA, SAN FRANCISCO SCHOOL OF MEDICINE, SAN FRANCISCO, USA
2 UNIVERSITY OF CALIFORNIA, SAN FRANCISCO DEPARTMENT OF ORTHOPAEDIC SURGERY, SAN FRANCISCO, USA

Introduction

Meniscal tears are common knee injuries, representing 75% or more of all internal derangements of the knee [1]. The annual incidence of meniscal tears has been reported to be up to 66 cases per 100,000 persons per year [2]. Meniscal tears are more common in males, with a male to female ratio range from 2.5:1 to 4:1 [2, 3]. Peak incidence tends to be in men at 20 to 39 years of age, while in women, meniscal injuries appear at a relatively constant rate after the second decade of life [2]. Seventy-three percent of all meniscal lesions are associated with a traumatic knee injury [2]. Meniscal pathology in association with anterior cruciate ligament (ACL) injury has been reported in 41%-100% of cases [4]. In patients with acute ACL injury and meniscus injury, the lateral meniscus seems to be torn more frequently than the medial meniscus. However, in patients with chronic ACL-deficient knees, medial meniscus tears seem to prevail [5].

Injuries to the meniscus may be asymptomatic or cause marked physical impairment (pain, swelling, locking and loss of motion) to individuals. Under these circumstances a surgical intervention may be required. Historically, a total meniscectomy was the primary treatment for a torn meniscus, but a better understanding of the function of the meniscus has led to the development of new meniscus-preserving interventions. This chapter is dedicated to the treatment of meniscal injury.

Methodology

Studies were gathered using Medline and Cochrane library searches. A variety of keywords, in various combinations, including (but not limited to) 'meniscus', 'meniscectomy', 'meniscus repair' etc., were employed in our searches. In addition, supplementary information was gathered via cross-referencing. Studies identified were appraised for their methodology. The focus of these searches was on studies looking at assorted meniscal repair techniques.

Anatomy

The menisci are crescent-shaped, fibro-cartilaginous structures positioned between the round

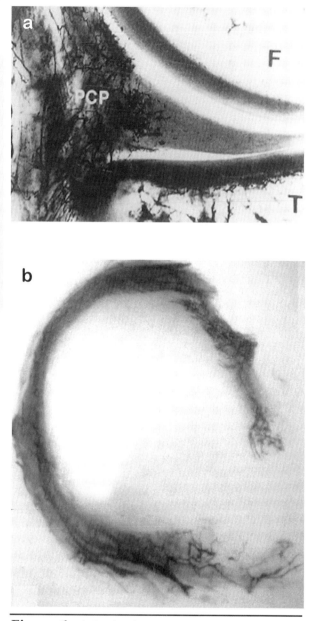

Figure 1. a) Sagittal and b) axial sections of the medial meniscus demonstrating the peripheral vasculature. Branching radial vessels from the perimeniscal capillary plexus (PCP) can be seen penetrating the peripheral border of the medial meniscus (F=femur, T=tibia). The central portion of the meniscus is avascular. *Reproduced with permission from Sage Publications Inc. Arnoczky SP, Warren RF. Microvasculature of the human meniscus. Am J Sports Med 1982: 10: 90-5.*

femoral condyle and the relatively flat tibial plateau. The medial meniscus has more of a C-shape compared with the circular shape of the lateral meniscus. Although the medial meniscus is larger than the lateral meniscus, it is much less mobile. It is this decreased mobility of the medial meniscus that may contribute to the higher incidence of medial meniscus tears.

Only the peripheral 10%-30% of the medial meniscus and the peripheral 10% to 25% of the lateral meniscus is vascularised [6]. Radial branches from the medial and lateral geniculate arteries provide the blood supply to the medial and lateral menisci, respectively (Figure 1) [6]. Thus, synovial fluid diffusion provides most of the nutrition to the relatively avascular menisci. The vascular anatomy of the meniscus has direct relevance in the treatment of meniscal tears.

Biomechanics

The primary function of the meniscus is to improve weight distribution across the knee joint. Early biomechanical studies have shown that the medial meniscus transmits 40%-50% of the compartment load, whereas the lateral meniscus transmits 65%-70% of the load in the lateral compartment [7]. Following partial and total meniscectomy, the biomechanics of the knee joint are altered [7-9]. A study by Baratz *et al* noted a nearly four-fold increase in peak contact forces in cadaveric knees who had undergone total meniscectomy when compared to those that had undergone partial meniscectomy [8]. A further cadaveric study found that removal of as little as 16% of the meniscus resulted in a 350% increase in articular contact forces [10].

The medial meniscus is also an important stabiliser of the knee and many authors have demonstrated the importance of the medial meniscus in limiting anterior tibial translation in response to anterior tibial loads in the ACL-deficient knee [11-14]. In the ACL-deficient knee, the posterior horn of the medial meniscus acts as a secondary restraint to anterior tibial translation. A recent cadaveric study demonstrated that the resultant force in the medial meniscus of the ACL-deficient knee increased significantly when compared with the medial meniscus of the intact knee in response to an anterior tibial load [15].

In summary, biomechanical studies have revealed the importance of the meniscus. Altered biomechanics following meniscectomy are responsible for the early degenerative changes seen after meniscectomy.

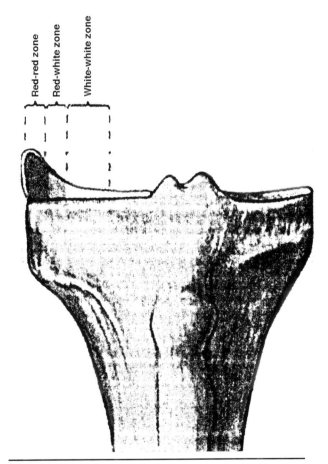

Figure 2. The location of the meniscus tear can be described by its vascular supply. A red-red tear occurs at the peripheral red zone of the meniscus where it is well vascularised. A red-white tear occurs at the transition zone where the meniscus becomes avascular. The white-white tear occurs at the central avascular white zone of the meniscus. *Reproduced with permission from Elsevier Inc. Miller MD. Sports Medicine. In: Review of Orthopaedics. Third Edition. Miller M, Ed. Philadelphia: WB Saunders 2000: 195-240.*

Meniscal tears

Meniscal tears can be divided into acute or degenerative tears. The tear pattern can further be characterised by its location, morphology and stability. The location of the tear is described by dividing the meniscus into posterior, middle and anterior thirds. The tear should also be distinguished with respect to the vascularity of the meniscus. The meniscus is commonly divided into a red-red zone, red-white zone and white-white zone (Figure 2). A red-red zone tear occurs in the peripheral, vascularised region of the meniscus close to the meniscal capsular junction. A red-white zone tear occurs in the middle part of the meniscus at the junction of the vascular and avascular portion of the tissue; these tears have decreased healing potential. The white-white zone tears occur in the central portion of the meniscus where there is no peripheral blood supply and markedly decreased healing potential. Accurate identification of the location of a meniscal tear is critical to determine whether repair or meniscectomy is indicated.

Meniscal tears are also characterised by tear morphology. Common tear patterns include longitudinal, radial and horizontal tears (Figure 3). Complex tears involve multiple cleavage planes. The tear pattern of the meniscus dictates the treatment options. Vertical longitudinal tears are more amenable to repair, while horizontal and complex tears are likely to require meniscectomy.

Treatment options

The treatment of meniscal injuries includes: non-surgical treatment, meniscectomy and meniscus repair. Recent efforts have also included meniscus transplantation or partial meniscus replacement.

Non-surgical treatment

The most common approach to meniscal injury historically has been either surgical removal or repair. The standard of care for non-surgical treatment, including the RICE protocol (Rest, Ice, Compression, Elevation), non-steroidal anti-inflammatory drugs (NSAIDs) and physical therapy, has usually been

Chapter 22

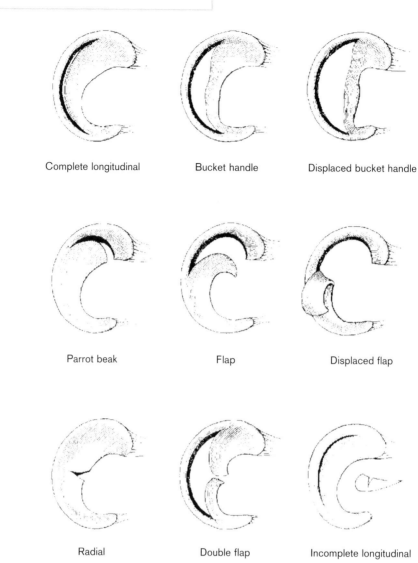

Complete longitudinal	Bucket handle	Displaced bucket handle
Parrot beak	Flap	Displaced flap
Radial	Double flap	Incomplete longitudinal

Figure 3. Common meniscal tear morphology. *Reproduced with permission from Elsevier Inc. Tria, AJ, Klein KS. An Illustrated Guide to the Knee. New York: Churchill Livingstone, 1992.*

found to be unsatisfactory. However, given recent advances in arthroscopy and an increased desire by clinicians to preserve as much meniscus tissue as possible, studies have focused on identifying meniscal injuries that can be left alone. A recent study treated all incomplete meniscal tears identified in conjunction with ACL injury with observation and found excellent knee function at two-year follow-up [16]. The average modified Lysholm score was 92.1 and the average Tegner activity score was five at two-year follow-up. Thus, given excellent knee function at two-year follow-up, short-term studies suggest that all partial

meniscus tears can be treated with observation at the time of ACL reconstruction **(III/B)**.

Other studies have also concluded that simple observation is sufficient treatment for short (10mm), full-thickness, vertical longitudinal tears that cannot be displaced 3mm with probing and radial tears measuring 5mm or less [17, 18] **(III/B)**. In a retrospective study looking at 189 lateral meniscus tears identified at the time of ACL reconstruction, Fitzgibbons and Shelbourne found that lateral meniscus tears, such as posterior horn avulsion tears, vertical tears totally posterior to the popliteus tendon, and other stable complete and incomplete lateral meniscal tears would remain asymptomatic if not repaired **(III/B)**. In their study, non-surgical treatment of lateral meniscus tears, in conjunction with ACL reconstruction, yielded excellent results; patients remained asymptomatic following a one to nine-year observation period [17].

In summary, several studies have demonstrated excellent clinical outcomes following non-operative treatment of several types of meniscal lesions. Studies to date suggest that partial-thickness tears, vertical longitudinal tears measuring less than 1cm that cannot be displaced more than 3mm, and radial tears measuring 5mm or less, can be left *in situ* [16-19] **(IV/C)**. Given the lack of randomised clinical trials comparing non-surgical and surgical interventions, more studies are needed to identify the best treatment of meniscal lesions. The clinician must use good clinical judgment, factoring in location and the age of the tear, patient age, the presence of secondary lesions or conditions, and the comfort level in dealing with meniscal lesions, when deciding to repair a meniscal tear.

Surgical treatments

Complete meniscectomy

Historically, complete meniscectomies were performed for internal derangements of the knee, but interventions now aim to preserve as much meniscus tissue as possible. In 1936, King [20] reported a direct correlation between the size of the meniscus segment removed and the subsequent extent of degeneration of the articular cartilage in a canine model. He also found that if meniscal tears extended into the vascularised zone of the meniscus, healing could occur [21]. Fairbank [22] later described changes in the knee joint following meniscectomy in humans, and various studies thereafter have documented the development of arthritis after total meniscectomy, and to a lesser extent, after partial meniscectomy [23-31].

In one retrospective study (10-30-year follow-up), patients reported satisfactory clinical results only 68% of the time and only 45% of men and 10% of women had symptom-free knees after total meniscectomy [31]. Another retrospective study (minimum ten-year follow-

up) looked at late clinical and radiographic results of total meniscectomy, and concluded that patients continued to have signs and symptoms relating to their initial meniscectomy 36% of the time and had radiographic changes 62% of the time [25]. Several studies on total meniscectomies have also documented that both radiological and clinical outcomes are worse after lateral meniscectomy than after medial meniscectomy [27, 32, 33]. One study reported that complete lateral meniscectomy resulted in satisfactory results in only 54% of the patients at early follow-up, and 16 out of 26 patients in that study developed late instability following complete lateral meniscectomy [33].

Studies clearly have demonstrated that long-term results (minimum ten-year follow-up) following a complete meniscectomy are disappointing and thus a complete meniscectomy should only rarely be performed [19, 25, 31] **(III/B)**. It was these studies, in addition to advances in arthroscopy and a better understanding of the importance of meniscal function, that provided the impetus for the development of partial meniscectomy for irreparable tears.

Partial meniscectomy

Several studies, with follow-up ranging from 2-14 years, report 85%-90% good to excellent results in patients with normal stability and no degenerative changes following an arthroscopic partial meniscectomy [30, 34-40]. However, a minority of authors have reported less favourable long-term results [41-43]. A large, retrospective study (minimum follow-up of ten years), which included 362 medial and 109 lateral partial meniscectomies in stable knees with no previous surgery or traumatic lesions, found that 95% of the patients were either completely satisfied or mostly satisfied with the result of their partial meniscectomy [36]. Furthermore, after a mean follow-up of 11 years, 85.8% of the medial meniscectomy group and 79.7% of the lateral meniscectomy group were normal or nearly normal according to the International Knee Documentation Committee (IKDC) scale. Though not statistically different, radiographs demonstrated a 21.5% increase in joint space narrowing in the medial meniscectomy group and a 37.5% increase in the lateral meniscectomy group.

Chapter 22

The authors concluded that a better prognosis can be predicted for a patient with an isolated medial meniscal tear with one or more of the following factors: age less than 35 years; a vertical tear; no articular cartilage damage; and an intact meniscal rim at the end of the meniscectomy. With an isolated lateral meniscal tear, a better prognosis can be predicted if the patient is young and has an intact meniscal rim at the end of the meniscectomy [43, 44] **(III/B)**.

A recent study of 40 patients with intrasubstance meniscal lesions found that partial meniscectomy had higher postoperative scores than other treatment modalities [45]. In the study, patients were randomly assigned to one of four groups: group A received conservative therapy (n=12); group B received arthroscopic suture repair with access channels (n=10); group C received arthroscopic minimal central resection, intrameniscal fibrin clot and suture repair (n=7); and group D received arthroscopic partial meniscectomy (n=11). Follow-up evaluation consisted of clinical examination with the findings recorded according to the IKDC protocol, radiographs and control MRI. After an average follow-up of 26.5 months, group D had the best results with 100% normal or nearly normal final evaluation at follow-up. Normal or near normal evaluation at follow-up for the other groups was: group A 75%, group B 90%, and group C 43%. These results indicate that performing partial meniscectomy can best treat intrasubstance meniscal lesions, but arthroscopic suture repair with access channels might give even better medium to long-term results because of preservation of meniscus. From the results of this study, conservative treatment is not satisfactory **(Ib/A)**. However, the treatment of intrasubstance meniscal lesions still remains controversial, as some clinicians would question the significance of these radiographic findings on clinical symptoms.

In summary, most studies report good long-term clinical and functional results following arthroscopic partial meniscectomy in knees with normal stability and no significant degenerative changes **(III/B)**. Most studies find evidence of radiographic deterioration after partial meniscectomy at follow-up **(III/B)**. Some studies have found correlation between radiographic findings and clinical results [14, 23, 29, 41-43, 46]. However,

other studies have found no correlation between radiologic and clinical results [43, 44]. Only when a meniscus tear is not likely to heal or when the patient's lifestyle and demands prevent meniscus repair, a partial meniscectomy should be performed. **(IV/C)**. All isolated degenerative or complex tears may be considered for partial meniscectomy **(IV/C)**.

Meniscus repair

Based on the established functions of the meniscus and the clinical results of meniscectomy, most clinicians advocate meniscal repair for all repairable tears. In a prospective study (six to ten-year follow-up) comparing the outcomes of partial meniscectomy vs. meniscus repair, Sommerlath found a statistically significant improvement in clinical outcome scores and decreased radiographic evidence of osteoarthritis in ACL-stable knees that had undergone meniscus repair, as compared to knees that had undergone partial meniscectomy [47] **(IIb/B)**. At 13-year follow-up, Rockborn and Messner, however, found no difference between meniscus repair and partial meniscectomy in knee function, subjective complaints, physical examination findings and radiographic signs of arthrosis. They reported excellent results in both groups, with almost 90% of patients reporting no knee problems during daily activities [48] **(III/B)**.

Criteria for meniscus repair

Although individual cases vary, the most commonly accepted criteria for meniscal repair include:

- a complete vertical longitudinal tear greater than 10mm in length;
- a tear within the peripheral 10%-30% of the meniscus (or within 3mm or 4mm of the meniscocapsular junction);
- a peripheral tear that can be displaced greater than 3mm towards the centre of the plateau by probing, thus demonstrating instability;
- the absence of secondary degeneration or deformity;
- a tear in an active patient; and
- a tear associated with concurrent ligament stabilisation or in a stable knee [19] **(IV/C)**.

The success of a meniscal repair depends on the healing capacity of the meniscal tear, the stability of the repair, type of repair and selection of appropriate patients [19, 49]. The healing capacity of a meniscal tear depends on the location and chronicity of the tear. A tear in the red-red zone has higher healing potential than a tear in the white-white zone because of the limited vascularity in this area [50, 51]. An acute tear also has higher healing potential than a chronic tear with remodelling [52]. The tear pattern is also important: vertical longitudinal tears are more likely to heal than a complex or horizontal tear pattern. A meniscus that has intrasubstance degenerative changes also has inferior healing potential [19]. The stability of the repair depends on the type of repair and stability of the knee.

If the knee has a concomitant ligament injury that is not addressed, the meniscal repair is less likely to heal [50, 53]. Lastly, the type of repair and patient selection can influence the healing potential of a meniscal tear. Patients under the age 50 should be considered candidates for meniscal repair if the tear is amenable to repair because of improved healing rates [19, 53]. However, there are no absolute age limits for meniscal repair.

Meniscus repair in the avascular zone

Historically, repair was advocated only for single longitudinal tears located in the outer-third region of the meniscus, but recent studies have published encouraging results advocating that more complex lesions, including meniscal tears extending into the avascular region, can be repaired **(III/B)**. Rubman *et al* [54] followed a large group of patients (n=198) after undergoing meniscus repair for meniscal tears that extended into the central one-third avascular zone. At a mean of 42 months postoperatively, they reported that 80% of the 198 repairs were asymptomatic for tibiofemoral joint symptoms. Of the 91 repairs evaluated arthroscopically, 64% of the tears were either healed or partially healed. The authors concluded that even though the failure rate is higher when repairing tears in the avascular zone, they believed that the benefits of a potentially functional meniscus outweighed the risk of re-operation. A second study [55] exploring arthroscopic repair of similar lesions in patients 40 years of age or older found that 87% were asymptomatic at a mean follow-up of 24 months postoperatively. Seventy-two percent

of patients in this study had also undergone concomitant ACL repair. In this study, the authors recommended preservation of meniscal tissue regardless of age, basing indications for the procedure on current and future activity levels.

Studies have been able to improve healing in avascular zones by implementing additional techniques, such as rasping of meniscal tears and parameniscal synovium, trephination to create vascular access channels, the use of fascial sheath and a fibrin clot, and addition of a fibrin clot to the tear [52, 55-61]. The ability of a fibrin clot to stimulate and support a reparative response in the avascular portion of the meniscus was first elucidated in canine experiments. In canines, Arnoczky *et al* demonstrated that addition of exogenous fibrin clot could promote healing of full-thickness lesions in the avascular portion of medial meniscus (control lesions had no reparative response) [56]. The authors suggested that the exogenous fibrin clot may enhance the healing potential of the meniscus in the avascular portion by providing a scaffold for a reparative response. Serum-derived factors found in the fibrin clot may also improve meniscus healing. In humans, fibrin clot also seems to improve healing rates [52, 61]. Van Trommel *et al* reported successful repair and healing of five tears found in the posterolateral portion of the meniscus in the avascular zone using a fibrin clot [61]. It is strongly recommended that a fibrin clot be used to enhance the healing potential of isolated meniscal tears **(IV/C)**.

Displaced bucket-handle (DBH) meniscal lesions

Successful outcomes have also been reported following repair of locked bucket-handle meniscal tears, which are relative surgical emergencies that require immediate attention. O'Shea *et al* reported the results of staged repair of locked bucket-handle meniscus tears followed by delayed ACL reconstruction once full range of motion was obtained [62]. At the time of ACL reconstruction (n=55), 55% of the meniscal repairs appeared healed, 34% partially healed, and 11% showed no healing. Of 43 tears in the white-white zone, 21 appeared healed, 17 were partially healed, and five showed no healing. Of 11 in the red-white zone, eight appeared healed, two were partially healed, and one showed no healing. One meniscal tear in the red-red zone appeared healed. At an average follow-up of 4.3 years, 84% of white-white meniscal repairs remained asymptomatic; all repairs in the other zones were asymptomatic. The authors concluded that locked bucket-handle meniscal tears heal at a high rate when repaired as an isolated procedure, even when full weight-bearing and activity before ACL reconstruction is allowed and when the tear is in the white-white zone **(III/B)**.

DBH meniscal tears should be repaired when encountered; however, whether DBH meniscal tears warrant a staged procedure is a matter of debate. Shelbourne *et al* recommend performing a two-stage procedure in which ACL reconstruction is delayed until the patient is fully rehabilitated after initial repair of the DBH meniscal tear, because they found a significant reduction in motion problems [63]. However, a larger retrospective analysis by Costouros *et al* has compared the return of extension in patients undergoing simultaneous ACL reconstruction and repair of DBH tears versus a control group of patients with non-DBH tears [64]. Although patients with simultaneous ACL reconstruction and DBH tears experienced a slower recovery to -5° and 0° of extension (22% and 35%, respectively), the results were not statistically significant. We recommend a one-stage procedure when encountering a DBH meniscal tear in an ACL-deficient knee. A one-stage procedure is sufficient in allowing patients with DBH tears to regain a functional knee to within 5° of full extension **(III/B)**.

Meniscus repair in conjunction with ligamentous injury

Meniscal injuries commonly occur in conjunction with ligamentous injury, and studies looking at meniscus repair in conjunction with ACL repair have reported successful outcomes. Cannon and Vittori reported successful results in over 90% of meniscal repairs performed in conjunction with ACL reconstruction, while only 50% of meniscal repairs in ACL-stable knees were successful when examined using arthroscopy or arthrography [50]. It is postulated that the greater success rate in patients undergoing concurrent ACL repair is due to:

 ◆ ligamentous stability afforded by the ACL reconstruction protecting against repetitive shear forces; and

 ◆ the presence of a haemarthrosis following ACL reconstruction, which may bathe the torn meniscus with a fibrin clot. This in turn might contain growth factors that contribute to enhanced healing [19].

Thus, it is recommended that all vertical longitudinal and displaced bucket-handle tears in an ACL-deficient knee be repaired in conjunction with ACL reconstruction. Other complex tears (such as radial tears, double bucket-handle tears or displaced bucket-handle tears) may be repaired with concurrent ACL reconstruction. However, one should expect lower healing rates **(III/B)**.

Rates of failure are also influenced by knee stability [1, 53, 65]. Steenbrugge *et al* followed 45 patients who had undergone a closed meniscus repair [1]. Twenty-three of those patients had their ACL intact (group 1), whereas in 22 patients (group 2), the ACL was deficient. After a mean follow-up of nine years, the ACL intact group (group 1) had 87% satisfactory knee scores, while only 64% in the ACL-deficient group (group 2) had satisfactory group scores. The success of meniscal repair performed in conjunction with ACL reconstruction has been reported to be greater than 90%, compared with reported 13%-40% failure rate when the ACL is not reconstructed [1, 50, 53, 65]. Based on these results, meniscal repair should only rarely be performed without concurrent ACL reconstruction, given higher failure rates **(III/B)**.

Surgical technique

Meniscal repairs should be performed after adequate preparation of the tear site. Any loose or frayed fragments of meniscus are removed and the tear edges should be abraded to stimulate bleeding. Abrasion of the local synovium and meniscal rasping may also be performed to improve healing [52, 60, 66, 67] **(III/B)**. Anatomic apposition of the tear edges is critical to ensure good healing potential and restoration of biomechanical function. Techniques for meniscal repair include either open or arthroscopic techniques (inside-out technique, outside-in technique and all-inside technique). A discussion of meniscal repair techniques is beyond the scope of this chapter, but suffice it to say that, historically, the inside-out arthroscopic meniscal repair has by far been the most

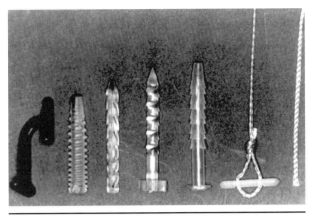

Figure 4. Various meniscal repair devices (left to right): Mitek Meniscal Repair System, Clearfix Screw, Arthrex Dart, Bionx Meniscus Arrow, Linvatec Biostinger, Smith and Nephew T-fix, 2-0 Ethibond suture. *Reproduced with permission from Elsevier Inc. Farng et al. Meniscal Repair Devices: A clinical and Biomechanical Literature Review. Arthroscopy 2004; 20(3): 273-86.*

suture captures the circumferential collagen fibres of the meniscus, giving it a higher pull-out strength than other suture orientations.

All-inside meniscal repairs are quickly becoming popular with the development of various implants, including meniscal arrows, darts, screws, as well as suture devices (Figure 4). All-inside meniscal repair devices are attractive as they do not require accessory incisions (reducing the risk of injury to popliteal structures) and can be time-saving. However, their effectiveness may be decreased when compared with traditional repairs. Biomechanical tests have shown that vertical repairs using sutures have the highest pull-out strength when compared with the all-inside meniscal repair devices [68-73] (Figure 5). A recent comprehensive literature review by Farng and Sherman of all-inside meniscal repair devices found that vertical sutures were superior or equivalent to most all-inside devices [74].

popular technique used worldwide, with the vertical mattress suture orientation being preferred. It is the ideal suture orientation because a vertical mattress

Early clinical results of meniscus repair with all-inside devices have been promising [75-79]. Studies have reported 80%-90% clinical success rates with

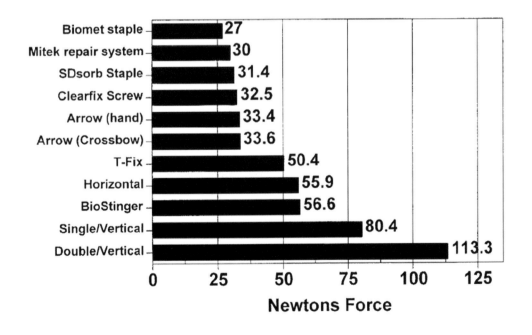

Figure 5. Load to failure strength of meniscal repair devices. *Reproduced with permission from Elsevier Inc. Barber FA, Herbert MA. Meniscal Repair Devices. Arthroscopy 2000; 16(6): 613-8.*

bioabsorbable arrows two to three years following repair [78, 80] **(III/B)**. However, complications have been reported with the use of all-inside devices. Friden and Rydholm reported a case of severe synovitis or foreign body reaction [81]. There have also been reports of damage to the overlying femoral condyle from prominent all-inside repair implants and reports of false positioning or inappropriate arrow size causing irritation to the posterior capsule or migration into the subcutaneous tissue [82-84]. Thus, care must be used to ensure that these implants are well seated in the meniscus and are not left prominent on the meniscus surface to avoid complications.

In summary, all-inside devices have been shown to be biomechanically inferior to vertical sutures. However, whether or not this is of clinical significance is yet to be determined. Short-term follow-up (two to three years) has yielded 80%-90% clinical success rates, but long-term follow-up is still necessary to assess the efficacy of these new devices **(III/B)**.

Future of meniscus repair

In the future, tissue engineering may offer new treatment modalities for either the regeneration of meniscus lesions or for the complete regeneration of a degenerated meniscus.

Tissue engineering techniques focusing on the regeneration of meniscus lesions involve the use of scaffold implants to support the generation of new meniscus-like tissue in meniscal lesions. Scaffolds have been constructed of various materials, but clinical studies have only been completed using collagen scaffolds [85-87]. Early *in vitro* and *in vivo*

investigations have demonstrated the safety and ability of collagen scaffolds (derived from Type I collagen fibres purified from bovine Achilles tendon with chemical treatment) to support tissue ingrowth in patients over a three-year period [85-88]. A decrease in pre-operative symptoms following a tissue-engineered collagen meniscus implant has been documented in eight patients (five to six-year follow-up) who have undergone reconstruction of one injured medial meniscus [86] **(III/B)**. Although these initial results are encouraging, further studies are needed to evaluate its use in clinical settings. A large US-based, randomised multicentre trial involving approximately 300 patients, comparing collagen meniscus implants with standard partial meniscectomies is nearing completion [86]. The outcome of this study will be instrumental in assessing the future of collagen-based scaffolds in meniscus repair.

Conclusions

The menisci are important structures with a role in load transmission and stability in the knee. Thus, it is important to preserve as much functional meniscal tissue as possible. Meniscal repair techniques are becoming more diverse, especially with the myriad of all-inside techniques. These new techniques, in addition to improvements in arthroscopy, have decreased morbidity and allowed repair for a wider range of meniscus tears. Tissue engineering techniques, such as collagen scaffolds, hold great promise and may play a significant role in the management of meniscal injuries in the future. With improvements in the treatment of meniscal injuries, early cartilage degeneration and morbidity associated with meniscal tears may be prevented.

Recommendations	Evidence level

Conservative treatment

- Partial thickness meniscal tears. — III/B
- Full thickness vertical longitudinal tears (<1cm and cannot be displaced >3mm). — III/B
- Radial tears (5mm or less). — III/B

Complete meniscectomy

- Rarely indicated and only acceptable when repair or partial meniscectomy is not possible. — III/B

Partial meniscectomy

- Isolated degenerative or complex tears. — IV/C
- Intrasubstance meniscal tears. — Ib/A

Repair (technique via discretion of surgeon)

- Complete vertical longitudinal tear greater than 10mm in length. — IV/C
- A tear within the peripheral 10%-30% of the meniscus and tears extending into the avascular zone. — III/B
- A peripheral tear that can be displaced towards the centre of the plateau by probing, (thus demonstrating instability). — III/B
- DBH and all vertical longitudinal tears in an ACL-deficient knee, in conjunction with ACL reconstruction. — III/B
- A tear in an active patient with a stable knee. — IV/C

References

1. Steenbrugge F, Van Nieuwenhuyse W, Verdonk R, *et al*. Arthroscopic meniscus repair in the ACL-deficient knee. *Int Orthop* 2005; 29: 109-12.

2. Hede A, Jensen DB, Blyme P, *et al*. Epidemiology of meniscal lesions in the knee. 1,215 open operations in Copenhagen 1982-84. *Acta Orthop Scand* 1990; 61: 435-7.

3. Yawn BP, Amadio P, Harmsen WS, *et al*. Isolated acute knee injuries in the general population. *J Trauma* 2000; 48: 716-23.

4. Bellabarba C, Bush-Joseph CA, Bach BR, Jr. Patterns of meniscal injury in the anterior cruciate-deficient knee: a review of the literature. *Am J Orthop* 1997; 26: 18-23.

5. Wickiewicz TL. Meniscal injuries in the cruciate-deficient knee. *Clin Sports Med* 1990; 9: 681-94.

6. Arnoczky SP, Warren RF. The microvasculature of the meniscus and its response to injury. An experimental study in the dog. *Am J Sports Med* 1983; 11: 131-41.

7. Seedhom BB. Loadbearing function of the menisci. *Physiotherapy* 1976; 62: 223.

8. Baratz ME, Fu FH, Mengato R. Meniscal tears: the effect of meniscectomy and of repair on intraarticular contact areas and stress in the human knee. A preliminary report. *Am J Sports Med* 1986; 14: 270-5.

9. Kurosawa H, Fukubayashi T, Nakajima H. Load-bearing mode of the knee joint: physical behavior of the knee joint with or without menisci. *Clin Orthop Relat Res* 1980; 149: 283-90.

10. Seedhom BB, Hargreaves DJ. Transmission of the load in the knee joint with special reference to the role of the menisci. Part II: experimental results, discussion and conclusions. *Eng in Med* 1979; 8: 207-19.

11. Bargar WL, Moreland JR, Markolf KL, *et al*. *In vivo* stability testing of post-meniscectomy knees. *Clin Orthop Relat Res* 1980; 150: 247-52.

12. Bonnin M, Carret JP, Dimnet J, *et al*. The weight-bearing knee after anterior cruciate ligament rupture. An *in vitro*

biomechanical study. *Knee Surg Sports Traumatol Arthrosc* 1996; 3: 245-51.

13. Levy IM, Torzilli PA, Gould JD, *et al.* The effect of lateral meniscectomy on motion of the knee. *J Bone Joint Surg Am* 1989; 71: 401-6.

14. Shoemaker SC, Markolf KL. The role of the meniscus in the anterior-posterior stability of the loaded anterior cruciate-deficient knee. Effects of partial versus total excision. *J Bone Joint Surg Am* 1986; 68: 71-9.

15. Allen CR, Wong EK, Livesay GA, *et al.* Importance of the medial meniscus in the anterior cruciate ligament-deficient knee. *J Orthop Res* 2000; 18: 109-15.

16. Zemanovic JR, McAllister DR, Hame SL. Nonoperative treatment of partial-thickness meniscal tears identified during anterior cruciate ligament reconstruction. *Orthopedics* 2004; 27: 755-8.

17. Fitzgibbons RE, Shelbourne KD. 'Aggressive' nontreatment of lateral meniscal tears seen during anterior cruciate ligament reconstruction. *Am J Sports Med* 1995; 23: 156-9.

18. Weiss CB, Lundberg M, Hamberg P, *et al.* Non-operative treatment of meniscal tears. *J Bone Joint Surg Am* 1989; 71: 811-22.

19. Belzer JP, Cannon WD, Jr. Meniscus tears: treatment in the stable and unstable knee. *J Am Acad Orthop Surg* 1993; 1: 41-7.

20. King D. The function of semilunar cartilages. *J Bone Joint Surg* 1936; 18: 1069-76.

21. King D. The healing of semilunar cartilages. *J Bone Joint Surg* 1936; 18: 333-42.

22. Fairbank TJ. Knee joint changes after meniscectomy. *J Bone Joint Surg Br* 1948; 30: 664-70.

23. Appel H. Late results after meniscectomy in the knee joint. A clinical and roentgenologic follow-up investigation. *Acta Orthop Scand Suppl* 1970; 133: 1-111.

24. Cox JS, Nye CE, Schaefer WW, *et al.* The degenerative effects of partial and total resection of the medial meniscus in dogs' knees. *Clin Orthop Relat Res* 1975; 109: 178-83.

25. Gear MW. The late results of meniscectomy. *Br J Surg* 1967; 54: 270-2.

26. Jackson JP. Degenerative changes in the knee after meniscectomy. *Br Med J* 1968; 2: 525-7.

27. Johnson RJ, Kettelkamp DB, Clark W, *et al.* Factors affecting late results after meniscectomy. *J Bone Joint Surg Am* 1974; 56: 719-29.

28. Krause WR, Pope MH, Johnson RJ, *et al.* Mechanical changes in the knee after meniscectomy. *J Bone Joint Surg Am* 1976; 58: 599-604.

29. Maletius W, Messner K. The effect of partial meniscectomy on the long-term prognosis of knees with localized, severe chondral damage. A twelve- to fifteen-year follow-up. *Am J Sports Med* 1996; 24: 258-62.

30. Northmore-Ball MD, Dandy DJ. Long-term results of arthroscopic partial meniscectomy. *Clin Orthop Relat Res* 1982; 34-42.

31. Tapper EM, Hoover NW. Late results after meniscectomy. *J Bone Joint Surg Am* 1969; 51: 517-26 passim.

32. Abdon P, Turner MS, Pettersson H, *et al.* A long-term follow-up study of total meniscectomy in children. *Clin Orthop Relat Res* 1990; 257: 166-70.

33. Yocum LA, Kerlan RK, Jobe FW, *et al.* Isolated lateral meniscectomy. A study of twenty-six patients with isolated tears. *J Bone Joint Surg Am* 1979; 61: 338-42.

34. Andersson-Molina H, Karlsson H, Rockborn P. Arthroscopic partial and total meniscectomy: a long-term follow-up study with matched controls. *Arthroscopy* 2002; 18: 183-9.

35. Barrett GR, Treacy SH, Ruff CG. The effect of partial lateral meniscectomy in patients > or = 60 years. *Orthopedics* 1998; 21: 251-7.

36. Chatain F, Adeleine P, Chambat P, *et al.* A comparative study of medial versus lateral arthroscopic partial meniscectomy on stable knees: 10-year minimum follow-up. *Arthroscopy* 2003; 19: 842-9.

37. Chatain F, Robinson AH, Adeleine P, *et al.* The natural history of the knee following arthroscopic medial meniscectomy. *Knee Surg Sports Traumatol Arthrosc* 2001; 9: 15-8.

38. Northmore-Ball MD, Dandy DJ, Jackson RW. Arthroscopic, open partial, and total meniscectomy. A comparative study. *J Bone Joint Surg Br* 1983; 65: 400-4.

39. Osti L, Liu SH, Raskin A, *et al.* Partial lateral meniscectomy in athletes. *Arthroscopy* 1994; 10: 424-30.

40. Steenbrugge F, Verdonk R, Verstraete K. Long-term assessment of arthroscopic meniscus repair: a 13-year follow-up study. *Knee* 2002; 9: 181-7.

41. Englund M, Roos EM, Lohmander LS. Impact of type of meniscal tear on radiographic and symptomatic knee osteoarthritis: a sixteen-year follow-up of meniscectomy with matched controls. *Arthritis Rheum* 2003; 48: 2178-87.

42. Hoser C, Fink C, Brown C, *et al.* Long-term results of arthroscopic partial lateral meniscectomy in knees without associated damage. *J Bone Joint Surg Br* 2001; 83: 513-6.

43. Jaureguito JW, Elliot JS, Lietner T, *et al.* The effects of arthroscopic partial lateral meniscectomy in an otherwise normal knee: a retrospective review of functional, clinical, and radiographic results. *Arthroscopy* 1995; 11: 29-36.

44. Burks RT, Metcalf MH, Metcalf RW. Fifteen-year follow-up of arthroscopic partial meniscectomy. *Arthroscopy* 1997; 13: 673-9.

45. Biedert RM. Treatment of intrasubstance meniscal lesions: a randomized prospective study of four different methods. *Knee Surg Sports Traumatol Arthrosc* 2000; 8: 104-8.

46. Benedetto KP, Rangger C. Arthroscopic partial meniscectomy: 5-year follow-up. *Knee Surg Sports Traumatol Arthrosc* 1993; 1: 235-8.

47. Sommerlath KG. Results of meniscal repair and partial meniscectomy in stable knees. *Int Orthop* 1991; 15: 347-50.

48. Rockborn P, Messner K. Long-term results of meniscus repair and meniscectomy: a 13-year functional and radiographic follow-up study. *Knee Surg Sports Traumatol Arthrosc* 2000; 8: 2-10.

49. DeHaven KE. Decision-making factors in the treatment of meniscus lesions. *Clin Orthop Relat Res* 1990; 49-54.

50. Cannon WD Jr, Vittori JM. The incidence of healing in arthroscopic meniscal repairs in anterior cruciate ligament-reconstructed knees versus stable knees. *Am J Sports Med* 1992; 20: 176-81.

51. Scott GA, Jolly BL, Henning CE. Combined posterior incision and arthroscopic intra-articular repair of the meniscus. An examination of factors affecting healing. *J Bone Joint Surg Am* 1986; 68: 847-61.

52. Henning CE, Lynch MA, Yearout KM, et al. Arthroscopic meniscal repair using an exogenous fibrin clot. Clin Orthop Relat Res 1990; 64-72.

53. Warren RF. Meniscectomy and repair in the anterior cruciate ligament-deficient patient. Clin Orthop Relat Res 1990; 55-63.

54. Rubman MH, Noyes FR, Barber-Westin SD. Arthroscopic repair of meniscal tears that extend into the avascular zone. A review of 198 single and complex tears. Am J Sports Med 1998; 26: 87-95.

55. Noyes FR, Barber-Westin SD. Arthroscopic repair of meniscus tears extending into the avascular zone with or without anterior cruciate ligament reconstruction in patients 40 years of age and older. Arthroscopy 2000; 16: 822-9.

56. Arnoczky SP, Warren RF, Spivak JM. Meniscal repair using an exogenous fibrin clot. An experimental study in dogs. J Bone Joint Surg Am 1988; 70: 1209-17.

57. Fox JM, Rintz KG, Ferkel RD. Trephination of incomplete meniscal tears. Arthroscopy 1993; 9: 451-5.

58. Henning CE, Yearout KM, Vequist SW, et al. Use of the fascia sheath coverage and exogenous fibrin clot in the treatment of complex meniscal tears. Am J Sports Med 1991; 19: 626-31.

59. Okuda K, Ochi M, Shu N, et al. Meniscal rasping for repair of meniscal tear in the avascular zone. Arthroscopy 1999; 15: 281-6.

60. Uchio Y, Ochi M, Adachi N, et al. Results of rasping of meniscal tears with and without anterior cruciate ligament injury as evaluated by second-look arthroscopy. Arthroscopy 2003; 19: 463-9.

61. van Trommel MF, Simonian PT, Potter HG, et al. Arthroscopic meniscal repair with fibrin clot of complete radial tears of the lateral meniscus in the avascular zone. Arthroscopy 1998; 14: 360-5.

62. O'Shea JJ, Shelbourne KD. Repair of locked bucket-handle meniscal tears in knees with chronic anterior cruciate ligament deficiency. Am J Sports Med 2003; 31: 216-20.

63. Shelbourne KD, Johnson GE. Locked bucket-handle meniscal tears in knees with chronic anterior cruciate ligament deficiency. Am J Sports Med 1993; 21: 779-82; discussion 782.

64. Costouros JG, Raineri GR, Cannon WD. Return of motion after simultaneous repair of displaced bucket-handle meniscal tears and anterior cruciate ligament reconstruction. Arthroscopy 1999; 15: 192-6.

65. Hanks GA, Gause TM, Handal JA, et al. Meniscus repair in the anterior cruciate-deficient knee. Am J Sports Med 1990; 18: 606-11; discussion 612-3.

66. Ochi M, Uchio Y, Okuda K, et al. Expression of cytokines after meniscal rasping to promote meniscal healing. Arthroscopy 2001; 17: 724-31.

67. Tetik O, Kocabey Y, Johnson DL. Synovial abrasion for isolated, partial-thickness, undersurface, medial meniscus tears. Orthopedics 2002; 25: 675-8.

68. Asik M, Sener N. Failure strength of repair devices versus meniscus suturing techniques. Knee Surg Sports Traumatol Arthrosc 2002; 10: 25-9.

69. Barber FA, Herbert MA. Meniscal repair devices. Arthroscopy 2000; 16: 613-8.

70. Kohn D, Siebert W. Meniscus suture techniques: a comparative biomechanical cadaver study. Arthroscopy 1989; 5: 324-7.

71. Post WR, Akers SR, Kish V. Load to failure of common meniscal repair techniques: effects of suture technique and suture material. Arthroscopy 1997; 13: 731-6.

72. Rimmer MG, Nawana NS, Keene GC, et al. Failure strengths of different meniscal suturing techniques. Arthroscopy 1995; 11: 146-50.

73. Walsh SP, Evans SL, O'Doherty DM, et al. Failure strengths of suture vs. biodegradable arrow and staple for meniscal repair: an in vitro study. Knee 2001; 8: 151-6.

74. Farng E, Sherman O. Meniscal repair devices: a clinical and biomechanical literature review. Arthroscopy 2004; 20: 273-86.

75. Barrett GR, Treacy SH, Ruff CG. Preliminary results of the T-fix endoscopic meniscus repair technique in an anterior cruciate ligament reconstruction population. Arthroscopy 1997; 13: 218-23.

76. Escalas F, Quadras J, Caceres E, et al. T-Fix anchor sutures for arthroscopic meniscal repair. Knee Surg Sports Traumatol Arthrosc 1997; 5: 72-6.

77. Gill SS, Diduch DR. Outcomes after meniscal repair using the meniscus arrow in knees undergoing concurrent anterior cruciate ligament reconstruction. Arthroscopy 2002; 18: 569-77.

78. Jones HP, Lemos MJ, Wilk RM, et al. Two-year follow-up of meniscal repair using a bioabsorbable arrow. Arthroscopy 2002; 18: 64-9.

79. Laprell H, Stein V, Petersen W. Arthroscopic all-inside meniscus repair using a new refixation device: a prospective study. Arthroscopy 2002; 18: 387-93.

80. Ellermann A, Siebold R, Buelow JU, et al. Clinical evaluation of meniscus repair with a bioabsorbable arrow: a 2- to 3-year follow-up study. Knee Surg Sports Traumatol Arthrosc 2002; 10: 289-93.

81. Friden T, Rydholm U. Severe aseptic synovitis of the knee after biodegradable internal fixation. A case report. Acta Orthop Scand 1992; 63: 94-7.

82. Albrecht-Olsen P, Kristensen G, Tormala, P. Meniscus bucket-handle fixation with an absorbable Biofix tack: development of a new technique. Knee Surg Sports Traumatol Arthrosc 1993; 1: 104-6.

83. Calder SJ, Myers PT. Broken arrow: a complication of meniscal repair. Arthroscopy 1999; 15: 651-2.

84. Seil R, Rupp S, Dienst M, et al. Chondral lesions after arthroscopic meniscus repair using meniscus arrows. Arthroscopy 2000; 16: E17.

85. Rodkey WG, Steadman JR, Li ST. A clinical study of collagen meniscus implants to restore the injured meniscus. Clin Orthop Relat Res 1999; 367: S281-92.

86. Steadman JR, Rodkey WG. Tissue-engineered collagen meniscus implants: 5- to 6-year feasibility study results. Arthroscopy 2005; 21: 515-25.

87. Stone KR, Steadman JR, Rodkey WG, et al. Regeneration of meniscal cartilage with use of a collagen scaffold. Analysis of preliminary data. J Bone Joint Surg Am 1997; 79: 1770-7.

88. Stone KR, Rodkey WG, Webber R, et al. Meniscal regeneration with copolymeric collagen scaffolds. In vitro and in vivo studies evaluated clinically, histologically, and biochemically. Am J Sports Med 1992; 20: 104-11.

Meniscus repair

Chapter 23

Unicompartmental knee replacement

Nick London MA MD FRCS (Tr & Orth)
Consultant Trauma & Orthopaedic Surgeon [1]
Nagarajan Muthukumar D Orth FRCS (Tr & Orth)
Consultant Trauma & Orthopaedic Surgeon [2]

1 HARROGATE DISTRICT HOSPITAL, HARROGATE, UK
2 HULL & EAST YORKSHIRE NHS TRUST, HULL, UK

Introduction

The popularity of unicompartmental knee replacement, much like the mythological Phoenix, has risen in recent years.

McKeever and MacIntosh first introduced tibial plateau prostheses in the early 1950s for the treatment of unicompartmental osteoarthritis (OA). Since Marmor introduced modern unicompartmental knee replacement (UKR) in early 1972, its initial popularity was followed by skepticism, due both to the publication of some adverse reports of their performance and to the improvement in the results with total knee replacement. However, more recently, with better understanding of the indications, improved soft-tissue balancing and avoidance of peroperative over-correction, along with the development of better designs and materials, UKR has seen a resurgence in interest for its use. In this chapter we attempt to present the rationale and options in the treatment of unicompartmental osteoarthritis (Figure 1).

Methodology

A literature search was done on Medline and Pubmed using search words 'unicompartmental', 'osteoarthritis', 'knee', 'replacement', 'arthroplasty' and 'high tibial osteotomy'.

Pathomechanics of medial compartmental osteoarthritis (III/B, IV/C)

In the varus knee, primary knee osteoarthritis is thought to commence in the anterior part of the medial compartment of the tibiofemoral joint [1], high stresses occurring here due to the impact in the heel strike phase of the gait cycle. The progression to tricompartmental osteoarthritis may be the result of abnormal kinematics and instability of anterior cruciate ligament insufficiency due to impingement of intercondylar notch osteophytes. Incompetence of the anterior cruciate ligament results in progression of wear to the rest of the medial compartment and onwards to multi-compartmental osteoarthritis. The varus deformity only becomes fixed when this progression occurs. It is therefore thought that if anteromedial wear can be addressed early on in the disease, the progression of arthritis can be halted.

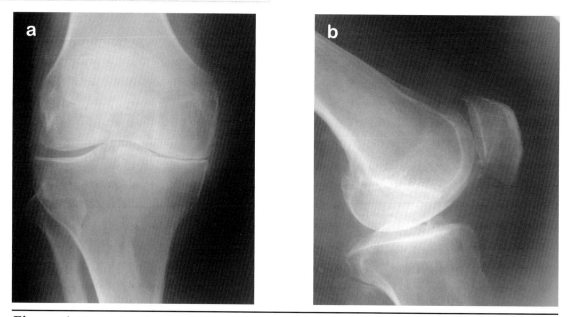

Figure 1. Typical radiograph of a knee with unicompartmental osteoarthritis. a) AP view. b) Lateral view.

Surgical options available for the treatment of unicompartmental OA

After exhaustion of conservative options, the surgical procedures which are available include:

- arthroscopic surgery;
- high tibial osteotomy (HTO);
- unicompartmental knee replacement (UKR);
- total knee replacement (TKR); and
- biological resurfacing methods.

Arthroscopic surgery

This may include lavage, debridement, chondroplasty and microfracture. It may result in temporary alleviation of symptoms. However, it does not address the pathology of the loss of ligamentous balance and loss of joint surface. This option will not be considered further in this chapter.

High tibial osteotomy (III/B, IV/C)

HTO is the traditional alternative to UKR [2-3]. Several reports describe deteriorating results with time.

Coventry [4] reported poorer results in patients with obesity and advanced patellofemoral arthritis. Alteration of knee anatomy can complicate future arthroplasty procedures. Conversion of a previous HTO to a TKR is difficult and the results are similar to revision knee arthroplasty [5-8]. There is a 28% failure rate by five years reported after converting a proximal tibial osteotomy to a UKR [9]. The indications for HTO have therefore narrowed. Improved patient selection, operative and rehabilitation techniques have been proposed as the keys to improve the outcome of this procedure. It still seems to have a place in treating medial gonarthrosis [10], especially in the young, physically active patients.

Unicompartmental knee replacement (III/B, IV/C)

UKR (Figure 2) has increased in popularity recently due to reports of ten-year survivorship comparable to TKR. Compared with HTO, UKR has been shown to provide more predictable pain relief and easier conversion to TKR. Weale and Newman [11] showed that the survival rate between the two procedures widens with time, with 90% for UKR and 76% for HTO at ten years and 88% for UKR and 65% for HTO at 15 years.

UKR is sometimes thought of as a 'pre-TKR' [12] or an 'arthritic bypass' [13]. It has been said that revision of UKR is often straightforward [14]. This, however, depends when failure occurs. Early failures due to loosening or mobile-bearing dislocation, as well as failures due to progression of arthritis, are easier to revise to TKR. Late failures with polyethylene wear, osteolysis and metallosis are more complex problems to revise and the results are probably comparable to revisions of TKR [15]. Vigilant follow-up is therefore essential to avoid less predictable results of revisions when significant bone loss has already occurred. Revision of UKR to another UKR and the addition of UKR in the contralateral compartment for progression of osteoarthritis has been shown to be associated with poor results [16].

Advantages of UKR

The main advantages include preservation of bone stock [15, 17-18], simpler revision surgery [15, 17, 19] and an increased range of motion [17, 20-22]. UKR is also associated with less blood loss during surgery [17, 23-27], simpler physiotherapy [17, 23-27] and decreased surgical cost [17, 21, 28]. Other benefits include subjective patient preference for the 'natural feel' of a UKR [17, 20-21], normal knee kinematics [29-30], a more normal gait,

better quadriceps function and knee flexion, as compared to TKR [31-32]. The results of UKR converted to TKR have been shown to be comparable to those of primary TKR [33-34].

Indications for UKR (IV/C)

Kozinn and Scott [17] suggested that UKR is indicated in patients who are >60 years old, <82kg in weight, lead a relatively sedentary lifestyle, have activity-associated pain and minimal pain at rest (rest pain might indicate an inflammatory component). Ideally, they should have a pre-operative arc of flexion of 90°, less than 5° fixed flexion contracture and an angular deformity ranging between 10° of varus and 15° of valgus, which must be passively correctable. With minor modifications, these various factors form the basis of current day practice in UKR.

Very small cartilaginous erosions in the non-weight-bearing areas of the contralateral compartment and patellofemoral joint are not contraindications.

Many surgeons consider a functioning anterior cruciate ligament and compartment-localised pain as pre-requisites for a UKR.

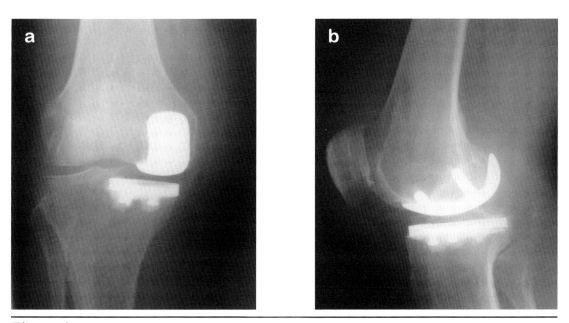

Figure 2. Unicompartmental knee replacement. a) AP view. b) Lateral view.

Contraindications for UKR

Exposed subchondral bone in the weight-bearing part of the opposite compartment, generalised inflammatory disease and recent infection are thought to be definite contraindications. Chondrocalcinosis or calcium pyrophosphate disease (because inflamed synovial tissue may increase the risk of secondary degeneration in the opposite compartment) and patellofemoral pain are relative contraindications.

Reasons for failure of UKR (III/B, IV/C)

Failure of UKR can be due to component loosening or infection, just as can occur with TKR. Specific factors associated with failure of UKR are progression of arthritis and polyethylene dislocation. Psychoyios *et al* [35] caution against revision of UKR without a clear diagnosis for pain. Revision of failed UKR should be to a total joint replacement.

Types of UKR

Fixed bearing

The earliest UKR were rather constrained (as were their TKR counterparts) polycentric prostheses. These failed due to subsidence of the narrow tibial component. They were followed by unconstrained designs (Marmor, St Georg Sled). The all-polytibial components of these prostheses were cemented to the cancellous bone within the cortical rim as inlay prostheses. This led to fracture of the surrounding cortex and subsidence of the tibial component.

The inlay designs were replaced by wider components that were implanted in an onlay fashion. Although the less constrained prostheses allowed dissipation of forces though the ligaments, new modes of failure emerged. Excessive delamination and wear of the polyethylene tibial component was caused by point contact stress and abrasion during the sliding and rollback of the femoral component on the polyethylene [36-37], which contributed to the high failure rate of these prostheses. The high rates of loosening of these early designs were attributed to the all-poly design being prone to deformation by creep or cold flow, which was thought to break up the cement-bone interface, causing micromotion and ultimately, clinical loosening [38].

Metal backing was introduced to eliminate this cold flow and also to allow the possibility of cementless fixation. The metal-backed tibial components also improved modularity and thereby facilitated alterations in the thickness of tibial components, allowing for more accurate knee alignment. The disadvantage of metal backing, however, was that it decreased the thickness of the polyethylene, which in turn increased the point contact stresses on the polyethylene by the femoral component [39]. Cementless fixation, which was made possible by metal backing, has also been shown to be associated with poor results [25]. A prospective, randomised study [40, 41] revealed no difference in the clinical results or migration of the tibial components of the same design when all-poly and metal-backed tibial components were compared.

Despite these changes, aseptic loosening of these prostheses continued to be a problem. It is now thought that the early high failure rates were due in part to the quality of the polyethylene, which is dependent on the manufacturing and sterilisation methods. In addition, a lack of understanding of the importance of under-correction of deformity, as well as inadequate balancing, contributed to poor results.

Mobile bearing

To offset the disadvantages of congruent, fixed-bearing prostheses (excessive shear forces) and less constrained fixed-bearing prostheses (increased point contact stress), a mobile polyethylene-bearing prosthesis was introduced [42]. This has the advantage of maintaining a large congruent contact area between the femoral component and the polyethylene, thereby reducing contact stresses. The shearing forces on the metallic tibial tray are also reduced as the polyethylene slides on the tray. The mobile-bearing prostheses are claimed to have reduced polyethylene wear [35, 43]. The backside surface of mobile-bearing knee replacements may tolerate the stresses and motions at that interface [44] better than modular fixed-bearing devices, thereby reducing backside wear.

The designers published an excellent cumulative survival rate of 98% at ten years [45], although this was for a group with retrospectively-developed selection criteria. Doubts have been cast on whether these results could be reproduced in an independent centre [16]. However, subsequently there have been encouraging reports from other units [46]. Despite this, it is suggested that the mobile-bearing UKR is a technically demanding prosthesis and the revision rate is influenced by the number of such operations the surgeon performs each year [47]. This observation is supported by data from the Swedish Joint Registry. There is no clear evidence to suggest that the results of mobile-bearing prostheses are any better than fixed-bearing prostheses at this stage.

Concerns have been raised with the mobile-bearing prostheses regarding the progression of arthritis in the lateral compartment and bearing instability, with occasional reports of dislocation of the polyethylene component.

Operative goals in UKR (III/B, IV/C)

It is important to aim for slight under-correction of the deformity, as overloading the contralateral compartment [17] (which is composed of articular cartilage that is inferior to that of age-matched controls [48]) may result in progression of the osteoarthritis [49]. Superior clinical results have been shown when the final mechanical axis was in the centre of the knee or slightly medial to the centre [50] in the varus knee. This position for the axis also improves the patellar tracking. Soft-tissue release to correct fixed varus is also not advisable.

Types of surgical approaches

Standard arthrotomy
This is the traditional method of performing a knee replacement and involves a wide exposure with patellar eversion.

Minimally invasive surgery (III/B)
The length of incision has been reduced, the patella is not everted, suprapatellar synovial pouch function is maintained and the extensor mechanism is not violated, thereby reducing postoperative morbidity and pain. This has permitted rapid recovery and early discharge from the hospital [51-52]. However, the basic principles of alignment and kinematics are paramount

and must not be compromised. Extramedullary instrumentation, with or without computerised surgical navigation techniques, might help to further reduce the morbidity of surgery.

Results of UKR (III/B)

Various series have demonstrated >90% long-term cumulative rate of survival of both the mobile-bearing and fixed-bearing unicompartmental knee replacements [45-46, 53-54], which compares favourably with the results of TKR.

Lateral compartmental UKR (III/B)

In general, most series of lateral UKR have smaller numbers and show poorer results than studies of medial UKR.

Greater translation of the lateral femoral condyle and elasticity of the lateral compartment ligaments increases instability and the risk of dislocation of the tibial insert in a mobile-bearing prosthesis [55]. It has also been suggested that valgus osteoarthritic knees may be associated with an abnormal anatomical shape of the lateral condyle. Access to the lateral compartment is technically more difficult through a limited incision. Patients with lateral compartment OA also tend to present later, as they usually have less pain. There is, therefore, a greater likelihood of instability and deformity, reducing the likelihood that UKR will be suitable.

These differences in kinematics, anatomical features and clinical presentation might explain the less predictable results [56-58] in the lateral compartment, as well as the suggestion that fixed-bearing prostheses might be more appropriate for lateral UKR [58].

Total knee replacement (III/B)

Long-term results of TKR have been well-documented with >90% survivorship at 15 years [22, 59-61]. The results in younger patients are, however, variable. Some papers quote only 76% survival at ten years in patients younger than 60 years [22]. However, excellent survivorship of cemented TKR is being reported in young patients [62-63]. It used to be thought that TKR was the most appropriate option for the elderly. However, more recently, it is widely accepted that UKR is the preferred option for treatment of unicompartmental osteoarthritis of the knee in the older patient, who is often sedentary and may have significant comorbidities. UKR is intended to be the last knee procedure needed for these patients.

Metallic hemi-arthroplasty (III/B)

This controversial option has been suggested for young patients with osteoarthritis who have unicompartmental arthritis of either the medial or lateral sides, in whom HTO is contraindicated by early opposite compartment disease or poor range of motion, and who are considered too young, too heavy, or too active for a TKR. It has also been suggested for patients who have a history of sepsis in the knee. It is thought to restore knee alignment and stability by replacing missing articular and meniscal cartilage with a single metallic implant. Pain relief is attributed to the redistribution of weight-bearing loads within the knee and to restored stability. However, recent reports of

the results of this procedure have not been encouraging [64].

Biological resurfacing methods

Various cartilage implantation trials are currently underway for localised cartilage defects. Whether these techniques would be applicable to the treatment of osteoarthritis in general remains to be seen.

In the future, treatment of early and established osteoarthritis is likely to involve developments in tissue engineering, gene therapy and pharmacology directed at the underlying pathological processes.

Conclusions

The better understanding of indications and surgical principles along with the development of improved designs and materials has led to both the excellent long-term cumulative rate of survival and the establishment of UKR as an effective option in the treatment of unicompartmental osteoarthritis.

Recommendations	Evidence level
◆ Pathomechanics of the progression of osteoarthritis is key to the underlying rationale of treatment.	III/B, IV/C
◆ HTO still appears to have a place in its management in the young, physically active patient.	III/B, IV/C
◆ Better understanding of indications, improved balancing, the avoidance of over-correction at the time of surgery, and the development of better designs and materials have been the key to the re-emergence of the popularity of UKR.	III/B, IV/C
◆ Excellent long-term cumulative rate of survival of both the mobile-bearing and fixed-bearing unicompartmental knee replacements have been reported.	III/B
◆ There is no firm evidence of any difference in results between metal-backed and all-polyethylene implants.	Ib/A
◆ There is no firm evidence of any difference in results between mobile-bearing and fixed-bearing implants as yet.	III/B

References

1. White SH, Ludkowski PF, Goodfellow JW. Anteromedial osteoarthritis of the knee. *J Bone Joint Surg Br* 1991; 73(4): 582-6.

2. Jackson JP, Waugh W. Tibial osteotomy for osteoarthritis of the knee. *J Bone Joint Surg Br* 1961; 43-B: 746-51.

3. Coventry MB. Osteotomy of the upper portion of the tibia for degenerative arthritis of the knee. *J Bone Joint Surg Am* 1965; 47: 984-90.

4. Coventry M, Ilstrup D, Wallrichs S. Proximal tibial osteotomy: a critical long-term study of eighty-seven cases. *J Bone Joint Surg Am* 1993; 75(2): 196-201.

5. Nizard RS, Cardinee L, Bizot P, Witvoet J. Total knee replacement after failed tibial osteotomy: results of a matched-pair study. *J Arthroplasty* 1998; 13(8): 847-53.

6. Haddad FS, Bentley G. Total knee arthroplasty after high tibial osteotomy: a medium-term review. *J Arthroplasty* 2000; 15(5): 597-603.

7. Mont MA, Antonaides S, Krackow KA, Hungerford DS. Total knee arthroplasty after failed high tibial osteotomy: a comparison with a matched group. *Clin Orthop* 1994; 299: 125-30.

8. Windsor RE, Insall JN, Vince KG. Technical considerations of total knee arthroplasty after proximal tibial osteotomy. *J Bone Joint Surg Am* 1988; 70(4): 547-55.

9. Rees JL, Price AJ, Lynskey TG, Svard UC, Dodd CA, Murray DW. Medial unicompartmental arthroplasty after failed high tibial osteotomy. *J Bone Joint Surg Br* 2001; 83(7): 1034-6.

10. Olin MO, Vail TP. High tibial osteotomy: will new techniques provide better results? *Curr Opin Orthop* 2001; 12: 8-12.

11. Weale AE, Newman JH. Unicompartmental arthroplasty and high tibial osteotomy for osteoarthrosis of the knee. A comparative study with a 12- to 17-year follow-up period. *Clin Orthop* 1994; 302: 134-7.

12. Romanowski MR, Repicci JA. Minimally invasive unicondylar arthroplasty: eight-year follow-up. *J Knee Surg 2002;* 15(1): 17-22.

13. Repicci JA, Hartman JF. Minimally invasive unicondylar knee arthroplasty for the treatment of unicompartmental osteoarthritis: an outpatient arthritic bypass procedure. *Orthop Clin North Am* 2004; 35(2): 201-16.

14. Marmor L. Unicompartmental knee arthroplasty 10- to 13-year follow-up study. *Clin Orthop* 1988; 226: 14-20.

15. Barrett WP, Scott RD. Revision of failed unicondylar unicompartmental knee arthroplasty. *J Bone Joint Surg Am* 1987; 69(9): 1328-35.

16. Lewold S, Robertsson O, Knutson K, Lidgren L. Revision of unicompartmental knee arthroplasty: outcome in 1,135 cases from the Swedish Knee Arthroplasty study. *Acta Orthop Scand* 1998; 69(5): 469-74.

17. Kozinn SC, Scott R. Unicondylar knee arthroplasty. *J Bone Joint Surg Am* 1989; 71(1): 145-50.

18. Marmor L. Unicompartmental and total knee arthroplasty. *Clin Orthop* 1985; 192: 75-81.

19. Marmor L. Unicompartmental arthroplasty of the knee with a minimum ten-year follow-up period. *Clin Orthop* 1988; 228: 171-7.

20. Laurencin CT, Zelicof SB, Scott RD, Ewald FC. Unicompartmental versus total knee arthroplasty in the same patient. A comparative study. *Clin Orthop* 1991; 273: 151-6.

21. Cameron HU, Jung YB. A comparison of unicompartmental knee replacement with total knee replacement. *Orthop Rev* 1988; 17(10): 983-8.

22. Rand JA, Ilstrup DM. Survivorship analysis of total knee arthroplasty. Cumulative rates of survival of 9200 total knee arthroplasties. *J Bone Joint Surg Am* 1991; 73(3): 397-409.

23. Thornhill TS, Scott RD. Unicompartmental total knee arthroplasty. *Orthop Clin North Am* 1989; 20(2): 245-56.

24. Broughton NS, Newman JH, Baily RA. Unicompartmental replacement and high tibial osteotomy for osteoarthritis of the knee: a comparative study after 5-10 years follow-up. *J Bone Joint Surg Br* 1986; 68(3): 447-52.

25. Lindstrand A, Stenstrom A, Egund N. The PCA unicompartmental knee. A 1-4-year comparison of fixation with or without cement. *Acta Orthop Scand* 1988; 59(6): 695-700.

26. Marmor L. Lateral compartment arthroplasty of the knee. *Clin Orthop* 1984; 186: 115-21.

27. Scott RD, Santore RF. Unicondylar unicompartmental replacement for osteoarthritis of the knee. *J Bone Joint Surg Am* 1981; 63(4): 536-44.

28. Robertsson O, Borgquist L, Knutson K, Lewold S, Lidgren L. Use of unicompartmental instead of tricompartmental prostheses for unicompartmental arthrosis in the knee is a cost-effective alternative. 15,437 primary tricompartmental prostheses were compared with 10,624 primary medial or lateral unicompartmental prostheses. *Acta Orthop Scand* 1999; 70(2): 170-5.

29. Robinson BJ, Rees JL, Price AJ, Beard DJ, Murray DM, OHKG. Oxford Hip and Knee Group. A kinematic study of lateral unicompartmental arthroplasty. *Knee* 2002; 9(3): 237-40.

30. Patil S, Colwell Jr CW, Ezzet KA, D'Lima DD. Can normal knee kinematics be restored with unicompartmental knee replacement? *J Bone Joint Surg Am* 2005; 87(2): 332-8.

31. Andriacchi TP, Galante JO, Fermier RW. The influence of total knee-replacement design on walking and stair-climbing. *J Bone Joint Surg Am* 1982; 64(9): 1328-35.

32. Chassin EP, Mikosz RP, Andriacchi TP, Rosenberg AG. Functional analysis of cemented medial unicompartmental knee arthroplasty. *J Arthroplasty* 1996; 11(5): 553-9.

33. Bohm I, Landsiedl F. Revision surgery after failed unicompartmental knee arthroplasty: a study of 35 cases. *J Arthroplasty* 2000; 15(8): 982-9.

34. McAuley JP, Engh GA, Ammeen DJ. Revision of failed unicompartmental knee arthroplasty. *Clin Orthop* 2001; 392: 279-82.

35. Psychoyios V, Crawford RW, O'Connor JJ, Murray DW. Wear of congruent meniscal bearings in unicompartmental knee

arthroplasty: a retrieval study of 16 specimens. *J Bone Joint Surg Br* 1998; 80(6): 976-82.

36. Blunn GW, Joshi AB, Minns RJ, Lidgren L, Lilley P, Ryd L, Engelbrecht E. Walker PS. Wear in retrieved condylar knee arthroplasties. A comparison of wear in different designs of 280 retrieved condylar knee prostheses. *J Arthroplasty* 1997; 12(3): 281-90.

37. Lindstrand A, Stenström A. Polyethylene wear of the PCA unicompartmental knee. Prospective 5 (4-8) year study of 120 arthrosis knees. *Acta Orthop Scand* 1992; 63(3): 260-2.

38. Ryd L, Lindstrand A, Stenström A, Selvik G. Cold flow reduced by metal backing. An *in vivo* roentgen stereophotogrammetric analysis of unicompartmental tibial components. *Acta Orthop Scand* 1990; 61(1): 21-5.

39. Engh GA, Dwyer KA, Hanes CK. Polyethylene wear of metal-backed tibial components in total and unicompartmental knee prostheses. *J Bone Joint Surg Br* 1992; 74(1): 9-17.

40. Adalberth G, Nilsson KG, Byström S, Kolstad K, Milbrink J. Low-conforming all-polyethylene tibial component not inferior to metal-backed component in cemented total knee arthroplasty. Prospective, randomized radiostereometric analysis study of the AGC total knee prosthesis. *J Arthroplasty* 2000; 15(6): 783-92.

41. Adalberth G, Nilsson KG, Byström S, Kolstad K, Milbrink J. All-polyethylene versus metal-backed and stemmed tibial components in cemented total knee arthroplasty. A prospective, randomised RSA study. *J Bone Joint Surg Br* 2001; 83(6): 825-31.

42. Goodfellow JW, O'Connor JJ. The mechanics of the knee and prosthesis design. *J Bone Joint Surg Br* 1978; 60-B(3): 358-69.

43. Argenson JN, O'Connor JJ. Polyethylene wear in meniscal knee replacement: a one- to nine-year retrieval analysis of the Oxford knee. *J Bone Joint Surg Br* 1992; 74(2): 228-32.

44. Callaghan JJ, Squire MW, Goetz DD, Sullivan PM, Johnston RC. Cemented rotating-platform total knee replacement: a nine to twelve-year follow-up study. *J Bone Joint Surg Am* 2000; 82(5): 705-11.

45. Murray DW, Goodfellow JW, O'Connor JJ. The Oxford medial unicompartmental arthroplasty: a ten-year survival study. *J Bone Joint Surg Br* 1998; 80(6): 983-9.

46. Svard UC, Price AJ. Oxford medial unicompartmental knee arthroplasty. A survival analysis of an independent series. *J Bone Joint Surg Br* 2001; 83(2): 191-4.

47. Robertsson O, Knutson K, Lewold S, Lidgren L. The routine of surgical management reduces failure after unicompartmental knee arthroplasty. *J Bone Joint Surg Br* 2001; 83(1): 45-9.

48. Obeid EMH, Adams MA, Newman JH. Mechanical properties of articular cartilage in knees with unicompartmental osteoarthritis *J Bone Joint Surg Br* 1994; 76(2): 315-9.

49. Tabor Jr OB, Tabor OB. Unicompartmental arthroplasty: a long-term follow-up study. *J Arthroplasty* 1998; 13(4): 373-9.

50. Kennedy WR, White RP. Unicompartmental arthroplasty of the knee. Postoperative alignment and its influence on overall results. *Clin Orthop* 1987; 221: 278-85.

51. Beard DJ, Murray DW, Rees JL, Price AJ, Dodd CA. Accelerated recovery for unicompartmental knee replacement - a feasibility study. *Knee* 2002; 9(3): 221-4.

52. Price AJ, Webb J, Topf H, Dodd CA, Goodfellow JW, Murray DW, Oxford Hip and Knee Group. Rapid recovery after Oxford unicompartmental arthroplasty through a short incision. *J Arthroplasty* 2001; 16(8): 970-6.

53. Deshmukh RV, Scott RD. Unicompartmental knee arthroplasty: long-term results. *Clin Orthop* 2001; 392: 272-8.

54. Berger RA, Meneghini RM, Jacobs JJ, Sheinkop MB, Della Valle CJ, Rosenberg AG, Galante JO. Results of unicompartmental knee arthroplasty at a minimum of ten years of follow-up. *J Bone Joint Surg Am* 2005; 87(5): 999-1006.

55. Gunther TV, Murray DW, Miller R, Wallace DA, Carr AJ, O'Connor JJ, McLardy-Smith P, Goodfellow JW. Lateral unicompartmental arthroplasty with the Oxford meniscal knee. *Knee* 1996; 3(1-2): 33-9.

56. Ohdera T, Tokunaga J, Kobayashi A. Unicompartmental knee arthroplasty for lateral gonarthrosis: midterm results. *J Arthroplasty* 2001; 16(2): 196-200.

57. Chakrabarty G, Ansari S, Newman JH, Ward AJ, Ackroyd CE. Lateral unicompartmental arthroplasty of the knee. *J Bone Joint Surg Br* 1997; 79-B (Supplement I): 115.

58. Ashraf T, Newman JH, Evans RL, Ackroyd CE. Lateral unicompartmental knee replacement survivorship and clinical experience over 21 years. *J Bone Joint Surg Br* 2002; 84(8): 1126-30.

59. Ranawat CS, Flynn Jr WF, Saddler S, Hansraj KK, Maynard MJ. Long-term results of the total condylar knee arthroplasty. A 15-year survivorship study. *Clin Orthop* 1993; 286: 94-102.

60. Keating EM, Meding JB, Faris PM, Ritter MA. Long-term follow-up of nonmodular total knee replacements. *Clin Orthop* 2002; 404: 34-9.

61. Ritter MA, Berend ME, Meding JB, Keating EM, Faris PM, Crites BM. Long-term follow-up of anatomic graduated components posterior cruciate-retaining total knee replacement. *Clin Orthop* 2001; 388: 51-7.

62. Duffy GP, Trousdale RT, Stuart MJ. Total knee arthroplasty in patients 55 years old or younger: 10- to 17-year results. *Clin Orthop* 1998; 356: 22-7.

63. Diduch DR, Insall JN, Scott WN, Scuderi GR, Font-Rodriguez D. Total knee replacement in young, active patients. Long term follow-up and functional outcome. *J Bone Joint Surg Am* 1997; 79(4): 575-82.

64. Sisto DL, Mitchell IL. Unispacer arthroplasty of the knee. *J Bone Joint Surg Am* 2005; 87(8): 1706-11.

Chapter 24

Clinical gait analysis

Rami J Abboud BEng MSc PhD MIEEE ILTM
Deputy Head of Division and Director of IMAR
Sheila Gibbs SRP MSc MRCSHC
Senior Clinical Gait Analyst
David I Rowley B Med Biol MD FRCS
Professor of Orthopaedics

INSTITUTE OF MOTION ANALYSIS & RESEARCH (IMAR), DIVISION OF SURGERY & ONCOLOGY, TAYSIDE ORTHOPAEDIC & REHABILITATION TECHNOLOGY (TORT) CENTRE, NINEWELLS HOSPITAL & MEDICAL SCHOOL, DUNDEE, SCOTLAND

Introduction

An equal and opposite force, better known as ground reaction force (GRF), develops when the foot comes into contact with the ground. The GRF changes in direction and magnitude as the body propels itself forwards (or backwards) (Figure 1). The foot must also be relatively compliant to cope with uneven ground, both bare and shod, yet simultaneously maintain its functional integrity. Foot function reverses the convention that a muscle is fixed at its origin and moves from its insertion during ground contact. In the foot, the conventional anatomical insertion is often fixed on the ground, and the origin in the heel or leg moves in relation to that fixed point. This provides both flexibility and stability during walking. The important mechanical structures of the foot include:

- bones, which together with the ligaments, provide relative rigidity and the essential lever arm mechanism required to maintain balance during standing and facilitate propulsion;
- joints and their axes of movement, including the structure and function of the arches, which provide flexibility;

- muscles, which in conjunction with their tendons, control foot movement.

Hence, the foot is the end part of the lower kinetic chain that opposes external resistance [1]. Normal arthrokinematics and proprioception within the foot and ankle influence the ability of the lower limb to attenuate the forces of weight-bearing (static and dynamic). The lower extremity should distribute and dissipate compressive, tensile, shearing, and rotatory forces during the stance phase of gait. Inadequate distribution of these forces can lead to abnormal movement, which in turn produces excessive stress, which can result in the breakdown of soft tissues and muscles. The normal mechanics of the foot and ankle result from the combined effects of muscle, tendon, ligament, and bone function. The co-ordinated and unified effect of these tissues within the foot, ankle, and lower extremity results in the most efficient force attenuation. This force is proportional to infinite discrete areas on the plantar surface of the foot when in contact with the ground and is described as foot pressure. Foot pressure is divided into two vectors: vertical and horizontal.

In healthy, normal feet, where there is no pain or any anatomical or functional deformity, normal plantar

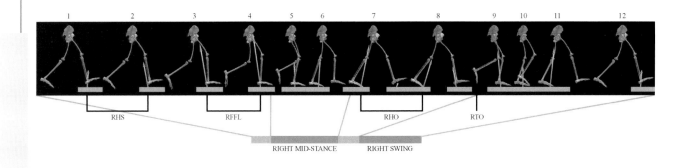

Figure 1. Normal gait cycle from the Polygon software (Vicon Motion Systems Ltd®, arrow is GRF). RTO = right toe-off , RHS=right heel strike, RFFL= right forefoot loading, RHO=right heel off.

pressure distribution exists under the load-bearing points of the foot (i.e. heel, metatarsal heads, and phalanges of the toes). Foot problems, however, range from the simple and obvious to the most subtle and complicated, which can often mislead clinicians and investigators in their assessment and subsequent treatment plan. Consequently, study of the distribution of pressure between the foot and the ground can often reveal valuable and otherwise unobtainable information about both the structure and function of the foot, and the postural control of the whole body. The use of this information varies; it may be utilised to assist the anatomical inspection of the foot, or the neuromuscular examination of the trunk and lower limb musculoskeletomotor system, as reflected from the characteristic loading patterns under the respective load-bearing points of the foot.

Foot ground force measurement (gait analysis) systems are mainly used to study the relationship of one part of the body relative to others by the use of special markers located over relevant anatomical landmarks. Unfortunately, there is a limit as to how much information they can reveal from underneath the plantar surface of the foot. The main advantage of these systems is in defining the relationship of one segment relative to another during walking, and in identifying the direction and orientation of the GRF line of action at each instant from heel strike to toe off. However, as force and pressure are inter-related, it is highly recommended to combine foot pressure and gait analysis systems, thus providing a comprehensive clinical biomechanical assessment of human motion

(IIb/B). Foot pressure and gait analysis systems are, therefore, of relevance to many different professional groups, including orthopaedic surgeons, prosthetists and orthotists, orthopaedic footwear manufacturers, physiotherapists, rehabilitation engineers, clinicians, and those involved in fundamental biomechanical research. In this chapter, we are mainly focusing on clinical gait analysis.

Methodology

The literature review was conducted utilising various search engines (Pubmed, Scopus, Recall and Google). The four engines allowed us to gather published relevant articles from the Index and non-Index Medicus. Key words used were: 'gait', 'pressure', 'foot', 'electromyography', 'proprioception', and 'motion'.

Gait analysis

At present, gait analysis laboratories are associated with the use of reflective markers and/or the utilisation of high technology equipment, such as low/high frequency cameras combined with compatible software for the analysis and presentation of motion (e.g. Vicon® system). The use of such systems, irrespective of their clinical outcome, has so far not been proven to be cost-effective and has been the topic of debate in recent national and international conferences [2, 3] **(III/B, IV/C)**. In addition, the mode of analysis depends on a number of factors such as the variety of equipment available, the expertise of the user and the space available. When considering the latter, a relatively large space is required to accommodate the cameras in a format to produce three-dimensional gait analysis. On average, up to 1½ hours is needed per subject to record gait data. In the last decade or so, new portable gait analysis systems (e.g. GAITRite®) appeared on the market, providing the user with an automated means of measuring the spatial and temporal parameters of gait. These systems complement the former generation and are portable and relatively cheap. They are extremely useful when dealing with patients with 'shuffling' gait and low assessment tolerance, (e.g. those suffering from Parkinson's disease). The primary disadvantage is, however, their incompetence in providing inter-segmental relationships, which is crucial when assessing patients with complex gait disorders, such as cerebral palsy.

Dhanendran [4] suggested that the first truly functional force plate was used by Amar in 1923, who used a combination of rubber balls and springs, which subsequent to their displacements, were able to measure the two horizontal components of force. This view was challenged by Lord [5], who nominated Basler's [6] harp-like instrument as the first ever device to carry out the above-mentioned objective by using a plate that was divided into ten beams, each of which was balanced and stabilised by a metal wire. This device, when subjected to force, would place tension on the wire, thereby changing the frequency emitted by the wire. The first modern form of force plate was most probably the one constructed using strain gauges mounted on each of four tubular aluminium columns, was able to measure directly all four components of force and the co-ordinates of the instantaneous centre of pressure [7].

Sakorecki and Charnley [8] constructed their system for measuring vertical components of force by using both mechanical and optical methods. This was designed originally to study the effect of hip replacements on the gait cycle. In a study by Grundy et al [9], the Sakorecki and Charnley plate was used to investigate the centres of pressures under the foot during walking. In 1972, a group of researchers from the Polytechnic of Central London also began to study foot pressure. This group [10] designed a force plate using 12 beams, each of 9.5mm wide and separated

by a 2mm gap, giving a 406mm by 140mm load-sensitive insert located in a 7m walkway.

This insert could be rotated through 90°, and a strain gauge method was used to record the vertical component of load on each beam during the stance phase of the gait cycle. By aligning the beams parallel to the direction of gait either the mediolateral or the anteroposterior distribution of the foot pressure could be selectively studied. A 12-channel UV recorder produced 12 simultaneous curves of force against a base of time. This device was further developed by Stokes et al [11].

While the London Polytechnic team continued to develop their strain gauge force plate, Dhanendran et al [12] described a variation on this beam technique, which involved the use of a full matrix force plate consisting of 128 cells in a 16 by 8 arrangement with each being 14mm square and supported by a strain gauge ring. A PDP 11/40 mini-computer was used for on-line recording of data and for immediate processing. Manley[13] also used the beam technique, but with 16 transparent parallel beams mounted in a walkway, aligned at 90° to the direction of walking. In order to calculate the total load and centre of pressure, force transducers were placed at the end of each beam. One camera was positioned to show the contact load of the foot during recordings, and a second camera was positioned to record information from the lateral aspect of the leg and foot. Using this same technique, Hutton and Dhanendran [14] investigated the mechanics of the hallux and four years later, Beverly et al [15] investigated silastic arthroplasty of the hallux.

A strain gauged load cell within two force plates was used by Pelisse and Mazas [16] in their study of the effectiveness of prosthetic knee and ankle joints, where they measured the vertical and two horizontal components of force and point of application.

In 1976, the Swiss company, Kistler, developed a piezoelectric quartz load cell capable of measuring three components of force simultaneously. In these load platforms special attention was paid to the use of stiff, light, top plates and provision of proper support for the force plate on a concrete base. The Kistler force plate was used to illustrate the types of data available [17]. Khodadadeh [18] described the use of a pair of force plates used to investigate gait dynamics in patients suffering form osteoarthritis. Lehmann [19] used the Kistler force plate to investigate the effect of ankle-foot orthoses (AFO) on subjects with lower limb muscle deficiency.

Draganich *et al* [20] reported a different approach combining a piezoelectric force plate measuring the three components of force, and a matrix of switches, the matrix being capable of measuring the foot contact area digitally via a sequence of switch closures. Despite this new innovation, West [21] questioned its use as a clinical tool.

Kistler Instruments Ltd emerged as the elite manufacturer in their multi-component measuring platform/load cell, which is made of piezo-instrumentation and is widely used in medical engineering applications. It can be used with the force platform and the Kistler system, as well as the pressure platform of optical dynamic pedobarographs (DPBG). It is capable of measuring forces and moments in three orthogonal directions by using four load cells positioned at each corner respectively. The accuracy, reliability and ease of calibration of this system have resulted in this being used worldwide in both research work and clinical studies investigating gait and foot pressure analysis [3] **(IIIB, IV/C)** [22, 23] **(IIa/B)**.

Based on the technology of force measurement platforms, Jin and Chizeck [24] described the development of a parallel bar system to obtain measurements of the forces exerted by the hands of a subject during standing, walking, stair climbing and descending. The data obtained from their modified system provided them with vital information on the magnitude and directions of hand support forces generated to assist them in the development of improved functional electrical stimulation (FES) systems for use with stroke and paraplegic patients.

Hirokawa and Ezaki [25] described the development of an automatic gait measurement system capable of collecting successive footsteps, both barefoot and shod. The apparatus consisted of a 12m walkway instrumented for signal acquisition and a microcomputer for data recording and processing. The walkway unit consisted of $1 \times 1 cm^2$ wire-latticed board 1.28m in length and 0.9m in width. Foot

contact was electrically detected by means of an x-y array of contact wires. This system was also used by Hirokawa [26], and Hirokawa and Matsumura [27] for the study of normal gait characteristics. As for its suitability for clinical use, it falls into the same category as with other available systems.

The ideal gait analysis system

Ideally, a gait analysis system should meet certain requirements: it must be supported by reliable software, hardware, load-cells and sensors (transducers) and should take into account:

- hygiene;
- comfort;
- repeatability;
- linearity of transducers;
- reproducibility of data in different formats;
- presence of reliable technical support;
- ease of use for both clinicians and researchers;
- time consumption; and finally
- cost.

Most of the existing systems satisfy at least one of these requirements but none meets them all as yet. When choosing a computerised system, the alternatives are rather wide and choice should normally be based on technical support as well as resource funding. At this stage, we can subdivide the precise need for such a system into: research and clinical applications.

If the system is reliable, repeatable with linear calibration, then it is suitable for motion analysis-related research; otherwise, it renders the system ineffective. In addition, support from graphical/numerical-oriented software may establish this as a clinical tool. The 'may' is added since the interpretation and relationships of obtained data to the clinical examination is greatly dependent on the expertise of the individual who undertakes the task.

This brings us inevitably to the conclusion that no matter how user friendly the system may be, it is essential for the operator to have a considerable background knowledge of biomechanics in order to carry out reliable assessment and therefore be able to achieve results as accurate as possible [28] **(IV/C)**. If they are truly to be of value, foot pressure and gait analysis systems must be used objectively in order to investigate and correlate the biomechanical examination of the foot and body inter-segmental relationships to the actual clinical condition, as accurately and meaningfully as possible **(IV/C)**.

Clinical assessment

In addition to clinical and biomechanical assessments, knowledge of various conservative modalities (e.g. functional orthoses and footwear mechanics) are important in providing a comprehensive treatment, not to mention that common sense should prevail. Gait is something that most of us take for granted. It is, in fact, one of the most complex and difficult motor tasks that we learn as humans, but how often do we take the time to appreciate this fact? The answer is - rarely, if at all. One of the considerations we should give some thought to, is the energy which is required in order for us to walk. Usually, the reason that we want to get from A to B is to undertake some task or other. If we were too tired to undertake the task then there wouldn't be much point in getting there. So, our gait must be efficient. In normal individuals the energy expended during gait is minimal and is the reason that we can pretty much walk (albeit on a level surface) for as long as we want to. The reason that we can achieve this is because our neuromuscular control is finely tuned such that our centre of mass moves minimally in all three planes; the forces which act across the joints are kept to a minimum; the muscle groups work in harmony transferring energy across the joints; and the range of motion of the lower limb joints is just enough for the foot to clear the floor during swing.

Since its inception in 1993, most patients seen at the Foot Pressure Analysis Clinic of the Institute of Motion Analysis & Research (IMAR) in Dundee, Scotland, irrespective of how minor or complex their problem, were using ill-fitting footwear with discrepancies in shoe width and size when compared to their feet. In some cases, there was a difference of up to three UK sizes and 4cm in width across the metatarsal head area, needless to say causing abnormal biomechanical forces and pressure through

the foot joints. The accumulative damage caused by footwear over the years goes, in most cases, unnoticed and gets ignored despite clear signs of pain and dorsal callous formation; the latter can only develop as a result of friction with the inner shoe. The damage becomes multi-compound with the use of high-heel shoes causing an instant forward shift of the centre of mass, resulting in increased pressure under the metatarsal heads and toes, abnormal joint and muscle function within the foot and lower leg and ultimately balance, proprioception and posture. It is always important to exclude footwear as a probable cause to the symptoms experienced when examining feet and lower limb pathology **(IV/C)**.

Case studies

Below are three cases recently treated at the Gait Analysis Laboratory of IMAR.

Pre and post-botulinum toxin

Botulinum toxin is a relatively new adjunct to the management of spasticity in children with cerebral palsy. It is not a panacea for the treatment of spasticity but it certainly has a role in understanding some of the abnormalities in complex gait disorders.

In the following case study, botulinum toxin was used to ascertain the influence of the short spastic plantar flexors on the gait pattern.

An understanding of the term 'ankle rockers' during the stance phase helps to understand this example (illustrated in Figure 2).

There are three rockers as follows:

- the first rocker is from initial contact until foot flat. During this phase the dorsiflexors control the motion of plantarflexion by contracting eccentrically (lengthening) (Figure 2 [1-2]);
- the second rocker is from foot flat until just prior to heel lift. During this phase the motion of dorsiflexion (progression of the shank over the foot) is controlled by eccentric action of the plantar flexors (Figure 2 [2-3]);

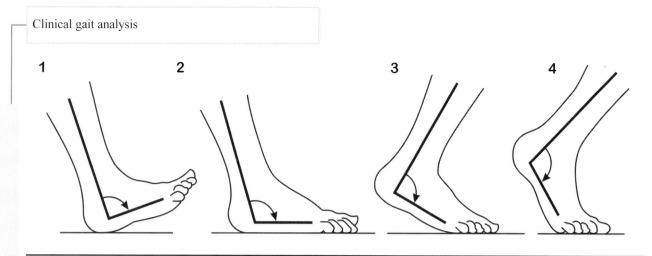

Figure 2. The ankle rockers during stance.

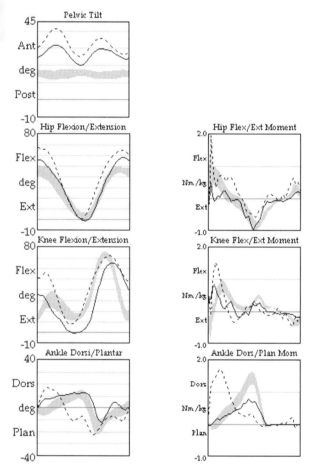

Figure 3. Sagittal plane kinematics and kinetics for the pelvis, hip, knee and ankle for the left side pre (dotted) and post (solid) injection of botulinum toxin. The shaded areas are normal averaged data.

♦ the third rocker is from heel lift to toe off and is the active push-off phase controlled by strong concentric action (shortening) of the plantar flexors (Figure 2 [3-4]).

The case involved a seven-year-old child with diplegic cerebral palsy, who presented with the difficulties of toe walking and early fatigue. Treatment intervention was with botulinum toxin into gastrocnemius bilaterally.

The graphs in Figure 3 show that although the botulinum toxin was injected into the plantar flexors bilaterally, the effects can be seen more proximally.

Points to note

Pre-injection, the foot makes initial contact on the toes followed by rapid dorsiflexion as weight is accepted (first rocker absent). This motion rapidly stretches the plantar flexors and initiates a spastic response resulting in early heel lift (seen in the graph as rapid plantarflexion [Figure 3], reversed second rocker and premature third rocker). This is the opposite of what should be occurring normally. In the kinetic data, there is a large dorsiflexion moment early in stance with a reversal of the normal pattern (i.e. with the largest peak in early stance rather than in late stance for push off). This results in very poor push off power as the lever arm over which the plantar flexors act is diminished.

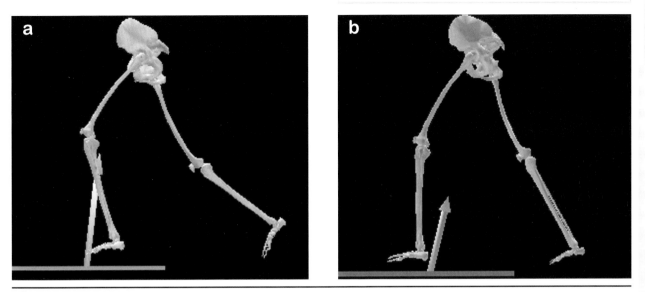

Figure 4. GRF a) pre and b) post-injection.

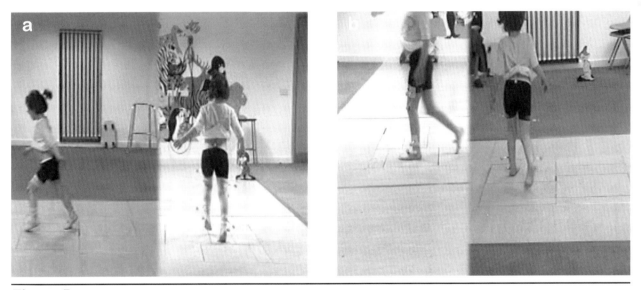

Figure 5. Video-captured images a) pre and b) post-injection.

Post-injection, the foot lands flat (first rocker still absent) with a gradual progression of the shank during stance (normal second rocker) but shows a delayed third rocker. The post-intervention kinetics (Figure 3) shows a more normal progression of the moment. This is also demonstrated in Figure 4 with the GRF under the fore-foot pre-intervention and at the rear of the foot post-intervention.

Pre-injection, the knee is significantly flexed at initial contact and it would be difficult to determine from

clinical judgement alone whether this was attributed to a limitation of the hamstrings or spasticity more distally.

Post-injection, the degree of knee flexion at initial contact has improved considerably, which indicates that it is the gastrocnemius that is limiting knee function. What is also interesting to note is that the knee hyper-extends when the gastrocnemius length is increased (albeit temporarily by the toxin reducing the spastic element) and this should sound warning bells

a

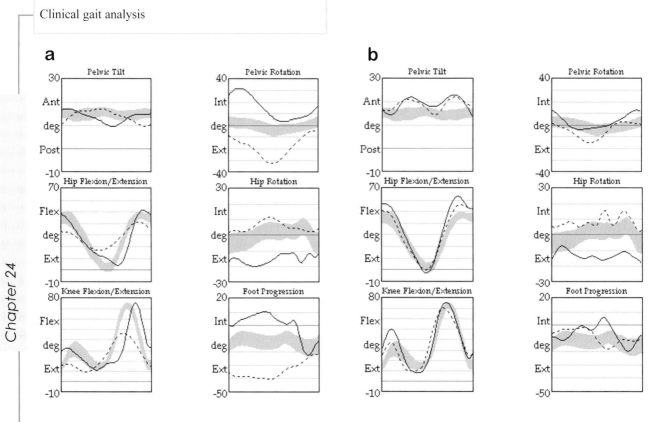

Figure 6. a) **Barefoot kinematics.** b) **AFO kinematics.**

as to what might happen if the muscle is surgically lengthened. The hyper-extension can be managed by an appropriate orthosis. The hyper-extension is secondary to the delayed third rocker.

At the pelvis, the most notable change is the lessening of anterior tilt. This can be better appreciated from the video-captured images in Figure 5, which reveal that the patient is no longer leaning forward at the trunk (a mechanism to keep the centre of mass over the feet). The hip also shows a more normal pattern post-injection.

In summary, this example shows how botulinum toxin can be used to assist in understanding the factors which result in complex walking patterns, the long-term aim being to minimise inappropriate surgery whilst maximising function **(IV/C)**.

With and without an ankle foot orthosis (AFO)

Ankle foot orthoses are commonly prescribed for individuals with neuromuscular disorders sometimes with little understanding of their complex biomechanical functions. It can easily be perceived that an AFO set at plantigrade will hold the ankle foot complex in this position to prevent contracture of the plantar flexors. However, by changing the biomechanics around the ankle, considerable improvements can be made at the more proximal joints. In the example shown below, changes were noted not only in the sagittal plane but also in the transverse plane.

This case involved a seven-year-old with a left hemiplegia. The presenting difficulty was frequent tripping, fatigue and inability to keep up with his peers at school.

In Figure 6, the left leg is represented by the dotted line and the right leg by the solid line.

Points to note

In the sagittal plane (far left column) the asymmetry between the limbs is obvious with the left, hemiplegic side, displaying restricted range of hip extension in terminal stance and poor knee flexion for swing. Clinically, these signs could be attributed to hip flexion contracture/spasticity in terms of the hip, and restricted hamstrings/rectus femoris function at the knee.

In the transverse plane the asymmetry is again obvious with the left side of the pelvis remaining retracted throughout the gait cycle.

When an appropriate ankle foot orthosis (AFO) is provided, the changes can be considerable. Figure 7 shows the obvious improvement of the foot position at initial contact. Also, in Figure 6b observe the much more symmetrical pattern between left and right and the improvement in the hip range of motion in terminal stance. Similarly, at the knee there is a more symmetrical pattern and no longer restriction in the degree of knee flexion for swing. This will improve foot clearance issues. Also in the transverse plane, observe the difference in pelvic rotation and foot progression. The pelvis is no longer retracted on the hemiplegic side. Foot alignment is no longer excessively external. In addition, improvements were also seen in the coronal plane (not shown) as he no longer hip-hitched on the left to facilitate foot clearance.

So, although the only intervention was an AFO, the improvements in gait are seen in all three planes and also in the temporal distance parameters (Table 1).

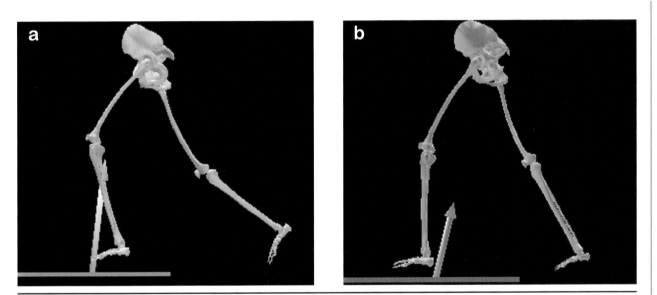

Figure 7. Left initial contact both a) barefoot and b) with the AFO.

Table 1. Temporal distance parameters barefoot and with an AFO [29, 30].

Temporal distance parameters	Barefoot		Normal	AFO	
	L	R		L	R
Walking speed	0.49		1.17	1.63	
Cadence	95		132	150	
Step length	35	33	54	0.60	0.71
Stride length	0.60	0.64	1.2	1.23	1.31
Single support	0.36	0.56	0.4	0.34	0.32
Double support	0.34	0.38	0.2	0.14	0.14

Walking speed has more than doubled and step length has almost doubled. This is the difference between being able to keep up with his peers or not. The time spent in single support has reduced on the unaffected side (i.e. he is more comfortable spending an equal amount of time on each limb in stance, whereas barefoot he was unwilling to spend much time on the hemiplegic side). In general, the gait pattern is much more symmetrical.

In summary, this case demonstrates that a detailed knowledge of the biomechanics of orthoses is needed to have an understanding of their effects on the gait pattern **(IV/C)**.

Pre and post-surgery

In some situations surgery is the correct option but it is not always immediately apparent which procedures are required to improve the gait pattern. Gait analysis can sometimes provide the additional information which can assist the clinician in making these decisions.

The following case examines the gait deviations, the patient's difficulties and the reasons why surgery was undertaken.

The subject was a 14-year-old girl whose main complaint was of frequent tripping and toe walking despite AFOs. She had previously undergone a left femoral derotation osteotomy and adductor tenotomy some eight years prior to the gait assessment. She attended mainstream school and managed to walk at least 200m unaided.

On clinical examination the following restrictions were noted:

Left:

♦ hip flexor contracture of ~15° with limited straight leg raise (~50°);
♦ popliteal angle of ~60°;
♦ restricted external rotation ~10° with excessive internal rotation ~80° associated with a femoral anteversion of ~75°;

♦ positive Duncan-Ely at ~45° with contracture of the rectus femoris at ~50° knee flexion in prone;
♦ dorsiflexion of the ankle 5° short of plantigrade with the knee extended;
♦ spasticity present in the hip flexors, rectus femoris, hamstrings, adductors and plantar flexors.

Right:

♦ ankle dorsiflexion to plantigrade with the knee extended;
♦ spasticity present in the adductors, and plantar flexors.

The initial pre-operative plan was to repeat the femoral osteotomy (to correct the rotational abnormality) and lengthen the plantar flexors (to correct the toe walking).

The gait analysis revealed a more complex situation. The rotational abnormality is obvious from the transverse plane graphs (to the right of Figure 8), with the hip internally rotated compared to normal and the foot alignment more internal than normal.

The ankle kinematics clearly demonstrate forefoot contact with rapid dorsiflexion as the weight is transferred to the limb (as seen in the previous example) followed by premature plantarflexion throughout the remainder of the stance phase.

The knee kinematics are more revealing with regard to the cause of tripping. Note the gradient of the normal curve prior to, and following, toe off (the vertical line). The gradient is steep and the knee reaches maximum flexion within the first third of the swing phase. The timing of this is critical in allowing clearance of the foot in early swing. Normally at this point, the ankle is plantarflexed, which leads to the limb being virtually longer causing the need for the knee to flex quickly enough to compensate. In this subject, note the change in the rate of flexion after toe off and the time taken to maximum flexion. The rate of flexion is reduced and the time to maximum flexion is delayed. The culprit - spasticity of rectus femoris.

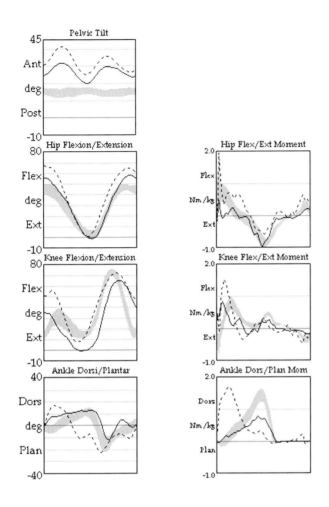

Figure 8. Sagittal and transverse plane kinematics for the left leg (dotted) and normal (shaded).

Figure 9 shows the inappropriate activity of rectus femoris during swing phase. If a derotation osteotomy was performed in isolation, it would be likely to cause an increase in tripping due to the fact that the foot would now be facing forwards rather than internally (effectively shorter) and clearance would be a greater issue.

The reason for initial contact being made on the fore-foot was thought to be spasticity of the plantar flexors in swing. However, electromyography (EMG) reveals no activity of any of the plantar flexors during swing, so this cannot be the cause for the fore-foot contact. Closer examination of the EMG reveals that the tibialis anterior is inactive during the second half of the swing phase, which contributes to the problem. There is another element which should be considered, namely, the inability to extend the knee in terminal swing due to spasticity and contracture of the hamstrings. If you are unable to extend your knee it is much easier to place the fore-foot down first than shorten the step length in order to get the heel down.

In terms of the treatment options it was decided to repeat the femoral osteotomy in conjunction with a transfer of the rectus femoris to gracilis, semitendinosus to biceps femoris and proximal release of gastrocnemius.

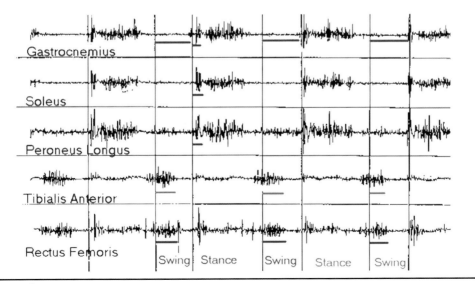

Figure 9. Surface EMG for the named muscles.

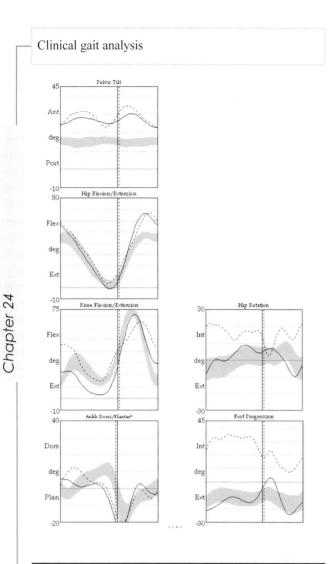

Figure 10. Sagittal and transverse plane kinematics for the left leg pre-operatively (dotted) and postoperatively (solid).

Figure 10 shows the differences between the pre- and postoperative kinematics. In summary, the rotational problems have been corrected, the knee is more extended at initial contact but now has a tendency to over-extend in mid-stance (possibly due to the gastrocnemius being slightly over-lengthened) and a better rate of flexion for swing with an earlier and greater maximum. The ankle did not show a normal pattern but was improved from pre-surgery. The knee ankle kinematics and hyper-extension were corrected with an AFO.

The subject was extremely happy with the outcome of her surgery.

Conclusions

Biomechanical assessment does not attempt to replace clinical examination, but rather it enhances the process by increasing the information upon which clinical decisions are made. This ensures the following:

◆ appropriate treatment;
◆ the avoidance of trial and error management;
◆ the identification of the primary cause of the problem;
◆ that the secondary symptoms are never treated without knowing the primary cause;
◆ that no detail is ignored, no matter how irrelevant.

Acknowledgement

The authors wish to thank Mr. Ian Christie for the illustrations.

Recommendations | Evidence level

Recommendations	Evidence level
◆ For a complete clinical overview of gait analysis, it is recommended to combine foot pressure and gait analysis when studying pathological cases.	IIb/B
◆ In order to effectively treat any part of the human musculoskeletal system, it is important to fully understand its biomechanics.	IV/C
◆ It is always important to exclude footwear as a probable cause to the symptoms experienced when examining feet and lower limb pathology.	IV/C
◆ If you are undertaking any intervention with patients suffering from complex gait pathologies then it is very advisable to use 3D gait analysis.	IV/C
◆ If you decide to purchase a gait or pressure analysis system make sure to address most of the points highlighted earlier for an ideal system and don't be misled by an impressive front, i.e. impressive software.	Ib/A, IV/C

Chapter 24

References

1. Donatelli RA. Normal anatomy and biomechanics. In: *The biomechanics of the foot and ankle.* Donatelli RA, Ed. FA Davis Company, 1990: 3-31.

2. Abboud RJ. If gait analysis is not cost effective in routine clinical practice, foot pressure analysis is. Presented at the International Society for Prosthetics and Orthotics (ISPO), 6th-7th November 1998, Dunblane, Scotland, UK. (This paper won the Conference Award Paper offered by Blesma.)

3. Abboud RJ, Betts R. Symposium on the role of pressure measurement in the management of foot disorders. 10th World Congress of the International Society for Prosthetics & Orthotics (ISPO), 1st-6th July 2001, SECC, Glasgow, Scotland, UK.

4. Dhanendran M. A minicomputer instrumentation system for measuring the force distribution under the feet. PhD Thesis, 1979, PCl.

5. Lord M. Foot pressure measurement: a review of methodology. *J Biomed Eng* 1981; 3: 91-9.

6. Basler A. Bestimmung des auf die einzehen sohlen bezirke wirkenden Teilgwitches des menschlichen Korpers. *Abderhalden's Hamduch* 1927; 5: 559-74.

7. Cunningham DM, Brown GW. Two devices for measuring the forces acting on the human body during walking. *Proc Soc Exp Stress Anal* 1952; 9: 75-90.

8. Sakorecki, Charnley J. The design and construction of a new apparatus for measuring the vertical forces executed in walking: a gait machine. *J Strain Anal* 1966; 1: 429.

9. Grundy M, Blackbum PA, Tosh RD, McLeish RD, Smidt L. An investigation of the centres of pressure under the foot while walking. *J Bone Joint Surg* 1975; 57: 98-103.

10. Hutton WC, Drabble GE. An apparatus to give the distribution of vertical load under the foot. *Rheum Phys Med* 1972; 11: 313-7.

11. Stokes IA, Stott JR, Hutton WC. Force distribution under the foot, a dynamic measuring system. *Biomed Eng* 1974; 9(4): 140-3.

12. Dhanendran M, Hutton WC, Paker Y. The distribution of force under the human foot - an on-line measuring system. *Measurement Control* 1978; 11: 261-4.

13. Manley M. Discussion contribution plus figure. In: *Disability.* Kenedi, *et al.* Macmillan, 1979: 185-90.

14. Hutton WC, Dhanendran M. The mechanics of normal and hallux valgus feet - a quantitative study. *Clin Orthop Relat Res* 1981; 157: 7-13.

15. Beverly MC, Horan FT, Hutton WC. Load cell analysis following silastic arthroplasty of the hallux. *Int Orthop* 1985; 9: 101-4.

16. Pelisse F, Mazas Y. A computer-directed measuring device to analyse pathological gaits. *C R Acad Sci Hebd Seanses Acad Sci D* 1975; 280: 2613-6.

17. Schoenhaus HD, Poss KD. The clinical and practical aspects in treating torsional problems in children. *J Am Podiatry Asso* 1977; 67: 620-7.

18. Khodadadeh S. Quantitative approach to osteoarthritic gait assessment. *Eng in Med* 1987; 16: 9-14.

19. Lehmann JF. Push-off and propulsion of the body in normal and abnormal gait, correction by ankle-foot orthoses. *Clin Orthop Relat Res* 1993; 288: 97-108.

20. Draganich LF, Andriacchi TP, Strongwater AM, Galante IO. Electronic measurement of instantaneous foot-floor contact patterns during gait. *J Biomech* 1980; 13: 875-80.

21. West PM. The clinical use of the Harris and Beath footprinting mat in assessing plantar pressures. *Chiropodist* 1987; 42: 337-48.

22. Abboud RJ. Temporal relationships between foot pressure and muscle activity during walking. PhD thesis, 1995, University of Dundee.

23. Kirtley C, Whittle MW, Jefferson RJ. Influence of walking speed on gait parameters. *J Biomed Eng* 1985; 7: 282-6.

24. Jin Z, Chizeck HJ. Instrumented parallel bars for three-dimensional force measurement. *Journal of Rehabilitation Research and Development* 1992; 29: 31-8.

25. Hirokawa S, Ezaki T. Development of a walkway system to measure distance and temporal factors of gait, and to

undertake gait-analytical study through the system. *Japan J Med Electron Biol Eng* 1983; 21: 9-16 (in Japanese).

26. Hirokawa S. Normal gait characteristics under temporal and distance constraints. *J Biomed Eng* 1989; 11: 449-56.

27. Hirokawa S, Matsumura K. Gait analysis using a measuring walkway for temporal and distance factors. *Med Bio Eng Comput* 1978; 25: 577-82.

28. Abboud RJ. Relevant foot biomechanics. *Curr Orthop* 2002; 16: 165-79.

29. Schuyler J, Miller F, Herzog R, *et al.* Predicting changes in kinematics of gait relating to age and velocity. http://www.motionanalysis.com/pdf/Abstract224.pdf.

30. Stansfield BW, Hazlewood ME, Hillman SJ, *et al.* Gait is predominantly characterized by speed of progression, not age, in 5 to 12 year. *Gait and Posture* 1999; 10: 57.